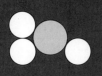

School-Based Group Counseling

Christopher A. Sink and Cher N. Edwards
Seattle Pacific University

Christie Eppler
Seattle University

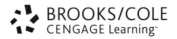

BROOKS/COLE
CENGAGE Learning™

Australia • Brazil • Japan • Korea • Mexico • Singapore • Spain • United Kingdom • United States

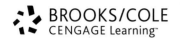

BROOKS/COLE
CENGAGE Learning™

School Based Group Counseling
Christopher A. Sink, Cher N. Edwards and Christie Eppler

Publisher/Executive Editor: Linda Schreiber-Ganster

Acquisitions Editor: Seth Dobrin

Assistant Editor: Naomi Dreyer

Editorial Assistant: Suzanna Kincaid

Technology Project Manager: Elizabeth Momb

Marketing Manager: Christine Sosa

Marketing Coordinator: Gurpreet Saran

Marketing Communications Manager:
Tami Strang

Senior Art Director: Jennifer Wahi

Print Buyer: Linda Hsu

Rights Acquisition Specialist (Text):
Dean Dauphinais

Cover Designer: Jeff Bane

Production Service: PreMediaGlobal

Content Project Management: PreMediaGlobal

For product information and technology assistance, contact us at **Cengage Learning Customer & Sales Support, 1-800-354-9706**

For permission to use material from this text or product, submit all requests online at **cengage.com/permissions**
Further permissions questions can be emailed to
permissionrequest@cengage.com

Library of Congress Control Number: 2011926941

ISBN-13: 978-0-618-57447-6

ISBN 10: 0-618-57447-6

Brooks/Cole
20 Davis Drive
Belmont, CA 94002-3098
USA

Cengage Learning is a leading provider of customized learning solutions with office locations around the globe, including Singapore, the United Kingdom, Australia, Mexico, Brazil, and Japan. Locate your local office at: **international.cengage.com/region**

Cengage Learning products are represented in Canada by Nelson Education, Ltd.

For your course and learning solutions, visit **www.cengage.com**

Purchase any of our products at your local college store or at our preferred online store **www.cengagebrain.com.**

Printed in the United States of America
1 2 3 4 5 6 7 15 14 13 12 11

We dedicate this book to the committed educational professionals who assist students to reach their goals through group counseling services.

Contents

Table of Contents

INTRODUCTION

Small-group counseling conducted in school settings is a highly effective way to reach children and youth where they most require support and care. If facilitated with one eye to theory and research and the other to best practice, professional school counselors will notice positive behavioral changes in students. The majority of new counselors who we have trained for the profession report that they enjoy leading groups. Other anecdotal data collected from more veteran school counselors, particularly those who have an established comprehensive school counseling program for 5 or more years, consistently indicate that group work is a highlight of their practice.

We realize that pre- and in-service school counselors desire immediate assistance with leading small groups in an ever-shifting educational climate. Whereas in the 1970s to the 1990s groups could be facilitated with a strong holistic emphasis ranging from personal growth to postsecondary transition groups, with the onset of this millennium and the massive academic press exerted on schools, counselors are finding it increasingly more difficult to obtain administrative and teacher support to conduct small groups with students who first and foremost must improve their achievement test scores. It seems odd that many educators fail to recall the key lessons of developmental psychology indicating that children must establish the basic personal/social, cognitive, and motivational building blocks essential to academic and educational developmental. Rather than releasing students for group participation, school counselors are repeatedly faced with, in our view, this shortsighted question: "What is this group going to do for my student's academic skill set?" Obviously, counseling professionals must have a plausible response to this inquiry.

RATIONALE AND FOCI

Although there are several fine texts available to counselors, in our view these options are neither firmly situated within the realities of school environments nor strongly grounded in current theory and research. As such, we offer this new text as a way to bridge what we perceive as a gap between current group counseling publications that focus largely on serving clients in clinical/mental health environments, paying little heed to the purview and concerns of school counselors, and those publications that are excessively practical, seemingly downplaying the need for a solid theoretical and research foundation underlying group counseling techniques and procedures. Specifically, despite what leading counselor educators (e.g., Gladding, 2008; Jacobs, Masson, & Harvill, 2009; Pérusse, Goodnough, & Lee, 2009) suggest—that theory is essential to effective group leadership—some group counseling books (e.g., Geroski & Kraus, 2010; Greenberg, 2003; Page & Jencius, 2009; Smead, 1995) targeting school counselors as their primary audience stress the pragmatics of group facilitation—"the how tos" of group work, omitting theoretical and research considerations.

Admittedly, treading a fine line between being overly academic and application oriented is easier said than done. We understand, and rightly so, that busy school counselors want the structure that highly practical books can provide. However, as alluded to earlier, counseling professionals, in this day and age of educational accountability, need to be able to defend the use of group counseling as an intervention apropos to school settings. It is not enough to outline the mechanics of group leadership and give some examples without providing a clear research-based rationale for the practice. Thus, in a genuine attempt to speak plainly to the need of school counselors-in-training and practitioners for best practice advice and address the recommendations of group counseling experts, we went into the field and canvassed at least 15 current professional school counselors across grade levels who regularly and effectively conduct small groups, asking for their time-tested ideas, suggestions, and examples. The school-based group counseling literature was also reviewed for research examples, content, direction, best practice illustrations, and so forth. Finally, salient theoretical orientations were carefully reviewed and synthesized, extracting only those that are germane to small groups conducted in schools. Each theory discussed herein had to (a) possess a strong research base and (b) be explicitly applied to educational milieus. In short, we believe this text is a well-balanced amalgam of school-based group counseling theory, research, and best practice.

TARGET AUDIENCE AND CHAPTER OVERVIEW

In particular, this text is written for use with graduate-level group counseling classes educating preservice and practicing school counselors. Each chapter is written in a counselor-friendly way, is relatively short, and includes supplemental material for further study and extended practice. Chapters 1 to 4 focus on setting the stage for actual in-school group counseling leadership. For example, chapter 1 explores the typical contemporary school counseling environment in which groups are conducted, while also addressing various definitional issues related to school-based small groups. The rationale for this crucial intervention is discussed and situated within comprehensive school counseling programs similar to the American School Counselor Association's (2005a) National Model. The types and formats for school-led groups are reviewed. Real-world group counseling examples dot the opening chapter as well as all that follow. Chapter 2 provides a robust theoretical and research foundation from which to develop and implement small groups in schools. Chapter 3 considers the basics of how school counselors prepare and conduct small groups, whereas chapter 4 addresses the professional issues (e.g., ethical and legal considerations) undergirding this service. Completing section 1, chapter 5 explains and illustrates the essential group facilitation skills. Section 2—Groups in Action—explores the processes and procedures for running groups in different school environments and with varying student populations. For example, chapters 6, 7, and 8 examine these issues from the perspectives of elementary, middle/junior high, and high school counselors, respectively. The remaining pair of chapters provides insight and concrete recommendations when conducting groups with students with special needs (chapter 9) and of color (chapter 10). Again, each chapter is replete with school-based examples and supplementary material.

CONCEPTUAL ORIENTATION

Some texts fail to clue readers in on the theoretical framework adopted by its authors. In our case, the book is written from a learner-centered, developmental perspective as well as from a systems approach (Stroh & Sink, 2002). These concepts are discussed in the initial section of the book, so suffice it to say here, small-group counseling is a vital prevention and intervention service of comprehensive school counseling programs (American School Counselor Association, 2005a, 2005b, 2008a) provided by school counselors to students from kindergarten to 12th grade.

More specifically, in our professional opinion, group counselors who desire to maximize their efficacy must view students in light of their status both as individual and social learners and as evolving human beings. Learning and development also occurs within a wider context, that is, the children's socio-ecological systems (e.g., Bronfenbrenner, 1977; Lerner, Lerner, Almerigi, & Theokas, 2005). Said differently, we encourage nascent and seasoned group counselors to perceive most students on a relatively normal developmental trajectory toward flourishing as mature adults. Of course, minor and major detours from students' healthy developmental pathways are also regular occurrences, but they do not determine final ends. However, depending on the severity of the child's background (e.g., familial, genetics, social environment), development for many youngsters living with learning challenges or in less than favorable conditions often occurs in fits and starts, and the stages are not as "clean" as some developmental psychologists would have us believe. Because learning is influenced by multiple factors including various socio-cultural-ethnic, developmental, and situational issues swirling in and around the student's life (see Moreno, 2010, for a detailed discussion), groups must account for these direct (e.g., psychobiological) and indirect (e.g., neighborhood safety) effects on student outcomes. Even with these potential obstacles to long-term healthy development, school-based group work should remain strengths based (Akos & Galassi, 2008) and proactive (Alvord & Grados, 2005), focusing on the students' developmental assets (Benson, 2003) rather than their deficiencies. In other words, most groups conducted in schools need not be remedial in nature and focus, aiming at "repairing" those key developmental competences students have yet to master. Instead, in our view, school counseling group work can be used to direct or redirect students toward positive goals and adding to their existing strengths. Finally, we believe group work in schools should be tied to educational aims. This does not mean, however, that groups must largely exist to improve *academic* outcomes; rather, educational goals are broad and encompass fundamental developmental domains, including, for example, personal/social, emotional, career/vocation, spiritual/moral, and academic.

SUGGESTIONS FOR READING AND PRACTICE

As you read and reread each chapter, do some reflection on the examples provided. Many chapters include self-reflection questions that will help you process and contextualize the content, particularly as it concerns school-based small groups. Practice the facilitation skills discussed in chapter 5 and throughout the subsequent ones. Start with a small group of peers or colleagues and have an impartial observer provide feedback on the processes and procedures used. If you are taking a group counseling class, ask the instructor to supply plenty of concrete feedback, including areas for improvement. Once you feel ready to facilitate a group in schools, do all the preparatory work outlined in chapter 3 and others. Obtain the necessary permissions and arrange for competent supervision. Whenever possible, record the group meetings and, on a weekly basis, process your group leadership experience with the supervisor. Evaluate yourself and ask the students to provide ongoing feedback. Once you have conducted a few groups, your skill set will solidify and the nerves will diminish. Because groups are difficult at first to facilitate, keep at it and your confidence level will increase with each session.

SUMMARY

In conclusion, as readers prepare for effective group leadership practice in the schools, there are several important prerequisites to work through. First, you will need to possess a strong grasp of group counseling theory, research, and the related pragmatic issues. Moreover, the developmental tasks associated with each stage of the group experience are essential to learn. Obviously, gaining the necessary group counseling skills is paramount to effective practice. Finally, high-quality supervised training both pre-internship (practicum experiences) and then during the school-based internship will round out your group counseling education. This text addresses each precondition and relevant supervision issues.

Please let us know what you think about this book and how the authors can improve each chapter for future editions. The lead author can be contacted at: Christopher Sink, Seattle Pacific University, School of Education, 3307 Third Avenue West, Seattle, WA 98155. Email: csink@spu.edu.

The authors wish to thank Seth Dobrin of Brooks/Cole Cengage Learning and his staff for making this book possible and shepherding it through the publication process. This text is dedicated to the professional school counselors who work selflessly each day to bring caring and healing to students and their families.

About the Authors

Sikhism = social justice faith.
= all people share common cause to humanity
+ .: right to equitable treatment, access to
resources + support for human rights.

CHRISTOPHER A. SINK Christopher Sink, PhD, NCC, LMHC, professor of counselor education at Seattle Pacific University (17+ years), has been actively involved with the school counseling profession for nearly 30 years. He has conducted small groups in K–12 schools and teaches the group counseling class. Prior to serving as a counselor educator, he worked as a secondary and postsecondary counselor. He has many years of editorial experience in counseling-related journals (e.g., ASCA's *Professional School Counseling* and ACA's *Counseling and Values*) and has published extensively in various areas related to school counseling and educational psychology. Chris is a strong advocate for systemic and strengths-based school-based counseling. Currently, his research agenda includes topics examining the outcomes of comprehensive school counseling programs, research methods in school counseling, and spirituality as an important feature of adolescent resiliency. Sink's (2011) latest book published by Brooks/Cole is called *Mental Health Interventions for School Counselors*. Dr. Sink also has a 3-year Visiting Professor/Scholar appointment in the Faculty of Education and Theology, York St John University, York, England.

What is going right in a person's life?

Factors
x 1) Physical health
2) Social support
3) Emotional resilience
4) Spiritual Outlook
5) Voc/Financial
6) Intellectual/Giftedness

CHER N. EDWARDS Cher Edwards, PhD, LPC, is an associate professor and chair of counselor education at Seattle Pacific University. She has taught group counseling and supervised preservice school counselors for over 10 years, and has focused her scholarly activities on issues relevant to the school counseling profession, specifically addressing cultural competency and social justice issues. Cher is currently serving as the vice president of Post Secondary Education for the Washington School Counseling Association and is the founding president of Washington Counselors for Social Justice. *— promoting a society to challenge injustice + valuing diversity*

eyes
what can I learn from this
what good can come from this?
what resources?
individuals can choose the way they think.

CHRISTIE EPPLER Christie Eppler, PhD, LMFT, is an associate professor of pastoral counseling at Seattle University. She was previously an associate professor at Seattle Pacific University in the Counselor Education program, an assistant professor at Seton Hall University in their Marriage and Family Therapy Program, and taught family nursing classes at the University of Michigan, Flint. Christie is a Licensed Marriage and Family Therapist (LMFT, Washington), and holds an approved supervisor designation from the American Association of Marriage and Family Therapists (AAMFT). Her clinical practice covers the complete age span of children, youth, and adults as demonstrated by 2 years of counseling with children and families in

Martin Seligman → ideas
1. 10 things I like about me
(what would friends say) — Daily visibility
2. Gratitude journal — the 10 events

xv

an elementary school setting, several years of clinical work with children, teens, and their families at community-based clinics, and work as a mental health counselor at a college counseling center. Christie is a member of the American Counseling Association (ACA), and is past president of the Washington State Association of Counselor Educators and Supervisors (WSACES). The Washington State School Counselor Association (WSCA) named her Counselor Educator of the Year in 2007. She has published in *Professional School Counseling, Psychology in the Schools*, and *Journal of Marital and Family Therapy*. Her future qualitative research will focus on the intersections of spiritual counseling and narrative therapy, resiliency, and issues of social justice.

[Handwritten annotations:]

ability to bounce back

non-blaming approach to asking clients to seek out values, knowledge + skill they have to effectively deal with life's problems.

problem separated from person to empower & offer collaborative counseling

give permission to be self-compassionate as view through lens how does it serve you

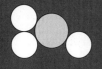

BEFORE THE ACTION STARTS

Landscape of Groups.

Exploration— Introduction to Small Groups in Today's Schools

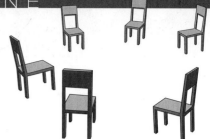

They that won't be counseled can't be helped. Without continual growth and progress, such words as improvement, achievement, and success have no meaning.[1]
—Benjamin Franklin (ca. 1705–1790)

The one person on the staff that every school needs is the COUNSELOR. Call her/him whomever you want, the reality is CHILDREN HAVE HUGE EMOTIONAL PROBLEMS AND THEY NEED SOMEONE TO TALK TO WHO IS A PROFESSIONAL.[2]
—Carol Parker (7/8 Teacher Drama, Film, Honors, and Regular Language Arts, May 14, 2010)

School counselors are highly qualified student support service professionals who can address these issues through individual, group *and/or classroom guidance lessons so that ALL students are serviced.*[3]
—Dr. Hardy (Administrator/Staff, May 14, 2010; emphasis added)

E ven when wise voices from the past and present see the importance of good counsel, many Americans still associate individual and group counseling with people who are emotionally or behaviorally disturbed (E. Miller & Reid, 2009). As a general rule, when parents are informally asked by educators about which students tend to meet with the school counselor, a common reply is "the kids with serious problems or the bad kids." This reveals a fundamental misperception. Particularly among young people, however, this perspective appears to be changing. Even if many parents do not know it, nearly all students in K–12 school systems have received some direct or indirect school counseling services. At a minimum, by middle/junior high school teens will have had a school

---

[1]Parker, P. M. (Ed.). (2008). *Counsels: Webster's Quotations, Facts and Phrases* (p. 1). San Diego, CA: ICON Group International.

[2]Retrieved from http://www.edutopia.org/school-counseling-importance-of-elias.

[3]Retrieved from http://www.edutopia.org/school-counseling-importance-of-elias.

counselor or two to assist them with various educational, personal/social, and career/life concerns. Not only are students supported by the school's general counseling activities, many children and youth are supported in small-group settings as well.

In doing our background research for this book, we visited numerous schools and spoke to multiple counselors and tens of students. With permission, we sat in on all types of small groups, ranging from those designed for shy kindergarteners to those for high school seniors planning for college. Our observations and conversations reinforced the general finding from school-based counseling research—that small groups are helpful on many levels for both the student participants and the counselors. Without much prompting, children shared about a variety of issues. One early elementary girl cried about losing the family pet and wondered "where dead dogs go." Sensing the little girl's pain, two of her group mates jumped up and gave her a heartfelt hug. A different member in another elementary small group needed assistance with friendship skills. Other children talked about not liking school and day care, and others shared how school was a safe place for them. Similarly, teenagers readily opened up about their concerns and goals. One middle-schooler, for example, indicated that she was thinking of joining a gang but was afraid. Students in diverse settings and groups spoke about their disengagement with school, how things were going in their lives, and how they could reinvent themselves. An 11th-grader spoke, for example, about her struggles with a physics class and the teacher, whereas others reported that they were failing in school and needed help with test taking and getting along with their teachers. Regrettably, we heard a common theme among older students in different settings: School was boring and irrelevant to their lives. Counselors did their best to counteract these perceptions with enjoyable activities, guiding the conversation toward positive outcomes.

Our overriding conclusions after these "real-world" observations suggested that the group counseling experience and peer interaction and feedback were rewarding to students and school counselors alike. In particular, school counselors appreciated the opportunity to make a genuine difference in students' lives by encouraging personal and social growth and effective problem solving. By and large, student participants reported learning new skills and enjoying the group experience.

This initial chapter provides a wide-angle view of school-based group work. Basic topics considered here include definitional issues, rationale for groups, and a description of different group types or formats. As readers move through the content, the need for a strong skill set and the importance of group work as an effective responsive service delivered within the context of operating a comprehensive school counseling program (CSCP; ASCA, 2005a, 2005b) will become more apparent. We hope this material will help fuel your desire to conduct small groups.

To avoid losing touch with actual practice, you will find many school-based examples sprinkled liberally throughout text. The following vignette, for instance, provides a glimpse at how a small group of several younger learners experiencing academic challenges was established. Here and elsewhere names are fictitious.

GROUPS IN PRACTICE

Scenario: Elementary School Small Group

Regularly, certain teachers at Booker Elementary School grouse to the school counselor and principal about the limited academic readiness skills of ELL children (English-language learners) who enroll at the start of each year from surrounding districts. For the past several summers when the statewide academic test scores were made public, these teachers noticed a worrisome trend: The new enrollees were on average at least one-half a grade level below the state mean scores for math and reading. Many of these low-scoring children came from modest-income families with limited English skills, whereas others seemed to be just unprepared for challenging schoolwork. Within the context of the school's Response to Intervention (RTI) program, teacher aides were then reassigned to various classrooms as a way to support the learning of new students. This practice was abandoned after little success. Other, more intensive interventions were considered.

In collaboration with the rest of the RTI team, Mr. Hernandez, the school counselor, decided to try a Level 2 intervention. He reviewed the school counseling literature and relevant websites for a "best practice" educational curriculum to direct the team's foci. He then developed a couple of content-focused small groups, first, to improve the children's academic skills, and second, to help them transition to the school. Some staff members voiced skepticism about the possible effectiveness of the groups, but the RTI team and principal approved of this intervention. Each teacher with a struggling transfer student was notified that the small groups were available. Later, Mr. Hernandez selected those children who most likely would benefit from a small group. The students' families were contacted to gain both parental consent for student participation and their support for this responsive service. After eight sessions, the counselor was able to document, from pre- to posttest, student improvement on targeted academic and psychosocial skills. The RTI team was impressed.

This scenario provides you with several insights on how groups get started in schools. First, there is a documented need. The students, teachers, and families realized that these ELL transfer students required additional educational support after the low-intensity classroom interventions did not work. The extra aide time with the students apparently was not focused enough to noticeably improve the targeted skills. One-on-one tutoring was also considered as a possible solution, but with so many students needing help, this remediation was viewed as too time consuming and inefficient. Second, as research has shown, quality consultation and collaboration between the school counselor and staff are essential to the success of focused interventions (Paisley & Milsom, 2007). Third, extra school and family support was solicited. Finally, rather than picking a group curriculum off the shelf, the school counselor began his preparations by looking for evidence-based materials best suited for ELL children.

Perhaps you have some relevant questions at this point. For instance, what is group counseling as conducted in schools? And how does this responsive service fit into the school's overall counseling program?

to fit needs of the commu ensu acade emo

Direct services formatted in a group setting working on a shared task/ to learn + develop supportive relationships issue

GROUP COUNSELING ROLE DEFINED

The Association for Specialists in Group Work (ASGW, 2000), a widely respected professional organization often cited by researchers and practitioners alike, refers to the practice of group counseling as "group work," suggesting that this term best represents the

> broad professional practice involving the application of knowledge and skill in group facilitation to assist an interdependent collection of people to reach their mutual goals which may be intrapersonal, interpersonal, or work-related. The goals of the group may include the accomplishment of tasks related to work, education, personal development, personal and interpersonal problem solving, or remediation of mental and emotional disorders. (pp. 2–3)

This portrayal is consonant with American School Counselor Association's (ASCA, 2008a) role statement on group counseling. ASCA describes this activity as "a small number of students working on shared tasks and developing supportive relationships in a group setting," adding that it "is an efficient, effective and positive way of dealing with students' academic, career, and personal/social/emotional developmental issue and situational concerns" (p. 1). In ASCA's role statement, group counseling is also viewed from a systems perspective, where this service is vital in the delivery of a component of a comprehensive school counseling program (CSCP; ASCA [2005a] National Model). Paisley and Milsom (2007) extended ASCA's (2008a) position, suggesting that

> school counselors must now be able to do more than facilitate groups of students. They must utilize skills and apply general principles of group work to effectively collaborate with adults in students' lives. A translation of what school counselors know about groups to teaming within the embedded communities of schools and societies may be critical to the success of school counseling programs. (pp. 10–11)

Essentially, school-based group counseling should be used to promote not only individual student behavior change but also systemic change. Over the long run, groups should foster the educational development of *all* students.

Another way to clarify the group counseling role is to make sure you understand what it does not include. For instance, when school counselors facilitate groups they are neither advice-giving leaders in the way physicians sometimes are for their ill patients, nor advice givers in the same way one might speak to a troubled friend or family member. Group counselors do not provide one-on-one counseling in a group format; they are working with all students as a unit, looking for ways to help members reach overall group objectives and each student's personal goals. In a well-functioning group, the counselor *facilitates* the action with the participants doing most of the "work." The learning process is active and engaging.

The group counselor has three primary functions as facilitator: to mobilize, model, and manage (the three "Ms") the members of the group. Counselors initially *mobilize* the group experience. They help group members to work through normal developmental issues as well as their home and school concerns. As the leader motivates and guides the group content and process, she also *models* how one behaves in a group setting. The students learn by watching the leaders in action, how they appropriately direct conversation and respond to each group member's contributions. (In chapter 2, you will read about Bandura's [2001] social learning theory and how observational learning works.) The last "M" relates to *managing* the group focus. In this role, group counselors guide the interactions among participants, cutting off and redirecting the focus when, for example, students stray too far from the topic, share confidential material about their families, or significantly disrupt the group experience. Sometimes you may feel like you are a parking lot attendant waving kids to certain areas, and other times like a sports team manager who steps back and lets the players play. Managing the group flow is obviously challenging, and well-developed skills are needed. Much of the time, you'll need to sensitively guide the group process so students to feel safe, "heard," and cared for; yet at other times, you'll want to be fairly directive so that members stay tuned in and on task. Each of the three "M"s is explained in more depth later in the text.

Small-group counseling is an important feature of the school counselor's role to enhance student development within the framework of a CSCP. Group counseling provides students with a positive and "protected" environment in which to share their lives, support their peers, and grow as young people and learners.

Comprehensive School Counseling Programs *(CSCP)* and Group Counseling

As alluded to above, small-group counseling, a responsive service, is generally described within the context of a systemic and operational structure to guide school counseling practice. For readers who may be unfamiliar with this programmatic approach, a short introduction is provided. Basically, although not ignoring students' immediate needs, CSCPs such as ASCA's (2005) National Model encourage school counselors to work from a *prevention* orientation, one that is proactive, comprehensive, and planned. Through the lens of CSCPs, school counselors view students within their particular sociocultural context. This broader perspective allows counselors to establish to some degree how the students' various subsystems (e.g., peers, family, community, religion, etc.) influence their educational/academic, personal/social, and career/life skill development.

More specifically, one of ASCA's (2005a) main goals is to advance school counselors' professional identity. With the publication of the *ASCA National Model: A Framework for School Counseling Programs*, school counselors have a serviceable blueprint to use to organize their practices. Although more than half of the states have their own versions, the National Model is now the leading "template" to guide the delivery of school counseling services. School counselors look to the National Model as they plan, implement, manage, and evaluate their work with students, faculty, and families.

The National Model's executive summary lists four primary objectives:

1. Establish the school counseling program as an integral component of the academic mission of the school.

2. Ensure every student has equitable access to the school counseling program.

3. Identify and deliver the knowledge and skills all students should acquire.

4. Ensure that the school counseling program is comprehensive in design and is delivered systematically to all students. (n.d., p. 2)

Retrieved from http://www.ascanationalmodel.org.

Beyond these four aims, the National Model has four supporting pillars. First, CSCPs need to be set up on a strong *foundation* that includes the program's underlying mission, beliefs, and philosophy statements. Based on the foundation, the *delivery system* is devised and implemented. This second pillar includes the activities, relations, and processes required to deliver the program to its constituents (e.g., educators, families, community members). The methods of service delivery involve classroom guidance (structured developmental lessons), individual planning (with counselor's assistance, students' formulate personal goals and develop life plans), responsive services (e.g., individual and group counseling services), and systems support (administrative and organizing activities keep the program functioning). The National Model's third pillar is the *management system*. Linked with the delivery system, it "incorporates organizational processes and tools to ensure the program is organized, concrete, clearly delineated and reflective of the school's needs" (ASCA, n.d., p. 2). Management activities include, for example, developing principal–counselor agreements, an advisory council, work calendars, data collection and analysis, and action planning. The last pillar is often referred to as *accountability*, where school counselors are charged with the responsibility to evaluate and document the efficacy of their work with students, families, and other educational processes.

In brief, the ASCA (2005a) National Model and other CSCPs are organizational frameworks for directing school counselors' practice. The Model endorses group counseling as an essential responsive service (ASCA, 2005a; Mason & Duba, 2009). Group work provides students an effective way to develop and maintain personal relationships and to improve targeted educational outcomes (Kayler & Sherman, 2009). Group counselors can also draw from ASCA's (2004a) National Standards for School Counseling Programs to devise their group objectives to align with specific educational/academic, career/life, and personal/social competencies.

RATIONALE FOR SMALL GROUPS

Groups are widely used in school settings for a number of reasons. First, as our introductory discussion suggests, there is plenty of anecdotal and empirical evidence indicating that despite all the challenges of school life, counselors see the value of small groups and generally like facilitating them. In their subjective view, groups help students mature, work out interpersonal problems, improve learning skills, and master important educational/academic, personal/social, and career/vocational competencies (for sample comments, see Table 1.1). The counselors' perceptions of the value of small-group counseling are also corroborated by multiple years of survey data gathered from a large, inner-city Washington State school district, where more than 1,200 elementary students showed in knowledge-based posttests that they had learned important personal/social information after participating in groups (e.g., Sink, Thompson, & Risdal, 2007). Because group counseling efficacy research is a foundation of our understanding of group work, this material is reviewed in chapter 2.

TABLE 1.1 | Practicing School Counselors Commenting on the Value of Group Work

Ms. Jinna Risdal
School Counselor at Southern Heights Elementary, Seattle, WA
Elementary Counseling Program, McKinney-Vento Homeless Student Education Program

"Many elementary schools use a screening instrument such as Systematic Screening for Behavior Disorders (SSBD) as well as staff input to identify students who need targeted interventions for behavioral and /or socio-emotional concerns. One of the most impactful interventions is the small support groups (6–8 students) led by elementary school counselors. The groups are predominantly social skills groups, but also include topics such as relational aggression, anger management, changing families, and transitions. The groups provide students with an environment where it is safe to discuss and share ideas and experiences.

The students participate in activities related to developing and practicing relationship skills. They have opportunities to role-play with their peers various situations that might be difficult for them in real life.

Pre- and posttests are administered to determine the effectiveness of the groups. Teachers are informed of the group goals and the students' progress.

Parents are involved in that they have to sign permission slips for group participation. Parents have made comments like: 'My daughter shares what she is learning in group. She is excited to go every week. I see that she is learning to be a better friend.' Teachers report that students who have been in groups transfer the skills learned to the classroom setting. Students refer their friends ('My friend needs to be in your group').

Small-group counseling in elementary comprehensive guidance and counseling programs is an effective way to improve students' academic engagement. Teachers at one school were asked for observations of students who have been in small groups. Teachers reported that 80% of students in groups for introverted or shy students showed significant or very significant improvement. They reported: 'Student seems more alert and participates more readily'; 'He is more willing to share and seems more social with his peers'; 'Student talks more with peers and has a friend now'; 'Student is more ready to speak when I call on her'; 'He is opening up and asking other kids to play.'"

Ms. Carol Johnson
School Counselor at Alderwood Middle School, Lynnwood, WA

"Working with a large caseload and a diverse student population, there is no way to effectively reach the majority without implementing classroom guidance or groups. Every fall we run assessments or surveys through our classes and gather feedback from our students to find out what is most presently concerning them or catching their interest. The feedback from these surveys drives what our counseling program focuses on. Within these surveys we usually find clusters of students who have common concerns such as anger, grief, making friends, needing help getting organized, study skills, struggling with a divorce, etc.

The power of running a group differs so much from individual counseling. Within a group setting, the foundation can be set for all the lessons and interactions that take place outside of the curriculum being taught. Students are learning how to care for each other. They are learning how to listen, respond, share, trust, understand, risk, confront, comfort, and support each other. Students are part of a group that understands them in a way most likely no other cluster of peers has before. They are learning they are not alone in their struggles, and they are learning ways to address their concerns from a variety of insights and perspectives. Peers can take information shared and make it comprehensible to their circumstance and developmental stage in a way an adult cannot as effectively do. A group experience when done well can be one of the most powerful experiences for a student to be part of.

As an educator, the group experience also offers challenges and rewards that offer insights into the populations or individual I am working with. I am able to observe a student's strengths, processing methods, coping skills, social skills, cultural references, peer pressures, family influences, and developmental stages. In a shorter amount of time than before, I can learn more about my students and the place they are living. I am also able to be a part of real, meaningful conversations with 8 to 10 kids at a time. That is amazing on so many levels but especially in light of trying to positively impact as many kids as possible through a given year."

Ms. Annie Carmona and Ms. Vicki Clark
School Counselors
Edmonds-Woodway High School, Edmonds, WA

"Running counseling groups in the high school setting can be challenging, yet effective and beneficial for students, the counseling department, and staff.

As high school counselors, we often hear that there isn't enough time to run groups due to having a large caseload and so many responsibilities, such as tracking graduation requirements, helping students with college admissions, and addressing the unique needs of individual students. Besides not feeling like there is enough time to run a small group, the need to pull students out of class can also be challenging because of the high stakes in high school and the likelihood that the students who would be in a group are often not performing well in their classes.

However, with adequate planning, having staff support, and finding helpful curriculum and resources that meet the needs of your students, running groups in the high school setting can bring several benefits to the students, staff, and your counseling program. At Edmonds Woodway High School, at least one or two groups are run each year. Not only have these groups been a great network and support to the students in the group, but the counselors have noticed major social improvement, which ultimately spills into the classroom, and typically students need to see their counselor less frequently for individual counseling appointments. With the high school age group especially, sometimes it's hard to know exactly what the students are benefiting from by participating in the group, but that's why providing pre- and posttests to collect data and feedback is important—not only for yourself as an opportunity to personally grow as a group facilitator, but also to share with your staff and administrators the data you have showing the increase in skills based on the group interventions."

Note: Counselors' statements were provided in writing in May 2010.   © Cengage Learning

Not only do school counselors believe in group work, school-based psychologists report that group counseling is a valuable service (Little, Akin-Little, & Gutierrez, 2009). For instance, Venkatesh (2006), a practicing psychologist, explained that small groups can be more effective than individual counseling because the needs of 8–10 students

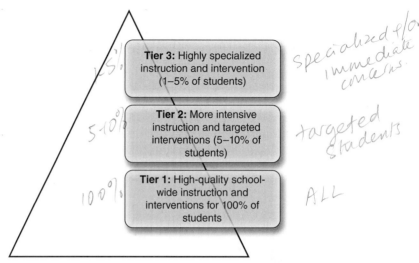

FIGURE 1.1 | Response to intervention—A multitiered approach to helping all learners succeed.

can be attended to at one time. Namely, they are time saving and efficient, and student issues can be simultaneously addressed. Groups are healthy environments in which students feel included, allowing for mutual learning, support, and sharing.

Group work also fits well within a school's Response to Intervention (RTI) plan as a targeted service (see Figure 1.1). To help struggling learners (e.g., students in special education) in a more collaborative and systemic way, school counselors have joined forces with teachers and other educators to implement RTI plans (for details, see Brown-Chidsey & Steege, 2005) and a complementary program called Schoolwide Positive Behavior Support (SWPBS; Curtis, Van Horne, Robertson, & Karvonen, 2010; see also http://www.pbis.org/ for resources). These interconnected, strengths-based approaches help students with differing levels of educational and psychosocial needs. Although group counseling is often implemented at Tier 1, this responsive service is considered most effective as a Tier 2 or 3 service (ASCA, 2008b; Marshak, Dandeneau, Prezant, & L'Amoreaux, 2009).

More specifically, whether students with learning challenges are participating in special education programming or not, all students within an RTI model are supposed to receive the appropriate level of targeted support. The RTI Action Network (Sugai, n.d.), a program of the National Center for Learning Disabilities and an informative resource for school counselors, exemplifies how the prevention/intervention process works: Tier 1 prevention attempts to meet all students' need to develop academic and social skills. Thus every student should receive a strong educational and prosocial behavior instruction and curriculum as a way to (a) avert the later development of problem behaviors, and (b) spot those learners whose behaviors indicate that they are not to be responding to conventional teaching. For those students who continue to struggle in school, Tier 2 involves more intensive academic and behavioral support (e.g., group counseling). Finally, Tier 3 entails even more specialized and concentrated educational and behavior support aimed at reducing learning barriers and the intensity level and/or severity of existing problem behavior.

Although we presented a few good reasons for doing groups, certainly there are obstacles to effective implementation. It is not uncommon for preservice and practicing secondary school counselors to ask a challenging question like this: "With all the hassles and limitations of schools today, do we really have adequate time and teacher and administrator buy-in to do group work well?" With the passage of the No Child Left Behind Act of 2001, and more recently, the "Race to the Top" (American Recovery and Reinvestment Act of 2009) legislation, most school counselors are doing their best to maintain quality services under stressful conditions where the pressure for improved academics can be overwhelming (McCarthy, Kerne, Calfa, Lambert, & Guzman, 2010; Wilkerson, 2009). Regrettably, many counselors, especially those who work in so-called "failing schools" and schools nearing this designation, have little desire to conduct groups. Some even push this essential service off their "to do" lists. Counselors, however, have to resist the temptation to give in to the prevailing climate of fear and the negative attitudes of some burned-out educators.

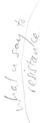

The reasons for conducting groups are important to keep in mind. For most educators and parents, a brief summary is all they require. Contrary to what you might hear in many hectic and academically focused schools, there still is adequate time for group work, and most students will benefit. However, in this day and age of results-based education and accountability, anecdotal evidence, such as that in Table 1.1, is simply not enough motivation for some administrators to make group work a priority service within schools. To counter the negativity, counselors need to implement small groups based on the national standards for counseling evaluation data (Astramovich & Coker, 2007; Sanders & Sullins, 2005) and efficacy research (see chapter 2 for a discussion). Counselors need to be able say with confidence to the skeptical: "Based on the solid evidence, group counseling *is* effective in changing student behavior and improving educational outcomes."

TYPES OF SMALL GROUPS

Once school counselors understand the value of small groups, they look forward to implementing them. To do so, counselors determine student needs, formulate group goals, screen potential members, and then decide on an appropriate group format. As you can probably imagine, the counseling literature offers group leaders multiple options. Thus school counselors attempt to match group members to the most appropriate group format, content, and process. They also need to consider whether the approach should be flexible and student driven, or one that is structured, curriculum centered, and counselor led. Sometimes educators and parents think the group sessions that are conducted in schools are psychotherapy sessions, raising red flags of concern. However, school counselors are not trained to use in-depth therapy techniques, and nor is the school an appropriate venue for them (Paisley & Milsom, 2007).

So what are the most appropriate group formats for school settings? To adequately answer this question, we summarize the major types (formats) of small groups discussed in the counseling literature. School-based groups are then compared with

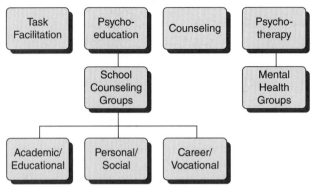

FIGURE 1.2 | Summary of key group designs (top level from ASGW, 2000; bottom level from ASCA, 2005a).

psychotherapeutic group sessions conducted in mental health/clinical settings. Next, school counseling groups are further differentiated into process- and content-oriented approaches. Finally, we overview content groups, which emphasize skill attainment related to academic/educational, personal/social, and career/vocational development.

Although there are many ways to categorize and define group types (e.g., M. S. Corey, Corey, & Corey, 2010; Pérusse, Goodnough, & Lee, 2009; Smead, 1995), the ASGW's *Professional Standards for the Training of Group Workers* (2000) lists four major approaches: (a) task facilitation, (b) psychoeducation, (c) counseling, and (d) psychotherapy. These are illustrated in Figure 1.2, and their defining characteristics, based on the ASGW Professional Standards, are listed in Table 1.2. Each group approach is suitable for off-campus mental health settings. However, psychotherapy groups and their target clientele (people experiencing severe and/or chronic maladjustment) are obviously incompatible with school environments (Paisley & Milsom, 2007).

Having similar features, the other three group options—task facilitation, psychoeducation (or psychoeducational), and counseling—are most commonly used in schools. These choices can address reasonably well students' developmental milestones (e.g., academic and career developmental groups) and their need for skill remediation (e.g., groups addressing issues that impede student learning and growth). Each approach can also be tailored to enhance the school climate (e.g., groups examining equity, diversity, or conflict resolution issues; Pérusse et al., 2009). Let's make some finer distinctions between group types.

School Counseling Groups versus Mental Health Psychotherapy Groups

To ensure that you understand why psychotherapy groups are inappropriate for school settings, this section briefly compares and contrasts the essential differences between school group counseling and groups conducted in mental health clinics, hospitals, and private practice (see Tier 2, Figure 1.1). Looking at Table 1.3, you will notice that school counselors conduct short-term, skill-based groups using a relatively structured curriculum,

TABLE 1.2 | Four Group Types Adapted from the ASGW (2000)

	Task or Work Group	Psychoeducational Group *(skill based)*	Group Counseling *aka (group therapy)*	Group Psychotherapy
Applies principles of	*normal* human development and functioning.			*normal* and *abnormal* human development and functioning.
Focuses on	educational, developmental, and systemic strategies	educational and developmental strategies.	cognitive, affective, behavioral, or systemic intervention strategies.	cognitive, affective, behavioral, or systemic intervention strategies.
Focuses on the context of	here-and-now interaction.			negative emotional arousal.
Promotes	efficient and effective accomplishment of group tasks.	personal and inter-personal growth as well as development and prevention of future difficulties.	personal and interpersonal growth and development as well as addresses personal and interpersonal problems of living.	personal and interpersonal problems of living, remediates perceptual and cognitive distortions or repetitive patterns of dysfunctional behavior, and promote personal and inter-personal growth.
Group members are people who may be	gathered to accomplish group task goals.	at risk for the develop-ment of personal or interpersonal problems or who seek enhancement of personal qualities and abilities.	experiencing transitory maladjustment, who are at risk for the development of personal or interpersonal problems, or who seek enhancement of personal qualities and abilities.	experiencing severe and/or chronic maladjustment.

Association for Specialists in Group Work. (ASGW). (2000). Professional standards for the training of group workers. Retrieved from http://www.asgw.org/training_standards.htm

13

TABLE 1.3 | Comparison of School-Based Groups and Clinic-Based Psychotherapy Groups

School-Based Groups	Clinic-Based Psychotherapy Groups
• Emphasize prevention and intervention activities and processes to support healthy student development and better coping with daily living challenges	• Emphasize remediation and treatment of clients' underlying mental health problems
• Designed for most K–12 students, including students who seek to enrich personal qualities and abilities; are experiencing short-term school, personal, interpersonal, or family concerns; and are at risk for more challenging problems (e.g., school failure)	• For most clients with potentially diagnosable long-term/chronic mental health problems (i.e., severe psychological and behavioral disorders)
• Group and student goals center around educational/academic, career/vocational, or personal/social goals, and helping students learn to reorient their feelings, thoughts, and behaviors toward healthy development and social interactions	• Group and client goals focus on re-structuring and reeducation to eliminate dysfunctional feelings, thoughts, and behaviors
• Stress the here and now, i.e., the present situation and conscious issues	• Stress current issues and past motivations (conscious and unconscious)
• Content and foci generally set by the group counselor based on student needs and group goals	• Content and emphases generally set by psychotherapist based on what she or he believes would be best for members' issues (diagnoses/needs)
• Conducted weekly for about 6–8 weeks (short-term)	• Conducted over the long term, that is, several or more months or even years
• Group counseling methods may include school-appropriate educational, developmental (emotional, cognitive, behavioral), and systemic strategies	• Group psychotherapy methods may include in-depth cognitive, affective, behavioral, or systemic intervention strategies

targeting student issues related to daily living (e.g., family and school stressors). Group psychotherapists, in contrast, address deeper and more persistent mental health problems over a longer period of time, and the actual group structure is often more dynamic, reflecting the clients' experiences and needs from session to session (Akos & Milsom, 2007; M. S. Corey et al., 2010). A quick word of caution though—some authors prefer the umbrella term *group therapy* rather than *group counseling* to denote any helping process occurring in a group setting such as support or skills training (e.g., anger management, mindfulness, relaxation training, or social skills training). Some use the label *psychoeducational* to identify skill-based groups (e.g., Montgomery, 2002).

Similar to mental health or psychotherapy groups conducted off campus, school-based groups require professional counselors to possess specific skills and competencies to successfully guide students as they work through commonplace developmental and situational issues (for details, see ASGW, 2000; Brigman & Campbell, 2003; Kayler & Sherman, 2009; Smead, 1995). Small groups in schools are generally most beneficial for students when organized to (a) develop more positive attitudes and better interpersonal skills, (b) support behavior change, and (c) transfer newly acquired skills and behavior to daily functioning (M. S. Corey et al., 2010; Paisley & Milsom, 2007).

Content versus Process Groups

Another way that is commonly used to distinguish group types is to look at their content and process. School- and clinic-based groups include both dimensions. As the term implies, content refers to what group members explore together, essentially the topic and curriculum of the group. Process relates to what the group leader does and says and what goes on within and between the group members. Strictly speaking, process involves the nature of the intra- and interpersonal dynamics occurring in groups (G. Corey, 2009; M. S. Corey et al., 2010). The psychotherapy and school counseling literature further differentiates process from content groups (Smead, 1995).

Process Groups—Practical and Theoretical Considerations

For at least 40 years now, most professional counselors are taught in their graduate programs that the important characteristics of counseling effectiveness are the attitudes, values, perceptions, and qualities of the helper as well as the processes (e.g., listening, modeling, facilitating cross-member discussion) underlying the counseling relationship (G. Corey, 2009; O'Hara, 2003; Pérusse et al., 2009; Ritter, 1978). So when the group's central theme and dynamics revolve around relationships, self-reflections, and exchanges among students and the counselor, the group tends to be more process focused (Smead, 1995). Counselors offer these groups for self-referred participants who desire to find out more about themselves and about what in their personal and social lives they would like to explore. Notably, as a therapist who regularly conducts process groups, Reeves (2008) likens them in part to the progressive stages of human development. The "therapeutic" group moves forward gradually from the initial "getting to know one other" phase to the final "consolidation of learning and growth" phase. Participants and the "group-as-a-whole" are supported by the leader (or coleaders) with guided feedback, process remarks, and nonverbal actions. If the process goes as intended, "the group inherently knits together with an abundance of experiences forming and emulating a social microcosm that bears its own unique culture and identity" (Reeves, 2008, n.p.).

Although process groups are relatively similar in design and practice, helping professionals use different descriptors reflecting the terminology used in their particular work setting. In a private practice, for example, psychotherapists may refer to them as personal growth or self-discovery groups, whereas in more public clinical settings or schools you will hear vague terms like *support group* or simply a *counseling group* (ASGW, 2000; M. S. Corey et al., 2010). Whatever they are called, if you observe a process group in a school or a mental health clinic, it generally appears to be free-flowing, lacking structure, and nondirective, emphasizing member interactions as well as individual member self-reflection and awareness. Encouraged by the ASCA (2008a), small groups such as these are particularly useful because they provide students an opportunity "to develop insights

Key to humanistic — *Experiencing — thinking, sensing, perceiving, feeling, remembering — subjective & free will, root to self growth + taking responsibility*

16   SECTION 1   Before the Action Starts

into themselves and others, ... to achieve healthier personal adjustment, cope with the stress of a rapidly changing and complex environment and learn to communicate and co-operate with others" (p. 24). Reflecting ASCA's statement, Smead (1995) noted that "by focusing on process, group members [students] learn to express and hear feelings, give and receive feedback, and support one another in the here and now" (p. 10).

Process-oriented groups conducted in schools also need to be in part theory driven (see chapter 2). When reading the above descriptions of process-oriented groups, it is no coincidence that the embedded concepts and techniques may remind you of humanistic psychology. Along with elements of developmental psychology (e.g., Erikson's 1963 psychosocial stage theory), Rogers's (1961/1989) child-centered approach largely undergirds process groups. As discussed later, this humanistic approach emphasizes active listening.

— looking at the issue through the client
— people are innately good

Examples of School-Based Process Groups

For a variety of reasons, process or growth groups are not as widely practiced in schools today as in previous decades. Even though contemporary examples of process-oriented groups are difficult to find in the school counseling literature, these types of groups are still facilitated at all grade levels (see, e.g., Baggerly & Parker, 2005, for discussion of a successful elementary school group for African American boys). Bauer, Sapp, and Johnson (2000), for instance, demonstrated the efficacy of high school counseling support groups (and content-focused psychoeducational groups) for students at risk for dropping out. Using a Rogerian-type child-centered approach to improving student self-esteem, the well-trained support group counselors focused their leadership efforts with these therapeutic skills in mind: unconditional acceptance, active listening, reflection of feelings and meaning, clarification, and summarization. As you would expect, the groups were loosely structured and the topics varied according to the issues raised by the students. Members were encouraged to provide their peers with feedback and support as they wrestled with problems and possible resolutions. Moreover, school counselors encouraged the students to express and share their feelings related to negative school and home experiences. Looking at the student outcomes, general self-esteem scores rose considerably from pre- to posttesting. Because the groups did not emphasize academic issues, it is not surprising that the students' grade point averages and academic self-concept scores did not vary much over time. Important to note, however, the in-school detention rates for the group members decreased over time, from an average of 3.2 events over a 10-week period prior to the start of the group intervention to 0.64 events (measured over a 20-week period following the group intervention launch). Clearly, these promising results suggest that school counselors should find time to conduct growth groups.

Even more unlikely to see in schools these days, process groups are beneficial with younger students. Akos (2000) reported on an elementary school empathy development group. His rationale for such a group reflects a strengths-based developmental focus (see Galassi & Akos, 2007), arguing that "as children seek to connect with others, empathy provides the foundation and skills necessary to develop competent social interaction" (Akos, p. 217). Because they are safe, warm, and caring learning environments, process-oriented groups are ideally suited for exploring and trying out empathy-related skills. With younger children, kindergarteners through second-graders, group counselors will

empathy dev.

find that the use of puppets, artwork, clay, and games will encourage emotional responsiveness. Children are encouraged to identify their own emotions using simple nonverbal (e.g., smiley faces) and verbal expressions. One way to do this, Akos explained, is for school counselors to distribute colorful "kid-friendly" magazines and play an "I spy" game (or a "Where's Waldo"-type activity) to find a face depicting someone who, for example, is happy, angry, or surprised. Next, the children share their examples and the rationale for their selections, with the counselor helping them work through how the connections to particular feelings were made. To further help children learn to experience and recognize their own emotions, counselors can display big photographs or pictures to elicit particular feelings in group members. Group sharing about how the photo made them feel is encouraged. Another exercise is to ask the children about how their "tummies" felt when they were last upset. Using a prop such as a mirror, they can explore what their facial features look like when they express anger and love.

For children further along in elementary school, Akos's (2000) empathy groups would expand on the vocabulary of feelings learned in the earlier grades. Group members in this age range are encouraged to work through the emotional meaning of their daily experiences (e.g., playing on the playground, doing well on a test, or having a disagreement with a friend). Similar to running empathy groups with young members, the use of activities to stimulate discussion is helpful. Akos recommends the use of games (e.g., Connect Four, Chutes and Ladders, Jenga, Skip-Bo, Uno) during group to generate emotions. Team-building experiences that help children see how others are feeling during the activity can foster emotional awareness. Related to the members experiencing and sharing group emotionality, empathy growth groups include activities that target children's ability to take the perspective of other members of the group. Through team building, games, or other school experiences, students can use group as a place to learn to observe cues and ask peers about emotional experiences. In addition, school counselors can use the students and their own creativity to facilitate the group. Training students in drama is one of the more effective and fun ways for students to examine the emotions and perspectives of others. Using scripts that demonstrate context around emotional experiences provides valuable learning. Movies, stories, and television can even be material for discussion of actor perspectives. For additional ideas, one could consult, for example, Devencenzi and Pendergast's (1999) book addressing the issue of "belonging" and how school counselors might lead a self- and social discovery group for children and adolescents. In short, this process-oriented group format provides children with the opportunities to experience, practice, and gain useful feedback from their peers.

Finally, evidence suggests if the group process is facilitated well, the underlying "therapeutic" factors will contribute to positive group experiences and participant outcomes (Blocher & Wade, 2010). Through the social interactions, this type of small group can help students develop a stronger sense of personal meaning, cope better with daily stresses, and express more effectively their culture (Stroh & Sink, 2002). Students learn healthy ways to negotiate their world while at the same time enhancing their personal growth. Importantly though, counselors must devise these groups very carefully, and students must be at the appropriate cognitive and psychosocial developmental level to take full advantage of the experience. Thus the ultimate value of process groups is highly dependent on student willingness to be completely engaged and the counselor's authenticity, modeling, and facilitation skills (M. S. Corey et al., 2010).

Content Groups—Practical and Theoretical Considerations

Unlike process groups, content-driven groups are flourishing in schools. Numerous examples are documented in the school counseling literature and in this chapter's supplement. Analogous to traditional classroom teaching and large-group guidance activities, school counselors facilitate small groups around an existing curriculum. Naturally, content groups still are reliant on effective process, but they are far more planned, structured, and skill based. School counselors design and conduct them as educational experiences, where group members learn and practice new behaviors and skills related mainly to school success. Whereas process-growth groups tend to reflect individual differences and interpersonal dynamics among group members, school-based groups are more concerned with the members learning and demonstrating the skills embedded in the content (Bauer et al., 2000; Stroh & Sink, 2002). For example, content groups may have the students work on study and test-taking skills, cognitive and metacognitive skills (e.g., goal setting, time management, and planning), social skills (e.g., conflict resolution, anger management, verbal and nonverbal communication), and self-management skills (e.g., emotional regulation, achievement motivation) (e.g., Kayler & Sherman, 2009).

Content groups may also help students develop important life skills (Picklesimer, Hooper, & Gineter, 1998). For instance, such a group may revolve around the subject matter of "making positive career choices." Because career choices tend to strongly affect one's quality-of-life perceptions, students learning together in group settings are able to safely explore these and related issues. As with all content-oriented groups, school counselors craft relevant skill-building activities that might involve training in assertive behavior, empathic responding, appropriate self-disclosure, listening tactics, role playing, and practice assignments. Group counseling methods can also include short presentations, printed material, audiovisuals, role playing, role rehearsal, and so on.

Content-driven groups are often simply referred to as *psychoeducational* skill development groups (Kayler & Sherman, 2009). Unlike *psychotherapy* groups, psychoeducational groups, as the term implies, are small groups with clear educational and psychological goals. Although process and content groups are similar in that they both emphasize member participation and interrelationships, group dynamics, and processes, psychoeducational groups are designed to help students develop a particular skill set within a content area (N. W. Brown, 2004). Moreover, psychoeducational groups tend to operate under two basic assumptions: (a) They are appropriate for all ages and settings, and (b) the groups emphasize education or learning over self-awareness and self-understanding. Counselors tend to deemphasize at some level the emotional side (feelings, motivations) of the group experience in favor of the cognitive dimension (N. W. Brown, 2004). A variety of techniques are used by the leader to improve student learning, understanding, and retention, including, for example, the use of games, role plays, learning exercises, and homework. One such 9-week psychoeducational group using cognitive-behavioral techniques produced positive academic and self-esteem outcomes with rural high school students at risk for dropout (Bauer et al., 2000). This group focused on teaching students how to identify academic and behavioral goals and then strategies (e.g., challenging irrational beliefs, self-monitoring, goal setting, success inventories, contracting) to attain their goals.

For their conceptual grounding, counselors leading content groups rely heavily on a mixture of three key sources:

1. developmental psychology (e.g., Jean Piaget's [Piaget & Inhelder, 1966/2000] cognitive development; Lawrence Kohlberg's [Power, Higgins, & Kohlberg, 1989] moral reasoning stages; Erik Erikson's [1963] psychosocial development; and Donald Super's [1990] career development; see also Green & Piel, 2010, and Halverson, 2002, for summaries);

2. social-cognitive/self-efficacy theory (Albert Bandura, 2001); and

3. allied approaches to cognitive-behavioral therapy (CBT; e.g., A. Ellis's rational emotive behavior therapy; A. Beck's cognitive therapy; see Dobson, 2010, and Nelson-Jones, 2000, for extensive overviews).

A psychoeducational group focused on teaching students conflict resolution skills may use all three sources. Group planning involves creating developmentally appropriate "lessons" for each meeting, and the actual counseling techniques used in the group might include elements of social-cognitive theory and CBT methods. Because an adequate review of developmental psychology is beyond the scope of this book, we recommend that school counselors refresh their memories by reading a general text or two (e.g., Green & Piel, 2010).

Content Groups Using ASCA's (2004a, 2005a) Developmental Domains

Returning to the bottom level of Figure 1.1, you will notice that the school counseling-appropriate groups can then be divided into *content* areas, reflecting one or more of ASCA's (2004a, 2005a) developmental domains. Certainly, you are not limited to just these general areas or the competencies included in ASCA's (2005a) National Model and ASCA's (2004a) National Standards. Your district or school may want to use small groups to help students expand their multicultural, character, or spirituality-related skills.

Academic Content Groups   If school counselors are mainly concerned with fostering academic/educational development, then content groups tend to initially "implement strategies and activities to support and maximize each student's ability to learn" (ASCA, 2004a, n.p.). Specifically, student educational competencies to focus on might include academic self-concept, skills for improving learning and achieving school success, and goal setting and planning. However, each group will have additional competencies that relate to the content covered in the group. For instance, suppose you wanted to lead a group for chronic underachievers. Perhaps you might aim to improve students' attention and engagement in class, achievement motivation, interest in class subjects, school rules compliance, organizational skills, note taking, identification of personal strengths, and cooperation with peers and teachers (Myrick, 2002).

The empowerment groups for academic success (EGAS) model is an excellent example of an academic-centered group from the school counseling literature (Bemak, Chung, & Siroskey-Sabdo, 2005; Johnson & Johnson, 2005; see chapter 1 supplement for overview of EGAS). The model's aim is to reach students in public high schools, deploying various group traditional strategies and structures (e.g., using a coleader, having a set number of meetings, developing objectives, and creating group unity and support). However, EGAS goes further, "by building in a multicultural approach that is sensitive to the environmental elements that impact students living in urban settings and uses the strengths of an unstructured process group with clearly defined goals to develop individual student success" (Johnson & Johnson, 2005, p. 399). As you can see, school counselors can combine multiple group counseling techniques and formats to "deliver" the academic content.

Personal/Social Development Groups   Content groups supporting ASCA's (2004a) personal/social development domain "provide the foundation for personal and social growth as students progress through school and into adulthood" (n.p.). Group counselors focus on helping students learn about themselves and others, as well as how to apply this knowledge to their school and home lives. Among many others, another competency area might include helping students acquire personal safety skills. As mentioned above, each personal/social group will have its own specific set of student competencies. In a group looking to help students cope with personal grief, R. H. Meyer (2006) suggested that the counseling group examine topics such as: (a) the feelings associated with grief (e.g., isolation and aloneness, sadness, anger), (b) the need for support, (c) how life changes after the loss of a loved one, (d) the effects of grief on the body, (e) family rituals following the loss, (f) how to use memories to cope with loss, (g) stress reduction strategies, (h) restoring hope, and (i) moving on. A small group designed to support students while one or more of their families are deployed to a distant military base requires another set of topics and potential student outcomes (see Aydlett, 2008, for examples).

Career Development Groups   Career development groups are mainly skills based, providing "the foundation for the acquisition of skills, attitudes and knowledge that enable students to make a successful transition from school to the world of work, and from job to job across the life span" (ASCA, 2004a, n.p.). They also overlap with other school-based counseling groups in many regards. For instance, they are largely similar in their information sources, the group processes used, and the desired outcomes (Pyle, 2007). Obvious differences include the group content. Group career counseling topics are narrowed primarily to career and vocational issues. Leaders use the participants' self-knowledge as well as external information about educational and occupational choices to guide the discussion. They help students through structured exercises to develop career awareness and employment readiness, as well as to gain career-related information and identify career goals. Moving from knowledge to application, group counselors also support the development of skills needed to achieve career goals. Action plans are created, so students operationalize their learning. One such career-focused high school small group might address ways to (a) actively search out colleges and plan for one's career, (b) determine the realities of one's chosen career, and (c) accurately estimate the financial cost of a college education (Gibbons, Borders, Stephen, & Davis, 2006).

Examples of Content Groups

Unlike the process-focused groups, exemplars of successful structured groups are well documented in the school counseling literature. Good models can be located in the group counseling texts, journal articles, and online. If you search the Web using terms like *group counseling schools*, you will be amazed at how many useful psychoeducational group plans are available. Additional examples are available on ASCA's online resource center web page (see http://www.schoolcounselor.org/; e.g., Campbell & Brigman, 2005). For instance, one helpful document located at the ASCA website provides sample small-group counseling topics and objectives (see chapter supplement). Next, a couple of real-world examples of content/psychoeducational groups conducted in schools are summarized.

Our first model content group aimed at supporting elementary-age students with ADHD (Webb & Myrick, 2003) goes by the letters SSS. Using the student success skills (SSS) model as its central organizing principles, the authors designed a 6-week group with the underlying supposition that the SSS group counseling approach could increase children's understanding of their ADHD challenges and how they impact school performance. Furthermore, the authors posited that group counseling has the advantage of approximating real-life peer relationship situations. In particular, the group's long-term goal was to help the targeted students realize that their ADHD would not keep them from reaching their personal, academic, or career goals. Calling the group experience "The Journey," Table 1.4 summarizes each session's content and objectives. Evaluation tools showed promising student outcomes following the group experience.

A second exemplary content group called "Creating Healthy Relationships" was documented by Zinck and Littrell (2000). At first glance at the group's title, one would think that a process group might be more appropriate for this topic, but psychoeducational groups work just as well or better. This content-focused group was conducted with 35 adolescent girls who were involved in high-risk relationships with friends, boyfriends, family members, or loosely knit gangs. They were also at risk for dropping out, running away, criminal activity, pregnancy, abuse, and exploitation. This healthy relationships group centered on teaching students how to recognize and develop healthy relationships, and how to recognize and avoid unhealthy or unsafe relationships. The girls were also taught how to define their primary problem and to set behavioral goals related to coping and problem solving. Summarized in Table 1.5, each session had three components, involving educational, counseling, and skill development. The overall results of this group were positive, showing that relationship development skills can be readily explored with students in a more structured fashion.

FINAL THOUGHTS

To summarize, in our data-driven and outcomes-based schools, psychoeducational groups appear to be the group format of choice for most school counselors. Practitioners find that content-oriented groups are efficient and valuable ways for students to make progress toward mastering various academic, personal/social, and career developmental

TABLE 1.4 | Overview of the Journey: Group Counseling Intervention for ADHD Students

Session Number, Title, and Activity	Students Will
1. Our Journey. Activity: Map Quest	1. gain increased knowledge of ADHD 2. identify behaviors related to ADHD and the influence of these behaviors on school success 3. discuss ADHD diagnosis and express associated emotions
2. Pack It Up. Activity: Messy Bag	1. learn and practice strategies to help improve organization skills related to school success
3. Stop Lights and Traffic Cops. Activity: Signs Around Us	1. learn and practice behaviors related to attending 2. identify school situations where attending is important 3. identity school situations were attending is a challenge
4. Using Road Signs as a Guide. Activity: Reading Classroom Cues	1. learn to recognize, create, and use external cues in the classroom 2. increase awareness of the need for school success strategies
5. Road Holes and Detours. Activity: When Things Don't Go Right	1. identify school situations that are challenging 2. identify ways to improve challenging school situations
6. Roadside Assistance and Being Your Own Mechanic. Activity: Increasing Control of Our Success	1. identify school resources 2. experience the feelings of self-control 3. make connections between the practice of a skill with improvement of that skills 4. increased knowledge of medications used to treat ADHD

Source: Adapted from Webb and Myrick (2003, p. 111).

competencies outlined in the ASCA (2005a) National Model (McGannon, Carey, & Dimmit, 2005; Paisley & Milsom, 2007). Group curricula and sample activities are widely available in the counseling literature and online, allowing for quick access, adaptation, and planning. Student outcomes are relatively easy to assess with a pre- and

TABLE 1.5 | Overview of "Creating Healthy Relationships" Counseling Group

Component	Topics
Educational	• healthy relationships, unhealthy and unsafe relationships, personal boundaries, violence in relationships, communication in relationships, effects of chemical use upon relationships, managing anger and conflict, community resources
Counseling	• increased awareness and expression of feelings, recognition of and distinction between needs and wants, and development of an internal locus of control • confidence, assertiveness, and capacity for self-evaluation • modeling and development of empathy
Skills	• teaching students to recognize and avoid unhealthy relationships, defining and maintaining healthy boundaries, exiting dangerous situations, recognizing and exiting unhealthy communication triangles, developing personal safety plan • refusal skills and anger management

Source: From Zinck and Littrell (2000).

posttest. In the next chapter, we turn our attention to the foundational components of group counseling: the role of theory in planning and implementing small groups, and efficacy results supporting the use of groups in schools.

CHAPTER 1 SUPPLEMENTS

Supplement 1   Sample Elementary School Small-Group Counseling Topics and Objectives (Adapted from ASCA, 2006–2010)

Topics	Potential Group Objectives
Developmental Domain: Academic/Educational	
Doing Well in School	1. List goals and make a plan on how to accomplish them. 2. Monitor academic progress. 3. Develop study skills. 4. Develop organizational skills.
Developing Good Study Skills	1. Identify the best place and time to study. 2. Set short-term academic goals. 3. Develop organizational skills. 4. Learn processes to best utilize time. 5. Monitor academic processes.
Developmental Domain: Personal/Social	
Creating Positive Friendships	1. Analyze how to make new friends. 2. Identify important qualities of a friend. 3. Understand common friendship problems. 4. Learn how to manage conflicts. 5. Develop a plan to improve friendships.
Understanding Yourself and Others	1. Understand your characteristic traits and uniqueness. 2. Develop a positive self-image. 3. Identify strengths. 4. Improve relationships. 5. Understand behavior/misbehavior.
Developing a Healthy Self-Concept (K–2)	1. Emphasize uniqueness. 2. Identify feelings and appropriately express them. 3. Understand similarities with others. 4. Develop a positive self-image.
Helping New Students Adjust	1. Help student become comfortable in new school. 2. Become acquainted with school. 3. Build new friendships in and out of group. 4. Have a school buddy (special class friend/helper).
Understanding Our Family (Divorce/Separation)	1. Express feelings about changing family. 2. Understand that divorce/separation is not the child's fault. 3. Identify common problems associated with divorce/separation. 4. Understand positive ways family and group members can help in adjustment.

Topics	Potential Group Objectives
Managing My Anger	1. Identify factors that cause anger. 2. Understand the consequences of irrational behavior when angry. 3. Examine why some situations make everyone angry and others do not. 4. Identify different anger reduction techniques.
Making Good Choices (Drug and Alcohol Prevention)	1. Learn dangers of drugs and alcohol. 2. Understand and utilize the problem-solving model. 3. Learn refusal skills. 4. Identify ways to have fun and keep friends while staying out of trouble. 5. Develop a plan to handle peer pressure.
Coping with Loss (Grief)	1. Express feelings about loss. 2. Learn the stages of grief. 3. Discuss happy memories. 4. Identify ways to handle stress and loss.
Getting Along in Class (Classroom Behavior)	1. Understand behavior/misbehavior. 2. Identify causes for misbehavior. 3. Set short- and long-term goals. 4. Identify positive ways to get attention in the classroom. 5. Learn and implement effective behavior plan.
Dealing Better with Conflict	1. Identify feelings and appropriately express them. 2. Learn win/win resolutions. 3. Speak clearly. 4. Understand others' point of view (be empathic). 5. Learn how to talk out conflicts.

Supplement 2 Additional Examples of School-Based Groups Categorized According to ASCA's (2004a, 2005a) Developmental Domains.

Educational/Academic

Study Skills and Tutoring Combo (Edmondson & White, 1998)

- The combination of group counseling services and tutoring for at-risk secondary school students can be useful.
- The group's foci are: (a) improving self-esteem and (b) classroom behavior.
- One group of students in the study received 2 hours of academic tutoring each week. The second group received tutoring and also participated in a self-esteem group focusing on developing study skills. A third student group served as a control (no tutoring or counseling services were provided). Students in the group receiving academic tutoring and group counseling improved significantly in achievement, classroom behavior, and self-esteem, as compared to those who merely received academic tutoring.

Empowerment for Academic Success (EGAS; Bemak, Chung, & Siroskey-Sabdo 2005)

- Multicultural EGAS groups were implemented at an inner-city high school with high rates of expulsion and suspension, teen pregnancy, absenteeism, poverty, and poor academic records.
- Students chosen to participate in the group were at high risk of suspension, academic failure, and dropout.
- Group participants were allowed to choose the discussion topic for each group meeting, while the ultimate goals focused on academic achievement. This method facilitated thoughtful discussion about the group experience and the group member's lives and how external events affect school achievement. This group counseling approach empowers members by allowing them to talk about what is meaningful to them.

School Success Skills (Brigman, Webb, & Campbell, 2007)

- School counselors led a student success skills program on the academic and social competence of students. Students from Grades 5, 6, 8, and 9 from six schools were randomly compared using state achievement tests in math and reading and a measure of social competence.
- The goal of SSS is to teach academic, social, and self-management skills—both classroom and group counseling components.
- Specific skills targeted in group were goal setting, progress monitoring, and memory skills; interpersonal skills, social problem solving, listening, and teamwork skills; and managing attention, motivation, and anger.
- The intervention focused on cognitive, social, and self-management skills to improve academic achievement.

Personal/Social

Discovery Program for Problem Behavior (Brake & Gerler, 1994)

- Developed for fourth- and fifth-grade boys with a history of inappropriate classroom behavior, this group's aim was, in part, to promote moral development and improve school performance.
- Sessions included lessons on acquiring a repertoire of learning strategies, including higher-order thinking skills (i.e., members were challenged to think at a level slightly higher than their current developmental stage) and responsibility and role taking.
- A practical service learning component was added to the group experience, where the boys were taught and role-played the basic skills and attitudes required to assist in a kindergarten classroom. The boys worked with the children for 25 class sessions lasting 30 minutes each. After each session, they met with the group counselor to discuss, reflect, and gain support.
- In the end, the group experience and training helped the boys gain confidence in their own abilities as well as look at themselves from another's point of view.

Group Intervention for Students with Depression (Sommers-Flanagan, Barrett-Hakanson, Clarke, & Sommers-Flanagan, 2000).

- According to the authors, school-based settings are appropriate for depression prevention and intervention.
- The model involved a 12-week group designed for middle school students with subclinical, mild, or moderate depressive symptoms and those children who are at risk for depression.
- Before conducting the group, possible members were identified and screened for group compatibility. Students were administered a depression inventory (e.g., Children's Depression Inventory or Reynolds Child Depression Scale) to get a sense of their pregroup depressive symptoms and screen for suicide ideation.
- Each session had a theme and a home project for the following week. The themes addressed the thoughts, emotions, and behaviors listed below:
  a. understanding the spiral effect of a negative focus;
  b. learning the use of relaxation to combat tension and anxiety;
  c. learning basic problem-solving strategies in a group context;
  d. understanding the social effects of irritating habits versus. attempts to be friendly;
  e. goal setting; and
  f. communication skills.

Self-Esteem Development (Khattab & Jones, 2007)

- A small group called "Growing Up Girl" was developed for fifth-grade girls (ages 9–11) who were particularly prone to negative self-esteem issues. The primary intent was to have the girls learn about and discuss puberty, body image, and peer relationships. Additionally, it gave them the opportunity to learn and practice positive coping skills in a safe environment.
- The authors provided a strong rationale for facilitating the group, suggesting that for elementary school girls the developmental period is vital to forming a positive self-worth and enhancing personal resiliency.
- Group topics included: patterns of development, fundamentals of positive body images (challenging media influences), developing healthy life habits, eating well, and social skills relevant for making and keeping friends.

Career/Vocational

Postsecondary Planning (Carrier, 1992)

- The school counselor designed and conducted a group for high school seniors who had not yet decided what they wanted to do after graduation. Students were also provided individual guidance.
- Participants were solicited by the school counselor from her caseload. Students were asked about their plans for after graduation and completed a survey.
- The group experience explored a career-planning guidebook and also toured local training and employment sites.
- Group counseling was found to be more effective than individual counseling, because the group format introduced a strong peer influence element. Group members held each other accountable for any commitments made during their time together.

Choosing the Military as a Career (Ciborowski, 1994)

- This psychoeducational group is based on a decision-making model that focuses on exploring military recruitment information, lifestyle contrasts, and values clarification.
- The group is for adolescents (13–17 years of age) and provides a forum for students and counselors to openly discuss this career path as it relates to enlisting in the armed services.
- Counselors must be clearly knowledgeable about the military, personal values, and possible group activities, so further training may be required.
- The author suggests that three sessions held in the autumn and lasting for a class period should be sufficient.
- The content and foci of each group session are presented here:
  a. Session 1 (Goal: to allow time for the recruiters to clarify what military enlistment entails)
     - The counselor explains the exploration program and its foci.
     - The counselor then introduces representatives of the armed services. This may include the use of films, slides, and distribution of literature.
     - The group format allows for an open discussion and questions between the service representatives and the students.
     - Harassment and discrimination issues should also be explored.
  b. Session 2 (Goal: to explore student values and lifestyle and how they match with the military)
     - The counselor begins a discussion of military life issues, focusing on the challenges of military discipline and daily regimen.
     - Members then discuss the appropriateness of this lifestyle to their own situation and values.
     - High school graduates who are in the service or who have had some military experience could be invited to be a part of the conversation.
     - Note: The counselor ensures there is a balance of perspectives discussed.
  c. Session 3 (Goal: to explore the moral issues of conscientious objection status and lifestyle discriminations of the services)
     - The counselor facilitates a discussion of current laws.
     - The counselor includes, if need be, knowledgeable community members who could explain military terms, laws, and so on.
     - The group conversation according to Ciborowski (1994) should center on student "values" and students' beliefs and feelings about the armed services.
  d. Additional sessions (if desired)
     - Later meetings could be scheduled to address, for example, the views of military families.
  e. Individual follow-up session with school counselor
     - Participants have another opportunity to examine their own lifestyle, career goals, and moral perspectives.
     - The one-on-one meetings can be used to determine whether or not the group sessions were useful to the students' decision-making process.

School-to-Work (or Postsecondary Education/Training) Transition Groups for High School Students with Disabilities (McEachern & Kenny, 2007)

- The authors provided two models of psychoeducational groups that can help students with special needs to transition from school-to-work or to school-to-postsecondary training/education.
- Group 1, "Transition to Further Education," gives students with special needs the skills necessary to be successful in post–Grade 12 educational settings.
  a. The group focuses on mutual support, knowledge attainment, and skill building.
  b. Participants ideally should include students in their junior years (ages 16–18) who are planning to attend a 2- or 4-year college.
  c. The group experience can be conducted for a longer period of time on Saturdays or during the regular class period on school days.
  d. Group processes include role playing, discussion, questions and responses, etc.
  e. Conducted over nine sessions, the topics include: (1) awareness of self and others; (2) self-determination and self-advocacy; (3) making the right college choice; (4) understanding and navigating through admissions; (5) what I need to know about my legal rights; (6) assessing college support services; (7) choosing a college major; (8) making new connections; and (9) ending, yet getting started.
- Group 2, "Transition to Work," provides members with the needed support, knowledge attainment, and skill building required to be successful on the job.
  a. The potential group members are comparable to those appropriate for Group 1.
  b. Group processes and time frame are the same.
  c. Conducted over nine sessions, the topics reflect, in part, those presented in Group 1: (1) awareness of self and others; (2) self-determination and self-advocacy; (3) why work?; (4) finding the right job for me; (5) how much do I need to make?; (6) the application process; (7) the job interview; (8) making a plan and following it; and (9) ending, yet getting started.
- Evaluation of group and student outcomes is encouraged.

Supplement 3 Additional Resources

Barlow, S. H., Fuhriman, A. J., & Burlingame, G. M. (2004). The history of group counseling and psychotherapy. In J. L. DeLucia-Waack, D. A. Gerrity, C. R. Kalodner, & M. T. Riva (Eds.), *Handbook of group counseling and psychotherapy* (pp. 3–22). Thousand Oaks, CA: Sage. (Useful history of group counseling and psychotherapy)

Blum, D. J., & Davis, T. E. (2010). *The school counselor's book of lists* (2nd ed.). New York: Wiley. (See section on small-group counseling)

Hernandez, M. (Ed.). (2010). *Self-esteem across the lifespan: Issues and interventions.* New York: Taylor & Francis. (Addresses key issues relevant to group work)

Hughes, F. P. (2009). *Children, play, and development* (4th ed.). Thousand Oaks, CA: Sage. (Covers developmental issues from birth through adolescence)

Miller, E., & Reid, C. (2009). Counseling older adults: Practical implications. *The professional counselor's desk reference* (pp. 777–787). New York: Springer.

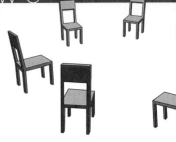

Foundations of School-Based Group Counseling

Frwsm research based ideas + techniques)

> *Theories help counselors understand the dynamics of human behavior and choose therapeutic approaches appropriate to specific clients and situations. Psychological theories come alive in the counselor's mind if they are seen as extensions of life experiences of various theorists.*
> —Victor J. Drapela (1990, p. 19)

The previous chapter provided an introduction to the landscape of group counseling. The types of small groups school counselors can offer students range from relatively free-flowing process-oriented groups to structured content-driven skills development groups. It would be expedient if this background information was all that was needed to run successful groups. However, before leaping wholeheartedly into small-group implementation, school counselors must first establish their practice on a solid foundation (Pérusse et al., 2009). The primary aim of this chapter, therefore, is to review the research-based counseling theories and associated techniques that are fundamental to effective group work in the schools. To begin our discussion, read over the following scenario. It offers a realistic glimpse of how a small group might be initiated in a middle school. Look for any clues that reflect the need to understand theory and research.

GROUPS IN PRACTICE

Middle School Boys Group

Ms. Fitz-Gibbon, a veteran middle school counselor, has several Grade 6 boys on her caseload with learning and behavioral challenges. They are in jeopardy of leaving middle school ill-prepared for high school. Each struggles to some extent with managing their behavior in stressful classroom situations as well as during unstructured time (e.g., lunch period). Because Ms. Fitz-Gibbon's school uses a Response to Intervention (RTI) plan for supporting all students, first-level classroom interventions were attempted on three occasions with no real change in the boys' behavior. Following the ethical

Source: The value of theories for counseling practitioners. *International Journal for the Advancement of Counselling, 13*(1), 19–26.

standards of the school counseling profession and in an attempt to head off further problems, she then decided to try a Level 2 intervention for each student. Ms. Fitz-Gibbon required parent and staff approval to move forward; so at the students' upcoming parent–teacher conferences and with the counselor's encouragement, the families and relevant teachers agreed that more intensive intervention was needed. The counselor outlined the various strategies she could provide, including individual or small-group counseling. In consultation with the school psychologist, who was also present at these particular meetings, the attendees decided that the boys needed to specifically improve their emotional regulation and self-management skills. Consensus was also found on a good way to achieve this aim. Because the boys would benefit from realistic feedback and positive peer modeling in a safe setting, the counselor would conduct a 6-week small group focusing on psychosocial skills development. Two other boys with stronger interpersonal skills would also be encouraged to join the group experience.

School counselors assist all students, including those with special needs and those at risk for school failure (ASCA, 2004c). If counselors do this well, they also support teachers and families. In reviewing the scenario, Ms. Fitz-Gibbon and the other educators believe that a small-group experience would be an advisable intervention for these challenging boys. She is committed to providing the students with a secure and caring place to obtain and accept the additional support they need. She hopes that the boys will gain the prosocial skills needed for educational success in middle school and beyond. Ms. Fitz-Gibbon also knows, within the context of the school's RTI plan and comprehensive school counseling program (CSCP), that small-group counseling is a useful strategy to foster the boys' educational and personal/social development.

The next step for Ms. Fitz-Gibbon is to frame the group experience on relevant theory and research. With this information, she can generate specific learning objectives, decide on the most suitable group format, plan the session content (curriculum) and activities, and devise an easy way to document student outcomes. As you will learn in the next chapter, the counselor will also work through the logistics of running a group (e.g., making the time schedule, obtaining parent and student consent). No matter how the group experience is designed and conducted, her ultimate group goals will be to help the boys to (a) overcome those behavioral, psychological, and situational obstacles adversely impacting their learning, and (b) extend their prosocial behaviors to their family lives (M. S. Corey et al., 2010; Smead, 1995).

WHY THEORY AND RESEARCH?

As you gathered from the above discussion, successful group practice is not as simple as doing what comes naturally to a leader or what the counselor "feels" is most appropriate for a particular set of students. Not surprisingly, however, some graduate students and practicing school counselors question the need for theory- and research-based groups. Sometimes after shadowing school counselors in the field, preservice counselors notice that seasoned group leaders tend to be more eclectic in their methods. During school-based or clinical classes, such as practicum and internship, beginning counselors may also express anxiety about learning and applying multiple theories on a group-by-group

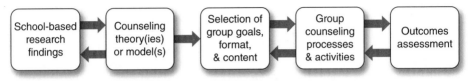

FIGURE 2.1 | Interrelationships among theory, research, best practice, and outcomes assessment.

basis. To be sure, strong group leadership takes substantial preparation, reflection, and adaptability.

Despite these concerns, counselor educators continue to advocate for the application of theory and research in group work (e.g., Capuzzi, 2003; Gladding, 2008; Jacobs, Masson, & Harvill, 2009; Pérusse et al., 2009). Some 50 years ago, Carl Rogers (1961/1989) affirmed that a useful theory allows the counselor to find patterns, order, and meaning in an otherwise seemingly chaotic world of emotions, thoughts, and behaviors. More recently, Gladding, like Rogers, suggested that without a sound theory to operate from, only confusion can result. A serviceable theory is like a naviga-tional tool. Practitioners not only have a sound and purposeful conceptual framework to conduct their groups, they also can utilize theory to formulate and refine their own individualized approach to counseling. Good theory provides insight into how groups evolve and how group members might behave from session to session.

Gladding (2008) further explained the usefulness of theory:

> The knowledge of theory generally helps group leaders formulate a specific approach for each group member. It is the leader-as-scientist's task to enhance the fit between the hypothetical group and the actual one. Theory allows for the making and testing of predictions about how the group member will behave in response to particular environmental conditions, including selected interventions. (p. 83)

Theory can also direct research efforts, allowing for ongoing improvements in group practices and processes. In turn, outcome assessments and evidence-based group prac-tice refine theory. This partnership between theory and research informs group plan-ning, organization, goals, and content, as well as shapes what occurs in the experience, its processes, and its activities. The interrelationships between theory, research, best practice, and assessment are represented in Figure 2.1.

Returning to the case study, Ms. Fitz-Gibbon could benefit from knowing some theory and research, specifically as a means to ground her middle school group. With this knowledge, tasks like goal and content/curriculum development, activity planning, and pre- and postgroup group assessments become easier to accomplish. By reviewing the professional literature, Ms. Fitz-Gibbon might come across, for example, Bandura's (1986) social learning theory and how children acquire prosocial skills through obser-vation, modeling, and role playing. She could incorporate these ideas into the group. Further, she might look for some useful ways to improve student self-control (e.g., Tice, Bratslavaky, & Baumeister, 2001). In her "spare" time, Ms. Fitz-Gibbon might also refresh her understanding of the developmental differences among student groups, and of the school's RTI model and how it can help coordinate various school counseling services and activities. No doubt, this background work is time consuming; however, by doing so you increase the likelihood that the group experience will lead to positive student outcomes.

WHAT COUNSELING THEORIES ARE MOST FITTING FOR SCHOOL-BASED SMALL GROUPS?

Needless to say, there is some debate among counselor educators about this ques-tion (e.g., Gladding, 2008; Jacobs et al., 2009), for the constellation of possible theo-retical orientations to select from can be daunting (Mobley & Gazda, 2006). Further complicating the issue, most counseling-related theories were initially applied to in-dividual psychotherapy and counseling and only later adapted to group work. Ideally, school counselors could draw from all 14 well-established theoretical orientations (see Table 2.1), developing an extensive collection of group counseling skills, but for obvious reasons this is an unrealistic expectation (Mobley & Gazda, 2006; Ripley & Goodnough, 2001).

To narrow your options to a reasonable number, we focus only on those perspec-tives where the research evidence supporting their use in school settings is fairly robust.[1] Of the 14 theories, 7 appear to be best suited for the basic group formats described in the previous chapter. They are reviewed below from the *least* counselor-directed alter-native (e.g., process-oriented groups using a humanistic/child-centered orientation) to the *most* directive alternatives (e.g., psychoeducational groups using behavior therapy or cognitive-behavioral therapy). Only the ideas central to each theory are highlighted. For extensive theoretical summaries, there are plenty of excellent resources avail-able (e.g., G. Corey, 2009; M. S. Corey et al., 2010; Gladding, 2008; Henderson & Thompson, 2010; Vernon & Davis-Gage, 2010). Later on, the criteria for selecting the "best" theory are tabled.

Each counseling theory has its own foci and aims, and so are not appropriate for all students. When relating theories to group work, it is therefore crucial that school coun-selors consider how each theory may or may not address important student differences and developmental patterns (Hughes, 2009). Piaget emphasized this point as well, suggesting that developmental theories must account for significant variations in chil-dren's social environments, cultures, languages, and communities (Piaget & Inhelder, 1966/2000). Similarly, counseling theories must be applied carefully to small groups, taking into consideration each group member's previous experiences and history. To illustrate this point, you may remember that cognitive-behavioral therapy and rational emotive behavior therapy target students' irrational thinking and decision making. When opting for this approach, you have already decided that the students' backgrounds and issues are appropriate for a cognitively focused group experience. To reiterate, students' cultural and ethnic backgrounds must be considered first before assuming a counseling theory is applicable to particular set of students.

---

[1]Other viable options are available (e.g., transtheoretical model of change and motivational interviewing), but these are yet to be widely used in school environments.

TABLE 2.1 | The 14 Dominant Theoretical Orientations at the Turn of the Millennium[a]

Counseling Theory	Seminal Theorist(s)
Analytic therapy	Carl Jung
Behavioral therapy	B. F. Skinner
Choice theory and reality therapy	William Glasser
Cognitive-behavioral therapy (CBT)	Donald Meichenbaum
Cognitive therapy	Aaron Beck, Judith Beck
Existential therapy	Viktor Frankl, Irwin Yalom
Gestalt therapy	Fredrick "Fritz" Perls
Individual psychology therapy	Alfred Adler, Rudolph Dreikurs
Multimodal therapy	Arnold Lazarus
Person-Centered therapy	Carl Rogers
Psychoanalytic therapy	Sigmund Freud
Rational-emotive behavioral therapy (REBT)	Albert Ellis
Social learning theory	Albert Bandura, John Krumboltz
Solution-focused brief therapy (SFBT)	Steve de Shazer and colleagues

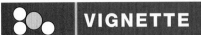

[a]Although narrative counseling (Winslade & Monk, 2007) is gaining in popularity with some counselors, due to its recency and the lack of supporting school-based research, it is not included in this discussion; however, for interested readers, the chapter supplement provides a summary.

Note: From Mobley and Gazda (2006). Mobley and Gazda did not include SFBT in their original discussion; it was added here because of its influence on contemporary school counseling practice.

Humanistic/Child-Centered Theory

We begin the theory discussion with the least directive approach to group leadership. Specifically, humanistic and positive psychologists focus on students' developmental assets and healthy life patterns rather than their personal limitations and problems.

VIGNETTE

Process Group for High School Girls

A number of freshman girls who are friends come into the counseling office, asking if they could be in a group to discuss their "personal and relationship problems." The girls want some fairly unstructured time to share their feelings. After deliberating on the various theoretical and group format options, the ninth-grade counselor decides to conduct a process-oriented group using humanistic counseling methods. Why did the leader opt for this approach over other alternatives?

To answer this question, we recap Carl Rogers's child-centered (person-centered) approach to counseling. If you recall, his perspective on counseling published in the mid-1900s was a radical departure from traditional notions of psychotherapy (e.g., Freudian and Jungian psychoanalysis; O'Hara, 2003). Instead of viewing themselves as the experts on and the directors of psychological healing, child-centered counselors aim only to be *facilitators* of their clients' personal growth (Rogers, 1951/2007, 1965). The client knows what he or she needs to do to get healthy. How children grow and change during the counseling experience is primarily enabled through the therapeutic bond nurtured over time between the student and counselor. The group counselor's role then is to create an encouraging, warm, and caring environment, where counselees feel free to express their conscious feelings, thoughts, and beliefs (Rogers, 1961/1989).

Not only are humanistic group leaders genuine and create a positive milieu for personal growth, they engage in the *active listening process* (Bent, 1996; Nelson-Jones, 2000). In reframing words and nonverbal actions, Rogerian group counselors echo back to students what they think reflects the original meaning of the students' comments. In other words, as a way of checking the counselor's understanding of a group member's emotional well-being, the counselor will mirror, without parroting, his or her under-standing of the student's words and nonverbal behaviors using succinct and poignant statements, voiced like gentle questions. For example, the counselor after hearing the student's story might tentatively say to the upset group member, "It sounds like you re-ally dislike your math class; am I hearing you right?" In response, the student, with a frown, might say in a hesitating way, "No, that's not what I mean." The counselor would continue to gently probe, verbalizing something like, "Well, perhaps you are just angry with the math teacher right now?" Of course, the counselor treads very lightly between providing the student words to express difficult or unrecognized feelings and putting words in the student's mouth. Counselors are not entitled to "force" change or their opinions, but instead must allow for self-discovery, even if this means students choose to "shut down" at particular times.

Child-centered group counselors do not explain or interpret their perspectives on students' emotions, behaviors, and thoughts, but listen actively to students' nonverbal and verbal communications. Nondirective group facilitation provides meaningful op-portunities and activities for personal sharing and self-reflection. In the process, students better connect to their present condition. Moreover, humanistic-oriented group experi-ences help students appreciate that they can change themselves. Personal growth does not require students to grapple with the causes of their problems or with their past mis-takes. Rather, the group experience focuses on improved self-awareness. Over multiple sessions, students begin to learn how they choose their own actions, thoughts, and feel-ings and how they can maximize their personal authenticity and psychological health.

Allied to Rogerian psychology, Maslow's (1965, 1968) humanistic-developmental model based on the "hierarchy of needs" provides further theoretical support for leading process-focused groups in schools (see also existential therapy; Coy & Kovacs-Long, 2005; Mobley & Gazda, 2006). Maslow urged counselors to help students move along the psy-chological path to self-actualization, a growth process toward experiencing day-to-day life more "fully, vividly, selflessly, with full concentration and total absorption" (p. 111). Group counselors support students in their journeys, encouraging them to reflect on their self-centeredness, self-consciousness, and personal defenses. Before counselors can focus on higher levels of functioning, growth groups must initially ensure students are meeting their basic survival and safety needs. Later, students' affiliation (belonging) and self-esteem needs can be explored. The all-important questions of life, such as "Who am I?," "Where am I going?," and "How do I fit into the world?," are processed in the group setting (Coy & Kovacs-Long, 2005; Guindon, 2010). Key student goals for growth groups are the development of self-confidence, self-worth, self-competence, and self-sufficiency, as well as a sense of being a productive and necessary person (Rogers, 1965).

To summarize, process groups based on humanistic psychology and child-centered therapy are conducted at the students' pace. They focus on the awareness of feelings, meeting personal needs, and developing a healthy view of self and others. Reflecting back on the opening vignette, a process group appears to be a good choice for the high school girls group. Naturally, before implementing a humanistic-oriented group, the high school counselor will want to interview the potential members to determine whether they possess the psychosocial skills needed for feelings-focused experiences and explorations. As a caveat to using this approach in schools, if students' motivation for change is unknown or limited, humanistic growth groups are probably not all that helpful. Finally, the research evidence for using Rogerian child-centered counseling techniques in small groups is fairly well documented. For example, child-centered play therapy can be used in a group format to help younger students more effectively handle their anger issues (Fischetti, 2010). Additional resources are available under the Examples of School-Based Process Groups section in chapter 1.

Adlerian Theory/Individual Psychology

🔵 | VIGNETTE

Psychoeducational Group for Middle School Boys

A physical education teacher reported that seven boys regularly misbehave in his over-enrolled gym class. Instead of asking the school counselor to get the "troublemakers" out of the class, the coach asks if something more positive can be done to improve the situation. The counselor suggests that a 6-week psychosocial skills group might be beneficial. The boys will be asked to voluntarily participate in a lunchtime small group. The way the counselor "sells" the group to the boys, five readily agree. Although perhaps not the best solution, the other two boys are reassigned to an alternate gym period where the coach has time for closer supervision.

The recommended psychosocial group for the boys is an ideal place for the application of Alfred Adler's (1927/2008, 1929/2004, 1929/2006) psychological theory as well as related interventions developed by Rudolf Dreikurs (1953/1989). Like Rogerian and Gestalt theories, school counselors operating out of the approach generally view students from a positive, humanistic, and holistic lens. Adlerian principles also reflect the theory and research related to the psychosocial development of children and youth (e.g., Erikson, 1968).

When conducting small groups using Adlerian and Dreikurs's principles, core dimensions of students' behavior are targeted. First, while assisting students with positive goal striving and goal setting, the group leader aims to improve their interpersonal skills as well. For example, during the goal-setting part of the first or second meeting, the counselor carefully listens to the students' stated goals (e.g., getting an A in a course, being a classroom nuisance, making good friends), noting any specific patterns in their comments. After the initial group meetings, the counselor reflects on what he or she heard, using such focusing questions as: Which students voiced negative and harmful goals? Which members set beneficial and future-oriented goals? How can the group process redirect negative goals to positive ones? How can the group reinforce students' healthy goals? What techniques could be used to foster the goal-setting process for those students who had trouble identifying any? Answers to these questions guide the direction of subsequent group meetings.

Because the goals students establish for themselves are strongly influenced by their style of life and social interest, as the group unfolds counselors are also on the lookout for these issues. Developing in early childhood, a student's style of life reflects, among other factors, his or her future life orientation, choices, social interest, and personal and cultural background. Social interest reflects one's desire to see beyond the self, to others and the wider world; for instance, after observing the boys, the group counselor tries to determine if they are motivated to support each other and receive peer feedback. If not, the students need to be shown how to appropriately give and receive feedback.

Moreover, Adlerian group leaders assist those members who are showing signs of inferiority. Showing little social interest, these individuals prefer "hand-holding" from others, particularly when faced with hardships. Feelings of inferiority also may lead to harmful long-term personal and social development. In a group setting, these self-defeating students may distance themselves from others, seek out negative attention from peers and the leader, or hesitate to attempt challenging group activities or conversations. When challenged with what is perceived as criticism, students with an inferiority complex may become so discouraged their self-worth plummets. Others may overcompensate, going overboard in their attempts to do group activities right or to look good to their peers. The group counselor's role is to address these issues with strengths-based activities and techniques (e.g., reinforcing and role playing of positive behavior; supporting team-building games).

Adlerian groups are flexible enough to combine other methods into the group process and content. Kern and Hankins (1977), for instance, included behavioral contracting to help resolve student issues (e.g., poor attendance, homework completion, notebook organization, playground behavior). Counselors can even fashion their groups around skill-building curricula such as the student success skills peer-coaching model (SSSPC; Campbell, 2003). The SSSPC approach incorporates certain Adlerian principles, offering counselors a research-based, step-by-step approach to facilitate group processes. Students first select a relevant and challenging situation for the group members to explore. Second, with the counselor's support and encouragement the crucial background details are reviewed. Third, to reveal unforeseen positive solutions for the problematic situation, students work through different promising scenarios and discuss their potential consequences. Fourth, students role-play and practice possible solution(s). During the last step, counselees give each other feedback on the proposed solution(s).

TABLE 2.2 | Mistaken Goals of Students' Misbehavior and Resulting Student and Adult Responses

Student Misguided Goals of Misbehavior	Student Observed Behavior	Adult Response to Student's Misbehavior	Student Response Following Adult Correction
Attention	Model student, overly sweet and amiable, or annoying, nuisance, indolent	Irritated, annoyed, frustrated	Generally stops for a short time
Power	Rebellious, arguing and fighting, stubborn, passive–aggressive behavior	Angered, challenged, defeated	Continues misbehavior even after asked to stop (sometimes intensifies misbehavior)
Revenge	Spiteful, aggressive/violent, vandalism, unkindness, passivity	Hurt, angered	Intensifies the misbehavior and turning to meanness
Feelings of helplessness/inadequacy	Hopelessness, discouragement, incompetence; gives up easily; lacks self-confidence	Despairing, feelings of "why continue trying" (i.e., start to limit their support of student), pull away	Restrained, limited, or no interaction

Note: Table content adapted from Bitter (2009, p. 138).

Another useful group application of Adlerian psychology is Dreikurs's social discipline model and its four goals of misbehavior (Dinkmeyer & Dreikurs, 1963/2001). Supporting a strengths-based approach to group work (Galassi & Akos, 2007), Dreikurs argued that there are no bad children, just discouraged ones. School counselors understand that children can be very irresponsible in their goals, leading potentially to ongoing problem behavior, unfulfilled wishes and dreams, and serious life consequences (e.g., psychosocial issues and identifiable mental disorders).

When students "misbehave," their actions fail to conform to the social norms of the school environment (Dreikurs, 1953/1989). As Table 2.2 elucidates, the *unconscious* goals of misbehavior may involve a student's need (a) for attention, (b) to seek revenge, (c) to obtain personal power, or (d) to "overcome" the feelings of helplessness and inadequacy (inferiority). Three lower-level *conscious* reasons why students misbehave include: to get something, to look important (self-elevation), or as an act of avoidance (Bitter, 2009). Groups can address these misguided goals through, for instance, building on students' strengths, never doing for students what they can do for themselves, encouraging students to understand themselves and how they interpret their actions and goals, and promoting group cooperation and social interaction (Linden, 2001).

In summary, Adlerian theory has much to offer school counselors. Studies have documented the utility of Adlerian groups with elementary (e.g., Brigman & Molina,

1999; Kern & Hankins, 1977; LaFountain, 1996; Stormer & Kirby, 1969), secondary school (e.g., Hoffmann, 1975; LaFountain, 1996; McKelvie, 1974), and Native American (Hunter & Sawyer, 2006) students. Its major concepts and techniques fit well with both process- and content-focused groups, providing a variety of effective methods to assist students in developing new goals, enhancing social interest, reducing feelings of inferiority, improving personal adjustment and social behavior, and so on. If you choose this approach for your group, the major ways to elicit behavior change are through student goal setting and monitoring, role playing and practicing social skills, peer feedback and dialogue, and self-awareness and strengths-building activities. Because we only scratched the surface of this approach, readers might want to consult other resources for additional ways individual psychology can be infused into school-based groups (e.g., Bitter, 2009; Campbell, 2003; Dinkmeyer & Sperry, 1999; Sonstegard, Bitter, & Pelonis, 2004; Stein, 2006; T. J. Sweeney, 2009).

Gestalt Theory and Therapy

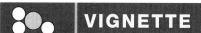

VIGNETTE

"College Readiness Group"

After performing a needs survey at the end the school year, the counseling team at Curtis High discovered that nearly 30 juniors expressed an interest in knowing more about college life and how to get into universities. Each teen was contacted and asked if he or she would like to be a part of a "college readiness group" to be offered in the fall semester of their senior year. Following the pregroup interviews with potential members, 16 students decided to participate. To accommodate all students, a couple of 4-week mixed-gender groups were conducted by two counselors.

Despite the fact Gestalt theory has powerful techniques to support student development, and change feeling, thoughts, and behaviors, this approach is not widely used in school-based group counseling (Glass, 2010). Perhaps this is because Gestalt psychology is a relatively complex perspective, requiring considerable background and training. Even so, Gestalt theory and group techniques merit a closer look. Research conducted in American and international schools is generally promising (e.g., Shen, 2007), showing, for example, improvement in students' emotional adjustment as well as the expansion of counselees' personal strengths. For additional information on Gestalt counseling theory, see Woldt and Toman (2005) and the other cited resources.

The central notions (e.g., closure, congruence and wholeness, disequilibrium, emotional health, personal choice, "unfinished business") and assumptions supporting Gestalt counseling are generally aligned with those of humanistic and developmental psychology (Mobley & Gazda, 2006; Mortola, 2001). The seminal theorists, Fritz Perls (1947/1969, 1976; Perls, Hefferline, & Goodman, 1951/1994) and Laura Perls, applied the Gestalt principles to individual mental health and psychotherapy, leaving their followers to apply the theory to group work (e.g., Polster & Polster, 1973). Not until the

1980s did Gestalt counseling techniques find their way into the school counseling literature and training procedures.

Assuming a school counselor wants to run a Gestalt-oriented group, what might it look like? First, the counselor would keep the proceedings in the "here and now," remaining present centered. Next, the counselor would gently probe the group members for their level of personal and social insight, hoping to break down their resistance to self-awareness and ultimately to change. All along, the process would focus on assisting students to develop more refined coping mechanisms (Kastner & Neumann, 1986). The counselor does this through self-awareness activities such as prescribed rituals and exercises (also called "experiments" in Gestalt language). Other appropriate techniques to improve self- and other-awareness are role playing of feelings; artistic depictions of feelings; "empty chairs" representing an absent feeling, person, or object; peer support expressions; and so on. Creativity using non-language-based activities is also encouraged, for verbalization of feelings is often not useful to emotionally "blocked" children and youth (Shen, 2007). The counselor brings art supplies to help students further develop their personal imagination. Group members are encouraged as an experiment to draw their house, significant others, and other relevant aspects of their lives. While processing their depictions and meanings, the counselor also makes sure the group stays in the Gestalt mode of "what is," rather than "what might be" or "what was." Leaders look for ways to bring wholeness to students' lives as well as to revitalize and build up their repertoire of personal strengths.

Returning to our vignette above, suppose a group member indicated that she has felt sadness, tension, and frustration on and off during the fall semester. When the group leader probes with an open-ended question, the senior discloses "how hard it has been to receive college rejection letters." The counselor suggests she has some "unfinished business" to work through; as such, the leader tries an open-chair exercise in the hope that it will facilitate some understanding and resolution of her negative feelings. After the exercise, the student reported experiencing a sense of satisfaction and relief. Later on, another group member indicates that he lost a parent early in life and feels like "he has to do the entire college search by himself." The counselor sees how the young man has bottled up his emotional pain. Rather than dealing openly with it, the student has rechanneled his emotions into becoming an overachiever. From a Gestalt frame of reference, the student with unresolved grief has "severed" an emotional part himself from his conscious awareness. To rectify the situation, the counselor through a nonverbal group activity helps this senior become more aware of the "aching part" of his self and his need for an adult mentoring relationship. As you can discern from these two examples, the students explored those areas of their lives that were incomplete, unresolved, and disconnected from daily awareness (A. R. Barlow, 1981). The counselor's role was to help the students become "unstuck" through various counseling techniques.

Here's a real-world example demonstrating how counselors can use Gestalt methods with distressed, inner-city elementary-age students (Woodard, 1995). The overall group goal was to increase the boys' self-esteem through self-awareness, self-responsibility, and self-assertiveness. After developing group rules, the leader focused on building group cohesion and personal character through "team spirit" activities or experiments. Group members were asked to set team goals and to make every effort

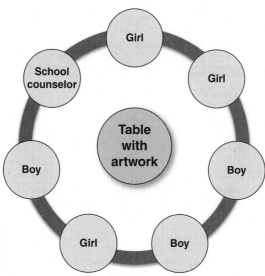

FIGURE 2.2 | Gestalt group as an art circle (Alexander & Harman, 1988).

to fulfill them. Team (group) rituals were established. Each session ended with a group huddle, including this final "ceremonial" chant: "Team, team, together—stay out of trouble!"

Earlier Alexander and Harman (1988) discussed how a school counselor conducted a Gestalt-oriented grief group with sixth-graders who were dealing with the unexpected loss of their well-liked peer. After doing whole-class meetings, there were several boys and girls who needed additional support and care. Adopting a Gestalt perspective, the counselor included these hurting children in a 3-month group utilizing several active and engaging techniques. Similar to what was used in Shen's (2007) Gestalt play-oriented groups with high school students, group activities were utilized to create an intense, supportive, and feeling-focused restorative process. For instance, with crayons the children drew symbols, pictures, and shapes on a large sheet of paper, communicating their emotions about their friend's passing (see Figure 2.2). With the counselor paying close attention to each picture, students were supported as they expressed their feelings of emptiness, loneliness, and confusion, and fears of suicide. In due course, the children were given the opportunity to achieve some closure. Another experiment involved students writing and drawing in a notebook their representations of the child who took his own life. The counselor directed those students who so elected to rip out the pages and then directed the children to tear up those evocative pages. The children were ridding themselves of grief, sadness, confusion, and so on.

To sum up, Gestalt-oriented groups are very useful for helping students regain personal and social wholeness. Students find closure to their problems and can progress toward healthy goals. However, some caution is warranted; to use this approach effectively, Gestalt group leadership requires a strong skill set.

Solution-Focused Brief Counseling (SFBC)

> ### ●●● VIGNETTE
>
> #### "Transitioning to Junior High" Group
>
> At the end of the school year, the elementary school counselor prepares the sixth-graders for junior high school. After several classroom guidance presentations overviewing junior high life, Mr. Shen noticed quite a few students who were very anxious about moving to the next level. He and the school psychologist decided to run two 4-week, mixed-gender groups for any student who wanted to talk further about transitioning to the new school. Because a couple of students with learning disabilities also chose to join a group, Mr. Shen consulted with the Resource Specialist at the junior high to ensure the group met these students' needs.

Since solution-focused brief counseling (SFBC) is relatively easy to do, is efficient, and has a strong research base, it is now widely used in schools (e.g., Brasher, 2009; Cooley, 2009; Mostert, Johnson, & Mostert, 1997). SFB group counselors focus on students' (a) past successes (when students were able to reach their goals) and exceptions to the problem (when students do not experience the problem); (b) existing skill set and healthy personal characteristics; and (c) preferred future (students specify what they want their future to look like). Thus change occurs not through rehashing the student's personal and social obstacles and deficiencies, but by the use of searching questions to access any and all resources available and to reframe goals in healthy, positive ways (LaFountain, Garner, & Eliason, 1996).

Similar to Rogerian psychology, solution-focused brief therapy (SFBT) theorists view people as possessing the necessary inner and outer resources and strengths to resolve their challenges (de Shazer, 1988; de Shazer & Dolan, 2007; Sklare, 2005). Counseling should "feel" like a positive experience in which students will notice small incremental behavioral changes, leading in time to bigger ones. Students in groups receive concrete, realistic, and honest feedback on what is needed for behavior change.

What areas do SFB group counselors focus on? Initially, they help students think through their beliefs about change. Leaders pay close attention to students' use of self-defining labels and absolutes that express vulnerability toward change. Through this ongoing process of reframing conversation, asking thought-provoking questions, and initiating thought-provoking activities (e.g., "What would you like to change in your life right now?" "If you acted differently, what would you do?"), group counselors help students develop realistic goals and solutions. Next, leaders encourage students to substitute their ineffective language with verb forms and qualifiers (LaFountain et al., 1996). For instance, when a student blurts out in the group, "I'm just no good at math," the counselor reframes the comment by replying, "You mean, sometimes you may find math really hard? Was there a time that you can remember when you did well on a math assignment?" Again, rather than dwelling on the students' problems, the aim is to inspire students to find new ways of developing appropriate solutions. Finally, age-appropriate SFB group counseling techniques are used (e.g., scaling, miracle question, finding exceptions, normalizing, homework), which are well described in relevant school counseling publications (e.g., Sklare, 2005).

The value of SFBC groups with K–12 students is well documented in the United States (e.g., Kress & Hoffman, 2008; LaFountain et al., 1996; W. Newsome, 2005; Springer, Lynch, & Rubin, 2000; Young & Holdorf, 2003) and internationally (e.g., Enea & Dafinoiu, 2009). For instance, LaFountain et al. discussed a psychoeducational group with nine middle school boys of mixed ethnicities. The specific session content, foci, and SFBC methods are summarized in Table 2.3. You will notice that the leader used common SFBC techniques such as goal setting, reframing language, interactive tasks, and looking for exceptions and strengths. Following the experience, LaFountain et al. reported that the SFBC small groups were generally successful. Students were able to largely achieve their goals, and reported higher self-esteem and more appropriate coping behavior with challenging emotions (e.g., anxiety and depression).

More recently, the value of school-based SFBC groups was further documented by Froeschle, Smith, and Ricard (2007). Based on aspects of ASCA's (2005a) National Model, the authors implemented a 16-week SFBC psychoeducational group for eighth-grade girls hoping to decrease their inappropriate drug use and improve their social skills. The school counselor also conducted two support meetings for the girls' parents. Each small-group meeting included various SFBC techniques and activities, including action-learning lessons, member discussions, and guest speakers. Weekly discussion topics involved goal setting, career exploration, drug information, peer-pressure resistance, decision making, and relationships. Positive results were found for participants. The girls reported less drug use, stronger negative attitudes toward drug use, increased use of socially competent behaviors, and higher scores on a measure assessing drug use knowledge.

In summary, SFB group counseling is an effective way to better students' behavior. The advantages are many, including its conceptual and implementation simplicity. The methods are strengths based and systems oriented, meshing well with the ASCA (2005a) National Model. School counselors will also appreciate that solution-focused groups can easily incorporate useful techniques from other group counseling approaches.

Glasser's Choice Theory and Reality Therapy

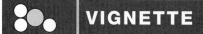 **VIGNETTE**

"Getting Ready for State Testing" Group

Tension among students and teachers at Snowbank Elementary is building in anticipation of the upcoming state achievement testing. At least 2 months before the big day, the school counselor conducts several in-class guidance lessons on test-taking skills. Certain students, however, voice their "hyper" nervousness. In response, Ms. Gray offers a short-term psychoeducational group for fifth- and sixth-graders to help these children work through their test anxiety. Another group is designed for five children in Grades 3 and 4.

TABLE 2.3 | Example of an SFBC Group Session by Session

Group Meeting	Activities
Pregroup Screening: Individual Meeting with Each Student	Counselor • asks student what he would like to change. • assesses student's willingness to share and his appropriateness for group.
Meeting 1: Forming	• Students are introduced and group guidelines are instituted. • An icebreaker activity is facilitated, encouraging interaction and getting to know one another. • Students share what they want to change in their lives. • Counselor ends the group by providing encouragement to the boys, saying "This week notice what happens to you that you want to continue to happen."
Meeting 2: Establishing Goals	• After review of homework, goal setting is introduced. • Hypothetical situation is introduced so that student can develop goals. Counselor says: "Suppose that tonight while you are asleep there is a miracle and the problem is solved. How would you know?" "What is the first thing you would be doing differently?" • Counselor processes student responses. • To get boys to set a realistic goal, the counselor remarks to the group: "Now that we have an idea of what you would like different and since miracles aren't likely, tell us what you will be doing to get that to happen." • Students share. • Counselor encourages the group and distributes the goal sheets, directing students to develop a goal for next week. The goal is to begin with "I will be …"

Meeting 3: Keys to Solutions	• Students share their process goals.
	• Counselor
	  • quietly assesses students' goals according to the criteria of a process goal and, as necessary, helps students to restate their individual goals to meet the criteria.
	  • presents a skeleton key and asks the students what skeleton keys are used for. (Counselor elicits the idea that one skeleton key can fit many locks.)
	  • explains various keys—exceptions, doing something differently, pretending, and so forth—and points out some keys that students are already using (and hands out a replica of a skeleton key to the students as each key is identified).
	  • encourages group members to point out keys that they notice each other using (while counselor continues to hand out the keys).
	  • after continuing to praise group members, directs students to look for the skeleton key (solutions) that they use toward their goal.

(continued)

TABLE 2.3 | Example of an SFBC Group Session by Session (*continued*)

Group Meeting	Activities

Meeting 4: Progress Toward Goals	• Counselor
	  • asks students what an obstacle course is and to share about progress toward goal.
	  • listens to students' comments, comparing them to such a course.
	  • processes the exercise and encourages.
	  • has boys review their individual directive for the week.

Subsequent Meetings	• Counselor develops following sessions around group needs.
Final Meeting	• Counselor asks students to share their progress toward meeting goal, encouraging boys to share feedback.

Note: Adapted from LaFountain et al. (1996). Some of the original text was revised.

William Glasser's (1965, 2000) choice theory (CT) and reality therapy (RT) are widely and effectively used in school counseling practice (e.g., Glasser, 1990; Mason & Duba, 2009; Wubbolding, 2007). To better understand how RT can be applied to small groups, CT's core axioms need to be first reviewed:

1. The only person whose behavior we can control is our own.
2. All we can give another person is information.
3. All long-lasting psychological problems are relationship problems.
4. The problem relationship is always part of our present life.
5. What happened in the past has everything to do with what we are today, but we can only satisfy our basic needs right now and plan to continue satisfying them in the future.
6. We can only satisfy our needs by satisfying the pictures in our Quality World (described below).
7. All we do is behave.
8. All behavior is Total Behavior and is made up of four components: acting, thinking, feeling, and physiology.
9. All Total Behavior is chosen, but we only have direct control over the acting and thinking components.
10. We can only control our feeling and physiology indirectly through how we choose to act and think. (Glasser, 1998, pp. 333–336)

Perhaps Axiom 6 ("satisfying the pictures in our quality world") requires further explanation. By at least adolescence, students have come to understand that their peers see the world differently from themselves. This life-changing realization emerges when the boundaries and parameters of their quality worlds expand. Interactions with the wider world generate a social awareness. Over time, students develop specific pictures (memories) that depict the most optimal ways to satisfy their fundamental needs for survival, belonging and love, fun, power, freedom or independence, and power or achievement. As Glasser (1998) further explained,

> What these pictures portray falls into three categories: (1) the *people* we most want to be with, (2) the *things* we most want to own or experience, and (3) the *ideas or systems of belief* that govern much of our behavior. Anytime we feel very good, we are choosing behavior so that someone, something, or some belief in the real world has come close to matching a picture of that person, thing, or belief in our quality worlds. Throughout our lives, we will be in closer contact with our quality world than with anything else we know. (p. 45)

As their worldviews are enriched, students try very hard to satisfy their needs, shaping and reshaping them according to their quality worlds. Those students, for instance, who desire more belonging and connectedness may put pictures of close relationships into their quality worlds. If those pictures work for them, then they will cling to them; if they seem unworkable, then the long, frustrating, and painful process of shedding those previously satisfying needs begins. At this point, group counseling can be supportive. Leaders help students view their quality world more clearly, allowing the students to reframe their pictures in response to real-world feedback and to meet their needs in new and productive and healthy ways.

As you will recall, a major goal of RT is to have students recognize that their present behavior is not meeting their core needs (Glasser, 1965, 2000). Similarly, the group experience is directed at motivating change by helping students realize that certain behaviors are ineffective at achieving important needs, and poor choices are partly to blame. By opting for new behaviors, students will in due course get what they really want; their needs will be satisfied in a constructive manner. Like all groups, leaders set a positive tone for each meeting. For students to genuinely open up and trust the leader to guide them to new behavior decisions and better self-management, the environment must feel safe, caring, empathetic, accepting, and so forth (Mason & Buba, 2009; Walter, Lambie, & Ngazimbi, 2008).

Once rapport and trust are established, RT-oriented group leaders nurture change by helping the students discover their wants and needs, providing direction and action, facilitating student planning to get those needs fulfilled, and fostering student self-evaluation (i.e., How are the new behaviors getting you what you want?). RT group counselors tend to be directive and action-oriented. Leaders start with asking probing and open-ended questions, and later switch to more coaching and teaching about goal setting, decision making, and action planning. Referring back to the vignette, for example, students in the upper elementary-age group are asked by the leader to state and explain what they really want (i.e., goal setting). One student might say, "I don't want to do badly on this stupid test!" The counselor may follow up with this probing question: "What are you doing right now to make this happen?" Depending on the student's response (e.g., "Nothing. I cannot do anything."), the leader might ask something like: "How is what you're doing getting you what you want?" Most of the time students are not doing things that help them achieve their goals; therefore, the leader's follow-up question might be: "What are you willing to do to get what you really want?" Assuming the student wants to do something productive to satisfy his or her need, the counselor and student make a specific action plan. In the ensuing group meetings, the action plan is reported on and evaluated, and any success is encouraged by the counselor and other group members. If the action plan needs reworking, the counselor and student again collaborate on making the appropriate changes. With each successive group meeting, this process is repeated as necessary.

There are multiple resources to consult as you plan and implement an RT group in schools (e.g., Comiskey, 1993; Duba & Mason, 2009; Pound, 2009; Walter et al., 2008). For example, suppose you have a bullying problem at your elementary school; running an RT group can be an effective prevention and intervention method. By combining both RT and CT, as well as training in social, self-control, and assertiveness skills, Jong-Un (2006) showed that a 10-week group with 8 fifth- and sixth-graders was successful in reducing harassment incidents. Table 2.4 provides a week-by-week overview of this antibullying group.

Finally, RT group counselors are cheerleaders for success, conveying encouragement, optimism, and a "never give up" attitude to members. Leaders can always supplement the group experience with non-RT methods (e.g., play, artwork, open-chair exercise) if they will help students meet their needs. In any case, RT group leaders (a) use open-ended questions to investigate students' total behavior and their wants, needs, and perspectives; (b) support students' positive actions for meeting goals and for their productive action planning; (c) provide analogies and metaphors to challenge students about their unrealistic actions; (4) use humor to nurture friendly student connections; (5) challenge group members to not give up and to not resort to excuse making; (6) reframe students' thought processes if they are nonconstructive; (7) try using paradoxical intentions, where the student is told to choose a symptom and act it out (Dalbech, 1981; Wubbolding, 2000).

Cognitive-Based Theories and Related Counseling Methods

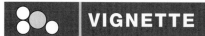 **VIGNETTE**

"Recovering from Parent Divorce" Group

A recent schoolwide needs survey showed that more than a few students are struggling with their parents' divorces. In response to the growing concern, Ms. Guerrero devised a 6-week psychoeducational group to address this issue. Promotional posters were placed in the hallways soliciting interest for the group. As a result, 5 seventh-graders and 2 eighth-graders volunteered. After pregroup interviews, each volunteer seemed appropriate for the group. Parent consent was obtained, and the group kicked off its first meeting with fun activity.

The structure and foci of many school-based psychoeducational groups are theoretically related to the principles of various cognitive-behavioral therapies (CBTs; Ingram & Siegle, 2010). CBT theorists and practitioners borrow heavily from the principles synthesized from cognitive psychology research and ancient Greco-Roman Stoic philosophy (e.g., Aurelius, ca. 150 CE/2006), where essentially, students' thoughts determine

TABLE 2.4 | Example of Choice Theory/Reality Therapy Antibullying Group Session by Session

Group Meeting	Activities
Meeting 1: The Feeling of Belonging	• Goal: to make new friends through group activity • Icebreaker: child selects nickname that is easily recalled by other members; children introduce themselves • Group rules and norms established (e.g., meeting time, attendance, session length, confidentiality, and termination)

Meeting 2: We Are Able to Choose Even Better Situations	• Goal: to facilitate group cohesion
	• Several activities were used to mobilize the group (e.g., matching game, finding the way, and stretching)
	• Counselor
	  • teaches choice theory
	  • asks students to share something about the feelings they chose when they experienced bullying from a bully or bullies.
	  • attaches Choice A (I am depressed) and Choice B (I am choosing to be depressed) to classroom floor.
	  • asks children present what they are doing and thinking.
	  • divides students into smaller groups, and encourages them to talk about their school life (e.g., good things, frustrations, bullying issues).

Meeting 3: Pictures of Reality	• Goal: to help children to recognize tangible problems they experience in peer relationships • Activity: students draw interpersonal relationship maps
Meeting 4: Five Basic Needs	• Goal: to have children learn the five basic needs • Counselor explains these needs • Goal-setting discussion follows in regard to basic needs • Children are taught assertiveness training, learning how to deal with bullying situations • Students practice new skills

Meeting 5: Total Behavior	• Goal: to learn about total behavior through use of a car metaphor
	• Counselor
	  • asks children to bring toy cars
	  • explains the Reality Therapy car and that four components make up total behavior: doing, thinking, feeling, and physiology
	  • asks children to complete an activity sheet
	  • asks them to present what they want and what they want to change in their life
	  • processes activities, asking children to share something they have learned

Meeting 6: Learning Self-Control Strategies	• Goal: to learn self-control techniques • Counselor first models self-control behavior • Children are then verbally guided through steps in enacting self-control behaviors. • Children are asked to perform self-control skills through realistic and relevant role-playing situations. • Counselor reinforces correct performance of desired self-control behavior and provides corrective feedback and additional modeling as needed

(continued)

TABLE 2.4 | Example of Choice Theory/Reality Therapy Antibullying Group Session by Session (*continued*)

Group Meeting	Activities
Meeting 7: Making and Cooperating on a Masterpiece	• Goal: to collaborate on creating something • Children put into small groups • Using art (e.g., drawing, mosaic, clay) as the medium • Counselor photographs artwork • Children exhibit their work and receive counselor and peer feedback and praise

Meeting 8: "I-Messages" to Get What I Want	• Goal: to allow children to respond appropriately when experiencing problems (e.g., other students cutting in line, leaving them out, bullying, and pushing)
	• Counselor explains how to use "I messages" when being bullied or teased
	  • provides children with an I-message activity sheet: "I feel … when you … and I want …"
	  • puts children in dyads in which they choose other conflict pictures and practice the "I-message" statements
	  • observes activity, providing additional tips, feedback, and encouragement

Meeting 9: Inviting Peers to Play	• Goal: to learn how to ask peers to play • Children in dyads role-play sample prewritten scripts related to bullying situations

Meeting 10: New Start and Saying Good-Bye	• Goal: to say goodbye and evaluate personal learning
	• Children write letters to themselves on how they have changed
	  • They read the letter out loud
	  • Other children give feedback and congratulations
	• To say goodbye and thanks, children write a short note
	• Before closing, children can make a short statement about their feelings about the group experience
	• Children receive a certificate of completion

Note: Adapted from Jong-Un (2006).

how they feel and act. Two major CBT approaches, rational emotive behavior therapy (A. Ellis & Wilde, 2001) and cognitive therapy (J. S. Beck, Liese, & Najavits, 2005) are conceptually very similar in their counseling methods.

More specifically, CBT/REBT practitioners assume that people's cognitions (thoughts, attitudes, and beliefs), not external agents like people, situations, and events, strongly influence their feelings and behaviors (National Association of Cognitive-Behavioral Therapists, 2009). Unlike humanistic approaches to counseling where the focus is on helping the students improve their emotional well-being, CBT/REBT practitioners help students challenge their negative thoughts so that they will revisit and modify their harmful behaviors. Thus students' irrational beliefs (e.g., "My father hates me or he wouldn't have divorced my mother.") can lead to detrimental reactions (e.g., depression and anxiousness).

Rational Emotive Behavior Therapy
ABCD[a] Worksheet

Step	Write My Responses Here
Step 1: What happened that upset me so much (A = *activating event*) and what was worst part(s) of it?	My A:
Step 2: Identify the *emotional consequence* (C_{EM}). (Based on A, identify your major distressing emotion, inappropriate behavior, warped subsequent thinking.)	My C_{EM}:
Step 3: *Identify and set goals.* (How would you like things to be?)	My Goals — Emotional: ___ Behavioral: ___ Thinking:
Step 4: Write down the *irrational* belief(s) (iBs) that are in your situation (iB).	My iB was:
Step 5: Write down any *alternative rational belief(s)* (rBs) that would help you reach your goals.	My rB was:
Step 6: *Dispute* (D) your **iBs**. (Identify a believable argument to convince yourself that your iBs are irrational and your rBs are rational.)	My D:
Step 7: *Reexamine* A and think about how reasonable my thoughts and behaviors were. What would be a more sensible way of looking at A?	My new view of A:

Source: Adapted from Dryden, Digiuseppe, and Neenan (2010, p. 253) for use with secondary school-age students.

[a]A = Activating event; B = Behavior you do as a result of A; C = Consequence (emotional) of B; D = Disputing belief to "undo" B and C.

FIGURE 2.3 | REBT worksheet.

However, despite the external conditions, students can positively change their garbled thinking and thus modify how they feel and act (Nelson-Jones, 2000). Potentially successful outcomes following cognitive-oriented group counseling include students' improving their sense of personal autonomy, self- and social-interest, and self-control, as well as their everyday functioning (e.g., Little, Akin-Little, & Gutierrez, 2009).

In practice, for instance, group counselors may have students' complete the ABCD worksheet (see Figure 2.3) as a structured learning tool to identify irrational beliefs and then change them. As you can see, this worksheet really addresses the student's underdeveloped or faulty cognitive skills. School counselors would first "teach" the ABCD process using group discussion and activities and then move to helping students work through their actual problem situations at school and at home. Through the CBT group

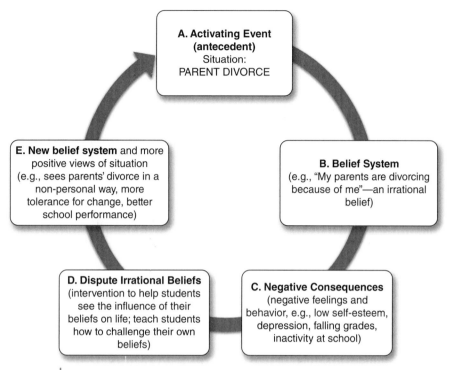

FIGURE 2.4 | REBT group counseling intervention framework for middle school students whose parents are divorcing (adapted from Bistaman & Nasir, 2009).

experience, students begin to understand their part in making themselves upset and how their negative thinking impacts subsequent emotions and behaviors.

A real-world example of how school counselors might visualize using REBT in a group setting is presented in Figure 2.4. Suppose a psychoeducational group was designed for middle school students whose parents were divorcing (see this section's opening vignette). Over 6 or so weeks, the group experience would gradually walk through REBT steps focusing on understanding the activating event and identifying irrational beliefs about that event and the accompanying negative consequences. Using the REBT worksheet (see Figure 2.3), students would then be taught how to dispute and challenge their own distorted beliefs about their parents' divorce. If done properly, the students would develop new, more positive views of the divorce situation and feel and behave accordingly. Follow-up activities can be facilitated individually with the students and in the classroom that reinforce the group learning experience and knowledge (e.g., provide students additional academic planning and "coping with change" skills).

Closely related to CBT is Bandura's (1986) social-cognitive learning model (also called social learning theory). Most content psychoeducational groups use Bandura's underlying learning principles to govern the group dynamics, foci, and activities. Albeit oversimplified, this approach to skill development is fundamentally based on observational or vicarious learning, where others (e.g., caregivers, peers, teachers) in a student's environment model behaviors, and in turn, the student imitates (practices) the observed behaviors (Nelson-Jones, 2000). Real learning however takes place only after the student first pays close *attention* to the key elements of the modeled action. Second, the student has to *retain* (code) the observed behavior in long-term memory for later retrieval. Third, for the behavior to be sufficiently reproduced, the imitator must learn and possess the requisite *motor* (physical) skills. The final step in observational learning is making sure the student has sufficient *motivation* to perform the demonstrated action. If the student *expects* to receive positive reinforcement when he or she imitates the modeled behavior, in all probability the desired behavior will be reproduced with increasing competence. So it is with learning to better cope with a parental divorce; the student must pay good attention to what is being modeled by the group leader or peer (e.g., how to express one's feelings in a healthy way), remember the modeler's actions and words, and want to learn the skill and try it out in the real world.

Similarly, Betz (2004) pointed out that the observational learning process used within a counseling relationship requires more than just good modeling to be effective:

> The counselor should be standing by with support and encouragement as the client tries these new activities and should be ready to provide extra doses of support if failure occurs. Although these will be the bases of the intervention, providing vicarious learning and modeling can be helpful when the counselor knows of, or can develop examples of, people who have succeeded in this activity. (p. 351)

Thus, in psychoeducational groups, it is imperative that the content to be learned and practiced in and outside the group be well explained, modeled, and supported by the leader.

Within Bandura's (1986, 1997) social-cognitive theory, the concept of self-efficacy also plays a major role in learning new behaviors. The term refers to a person's beliefs in one's own ability to effectively complete a desired task or behavior. Students' self-efficacy beliefs have a noticeable impact on learning key life skills, affecting, for example, their choices, goals, the level of effort expended on learning difficult skills, motivation to keep trying despite obstacles, how much stress they are willing to endure (coping and resiliency), and so on. Higher levels of self-efficacy are thought to foster approach rather than avoidance behavior. For instance, if students sincerely *believe* they can master the steps necessary to build strong relationships with the opposite gender, it is more likely that they will try to learn them reasonably well. Thus students with high levels of interpersonal self-efficacy tend to approach learning new social skills with less hesitancy than students with poor interpersonal self-efficacy.

Suppose you are conducting a small group on overcoming math anxiety with a handful of second-graders, wherein it is vital that the group focuses on improving the children's sense of math self-efficacy. Using Bandura's (1986) observational learning techniques, you will model how to approach calmly math problems and work through them. You will show them with fun activities how to ask for help and how to cope with anxiety. As they practice the demonstrated skills, the children should feel over time more competent in doing their math assignments.

The research on the value of CBT-related groups with K–12 students is promising (e.g., Little et al., 2009; Shen, 2007). Shen provided a useful example of how CBT groups can be effectively run with middle school students over 10 sessions, lasting

40 minutes each. The primary group goal was to enhance the students' behavioral and emotional assets. The CBT activities were drawn from an existing curriculum. For the purpose of brevity, only some of the content and foci of the group meetings are reviewed here. During the first session, for instance, students went over the group's ground rules and got acquainted. Additionally, in this meeting and those that followed, students were asked to share any current personal concerns. As a result of this personal sharing, students' self-perceptions (i.e., what they thought about themselves) were explored within the group. At the second meeting, each student had to hypothetically ask seven people (including at least two they liked and two they disliked) over for dinner and arrange how the guests would be seated around the table. Who the students invited over and their interpersonal relationships with classmates, friends, or family members were discussed by the group members and the facilitator. Any interpersonal challenges were acknowledged, unreasonable beliefs were disputed, and problem-solving strategies were taught. Skipping ahead to Meeting 6, students presented their individual "emergency plans" as a way to review any available supportive resources. Trust issues with family members, friends, and others were explored as well.

Another activity attempted in this CBT group was the "time capsule," where students wrote down their wishes that they'd like others to read 100 years later. These containers were thrown into an imaginary sea. The counselor then processed the students' comments, looking for better understanding of their thoughts and perspectives on life. Consistently, the group facilitator explored the "cognitive processes triggering the members to distinguish personal concerns, examine and dispute irrational thoughts, if any, establish rational concepts, and learn coping skills" (Shen, 2007, p. 292). For instance, one student indicated that she would put on her wish list, "I want to be a billionaire!" Clearly, the group leader would process with this student how she came to this goal, the likelihood of achieving it ("What makes this a realistic goal?"), and so on.

Behavioral Theory

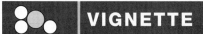

VIGNETTE

"Changing Negative to Positive Behavior" Group

There's no question based on the RTI discussions among faculty and administrator that certain "mean" girls are harassing other girls both in person and through Facebook postings. Using teacher referrals, 6 fifth-graders were encouraged to attend a highly structured prosocial skills–based group. The goal was designed to help the girls better manage and significantly reduce their inappropriate behavior toward peers.

B. F. Skinner's (1984) behaviorism,[2] also called operant conditioning, remains a significant force in American education and counseling (e.g., Allen, 2010; Ediger, 1991;

---

[2] There are too many behavioral traditions following in Skinner's theoretical footsteps to summarize in this chapter; however, refer to Sapp (2009) for an overview.

Heitzman-Powell, White, & Perrin, 2007). School counseling groups frequently deploy the highly directive and prescriptive behavioral techniques to facilitate student learning and change. A definitive rendering of behavioral theory is no longer possible, for its original principles have evolved into the more hybrid cognitive-behavioral counseling models referred to earlier (e.g., CBT; see Meichenbaum, 2007; Sapp, 2009). Small groups founded strictly on operant conditioning principles are not common practice. Instead, certain behavioral counseling techniques are used in groups without too much regard for underlying theory (Heitzman-Powell et al., 2007).

Notwithstanding, there are some fairly explicit principles that link the different strands of behaviorism. First, hard-core behaviorists see themselves as scientists and explain behavior–environment relationships in largely mechanistic terms (e.g., cause and effect; a stimulus leads to a response and then to a consequence). Student behavior like harassment is largely a function of the ecological context from which it occurs (e.g., home, school, the streets); that is, students' mean-girl actions are learned from external sources, rather than—as the other counseling theories might contend—a function of both internal and external mechanisms and processes.

Technically, behavioral counselors speak of operant conditioning as the process that shapes all behavior. The "power" of conditioning is influenced primarily by the student's immediate external reinforcement contingencies, where those proximal things in his or her world (family, peers, and events) will exert the most influence on current behavior. The consequences students receive for their responses (i.e., they are positively or negatively reinforced or punished) affect their current behavior. Behavior and its effects are associated with notions of frequency (how often), duration (how long), and intensity (magnitude).

In plain language, Skinnerian conditioning works something like this: A toddler begins to explore the kitchen. The child's "ineffective" parents consistently (frequency) and harshly (intensity) punish the toddler with a slap on the hand (negative consequence) each time he or she makes a mess after going through kitchen cupboards (behavior); as a result, over time the toddler's fear of punishment becomes conditioned and he or she becomes less and less inclined ("motivated") to seek out new experiences or try new tasks. To counteract this early negative conditioning, in all probability, the child will need behavioral intervention to "undo" the damage.

Perhaps, when the toddler goes to kindergarten, the elementary school counselor could put the child in a behaviorally oriented counseling group. How would behavioral principles be implemented in such a group context? Unlike the other theoretical models, where the rapport-building dynamics of the counselor–student relationship are vital for "recovery" to occur, the behaviorally oriented counselor aims to set up *reassuring* (non-negative) environmental conditions. Understandably, the group counselor must be well versed in the principles of operant conditioning and then apply them to the students' presenting issues. For students to modify their behavior, they do not need to be familiar with the "ins and outs" of the conditioning process and their personal learning histories. This is the job of group counselors, who are, in effect, behavior analysts attempting to consider in the therapeutic interchange all relevant conditioning variables. In Skinnerian-speak, the goal of group counseling is to modify "the control of stimulus-response patterns and contributing to a reduction in problematic behaviors in the client's life" (Heitzman-Powell et al., 2007, p. 579).

Returning to our "mean girls" vignette, during the initial group meeting the counselor collects observational data from the students' environment and their group behavior, determines the function of the girls' problem behaviors, and plans potential interventions. Specifically, the group counselor probes the students' experiences in attempt to understand *what* in the students' family, school, and community environments could be the events "triggering" the problem behavior (Heitzman-Powell et al., 2007). In other words, the group counselor analyzes the potential cause-and-effect relationships (students' unique learning histories) based on observable events their lives. To aid in this investigative work, the counselor may enlist the girls' teachers to conduct a functional behavior analysis (FBA) of their problem behavior wherever it occurs (e.g., lunchroom, classroom, hallway). Once these triggers and how they influence student behavior are well understood, the group works together so that each member learns to better cope with problematic situations or events. As the girls modify their negative behavior to positive behavior, significant people in their lives will in turn positively reinforce them.

Behaviorally oriented counseling methods are useful to implement in schools, particularly if the goal is to change or prevent negative behaviors. For instance, as a way to prevent bullying, Allen (2010) reported on a school-based comprehensive behavioral system, including individual counseling and small-group interventions. Like a good behavior analyst would do, the school's educators rigorously collected data in an attempt to understand bullying behaviors. The environment was carefully examined, with all problem behaviors coded and documented, and reports written. Behavior plans were instituted. Environmental modifications were made as needed, including (a) changing the student's (target or bully) seat, (b) putting the student (target or bully) in a different cooperative learning group, and (c) enlisting the support of one or two students in the class (or other activity) who will sit near (be near) the targeted student during class (or other activity) (Allen, 2010, p. 204).

To reiterate, even if most school-based groups don't strictly employ behavioral techniques, the "tools" can be successfully utilized in combination with other aligned counseling approaches (e.g., CBT and reality therapy). Group counselors can expand their repertoire of behavioral techniques by adding more sophisticated methods like behavioral rehearsal, systematic desensitization, visual imagery, stress management or relaxation techniques, token economies, behavior modification plans, and behavioral contracting (e.g., Alvord & Grados, 2005; Forehand, Middlebrook, Steffe, & Rogers, 1984; Watson & Gresham, 1998). At the very least, almost all groups deploy simple behavioral strategies as part of their general behavior management processes and procedures (e.g., issuing reinforcement for following directions, sharing, taking turns).

CRITERIA FOR CHOOSING THE "RIGHT" THEORY

After familiarizing yourself with the seven major conceptual approaches and their core elements associated with school-based group counseling, then you can select the most appropriate perspective or perspectives that match the group's aims, proposed format (e.g., psychoeducational group), and student needs. Although certainly not exhaustive, here are four "quality" indicators to think about as you consider which theoretical orientation(s) to base a group on (Erford, 2010; Gladding, 2008; Pérusse et al., 2009). You should view these as steps to follow.

Indicator 1 (Adjusts for Individual Differences)   Check to see if the theory (or theories) you plan to use for your group is adaptable and flexible to students' developmental differences. CSCPs are steeped in developmental theory and systems thinking; it follows that the counseling theory(ies) you select should be sensitive to the individual differences among group members, whether they are cognitive, emotional, social, or cultural. For instance, if you go with a content-focused conflict management group for middle school students, ask yourself whether the particular theoretical model is adaptable to a variety of student needs and abilities.

Indicator 2 (Strengths Based)   The next step is to consider whether the counseling theory(ies) supports and builds from existing student strengths, rather than merely remediating student deficits. Can the approach help students rekindle and expand their developmental assets?

Indicator 3 (Contextual Sensitivity)   Make every effort to ascertain whether the theory you might use is flexible enough to address external influences (peer, familial, and community) on students' welfare and functioning. In other words, Step 3 in theory selection is to determine whether the approach reflects contextual sensitivity: Is the milieu from which group members live and learn pertinent to the particular counseling orientation? A worthwhile counseling theory must be able to incorporate the students' subsystems into the group dynamics and processes.

Indicator 4 (Validity Issues)   The last step is check to see if the theory and its counseling methods have been validated in schools with the particular age and ethnic group you are targeting. It is the counselor's task to ensure the approach is evidence based and found to be relatively effective with school-age children.

In comparison with these four quality indicators (criteria), Table 2.5 provides a rough idea of how each counseling model fares. Notice that solution-focused brief and Adlerian approaches receive positive marks for each of the four standards. The Rogerian or child-centered approach appears to be a good place to begin if you are conducting a growth or support group. Cognitive-behavioral approaches tend to be helpful for psychoeducational groups that are skill based and intended for late elementary-age to secondary school-age participants. Although Gestalt group counseling has its advantages, this model tends to overaccentuate what's "wrong" with the students' feelings, thoughts, and behaviors. In terms of the level of counselor leadership skills, all the theoretical approaches require a strong skill set. Five of the seven perspectives tend to rely on a high level of counselor direction, requiring an additional layer of conceptual understanding and practical experience.

The differences between some theories are often more strategic than conceptual, so opting for a mix of similar approaches in one group makes sense. This is perhaps why many group counselors in the schools claim they are theoretically eclectic. For instance, a psychoeducational group that focuses on student emotions, self-awareness, and growth might use a combination of methods from Gestalt and Rogerian theories. Note, however, that a group utilizing Gestalt techniques is far more hands-on (counselor directed) than a traditional Rogerian-oriented group. To resolve this tension, school counselors can exploit Rogerian counseling methods to reveal the students' developmental

TABLE 2.5 | General Comparison of Major School-Based Group Counseling Approaches Using Level of Counselor Directedness and Quality Indicators

Indicator	Theoretical Orientation						
	Level of Counselor Directedness						
	Lowest	Moderate		High		Highest	
	Humanistic Child-Centered (Rogers, Maslow)	Adlerian[c] (Adler, Dreikurs)	Gestalt (Perls, Simick)	Choice Theory/ Reality Therapy (Glasser)	CBT (A. Beck, J. Beck); REBT (Ellis)	Solution-Focused Brief Therapy (de Shazer)	Behavioral[d] (e.g., Skinner)
Adjusts for developmental differences?	+	+	+	+	+	+	
Strengths based	+	+		+		+	
Considers context of student's world	+	+	+	+	+	+	+
Validated with K–12 students[a, b]		+[3]		+	+	+	+[4]

Note: CBT = cognitive-behavioral therapy; REBT = rational emotive behavior therapy.

[a]The Rogerian approach is useful for rapport building, but there is little solid evidence that this approach would work for the entire group experience. [b]None of these models are well documented for early elementary-age students (i.e., K–3). [c]Recent evidence of the effectiveness of Adlerian groups is limited. [d]Behavioral techniques are effective when coupled with other approaches to groups.

assets (strengths) and to establish group cohesion, and later make use of Gestalt techniques (e.g., role-playing and empty chair) to explore student issues at a deeper level. Alternatively, if a group counselor wants to conduct a psychoeducational group that aims at increasing student awareness of how cognitions and beliefs affect behavior, then the counselor might link congruent ideas from solution-focused brief counseling, CBT, REBT, and reality therapy. It is safe to say that you need to do your homework, for certain counseling approaches like the Adlerian and humanistic models do not mesh well with an approach that emphasizes behavioral principles (e.g., behaviorism emphasizes environmental modification to effect behavior change, whereas humanistic therapy situates behavioral change within the person). Sharply put, theoretical incompatibility should probably be avoided. In brief, the seven theoretical options are not mutually exclusive; some theories work far better together than others, and with the appropriate level of care, forethought, and planning, they can be interwoven into effective group practice.

RESEARCH SUPPORTING USE
OF SCHOOL-BASED GROUPS

As affirmed previously, all group processes, procedures, and activities should not only reflect a strong theoretical framework but must also be founded on quality research. Successful group leaders pay particular attention to counseling research, looking for well-documented group practices that can augment their student interventions. They try new methods and discard unsuccessful ones. To highlight the need for theory and research in his own counseling work, Rogers's (1961/1989) comments here are quite helpful:

> I have come to recognize that the reason I devote myself to research, and to the building of theory, is to satisfy a need for perceiving order and meaning ... There is only one sound reason for pursuing scientific activities, and that is to satisfy a need for meaning. *The facts are friendly.* (p. 25; italics in original)

Some readers may be tempted at this point to skip over this section, assuming that the research is readily available, and if need be, you can access it. True enough, but it is sensible to know this literature *before* facilitating a group. As pointed out by Ripley and Goodnough (2001), convincing overworked principals and busy teachers that schools need to provide group counseling as a way to enhance student learning often takes more than good intentions; it necessitates, as Rogers (1961/1989, p. 25) says, "friendly facts." School counselors must be accountability leaders, documenting to their constituents the importance of their responsive interventions, including group counseling (Carey, Dimmitt, Hatch, Lapan, & Whiston, 2008; Sink, 2009). In an effort to provide the "hard" evidence, key findings and conclusions from meta-analyses[3] spanning perhaps two decades of group counseling research with K–12 students are primarily summarized here.

Counselor education scholars are committed to researching the impact of group counseling on a variety of client/student outcomes. As result, the number of quality studies to wade through is staggering (Erford, 2010). Mercifully, there is also an assortment of quality literature reviews to draw conclusions from (e.g., Bemak et al., 2005; Hoag & Burlingame, 1997; Hoag & Burlingame, 1997; Whiston, Tai, Rahardja, & Eder, 2011; Whiston & Quinby, 2009; Whiston & Sexton, 1998). For additional resources, other good but less comprehensive summaries of group counseling studies are available (e.g., Dykeman & Appleton, 2002; Erford, 2010; Gerrity & DeLucia, 2007; McGannon et al., 2005; Paisley & Milsom, 2007; Pérusse et al., 2009; Whiston & Sexton, 1998).

Reaching back to the late 1990s, Hoag and Burlingame (1997) conducted a meta-analysis of 56 studies that examined the potential effects of group counseling on psychosocial outcomes of children and adolescents. Encouraging results were reported,

---

[3]Meta-analyses are conducted by researchers as way of quantitatively synthesizing multiple studies in a particular area of investigation (e.g., group counseling effectiveness research). See Sink and Mvududu (2010) for a discussion of ESs, statistical power, and sampling.

including a moderate overall effect size[4] ($ES_\Delta = 0.61$) for the group counseling studies conducted in school settings. Basically, a group difference index like a delta (Δ) involves calculating the magnitude of the mean difference between two samples (e.g., experimental and comparison), taking into account group size (n) and the distribution of scores (SD) (Sink & Mvududu, 2010). What an ES of 0.61 means in relatively nontechnical terms is: The students who participated in the group counseling intervention improved over one-half a standard deviation more than the students who did not receive this assistance. Another way to interpret this overall ES_Δ of 0.61 is to say that the average child or adolescent receiving a group intervention generated higher outcome scores (i.e., reported better functioning) than 73% of their peers in the control or comparison groups. The strongest effects were reported for these outcome variables: disruptive behavior, anxiety, adjustment to divorce, cognitive performance, social skills, and self-esteem. Middle-class students ($ES_\Delta = 0.79$) appeared to benefit more from group interventions than students from families who reported a lower socioeconomic status ($ES_\Delta = 0.29$).

As a caveat to the Hoag and Burlington's (1997) optimistic findings, Carey and Dimmitt (2005) pointed out a worrisome trend emerging from the meta-analysis. The ESs varied dramatically from study to study. Some group counseling investigations generated little or no effect (e.g., $ES_\Delta = -0.04$) on the group participants' outcome scores, whereas others reported very strong ESs (e.g., $ES_\Delta = 2.99$). Even though researchers conducting literature reviews prefer to find consistent ES trends across studies, Hoag and Burlington found that on average most students benefited from the small-group experience. As a caveat, however, group counseling did not seem to have the same level of efficacy with lower-level socioeconomic status students.

More than a decade later, Whiston and Quinby's (2009) quantitative review of school counseling outcome research indicated that group counseling interventions were again largely effective ($ES_\Delta = 0.35$). In real-world terms, a small to moderate effect size of 0.35 suggests that those students receiving group counseling scored higher than 64% of the control or comparison group students. Evidently then, from the late 1990s to 2009 the advantages of group counseling for students remain, but the downward ES trend is cause for some concern. Hence, counselors need to (a) follow the group counseling research closely and (b) evaluate group outcomes, ensuring that their groups use best practice.

To sum up, the research documenting the efficacy of school-based group counseling remains a "work in progress," but the overall trend of the results reported in American and British (R. Lee, Tiley, & White, 2009) studies is clearly positive. Psychoeducational groups using CBT techniques seem to be the most efficacious. Groups are typically successful for male and female students across grade levels, and for students with learning challenges, those at risk for school failure, and those representing the major ethnicities.

---

[4]Effect sizes (ESs) represent the practical significance of statistical findings, generally ranging from 0.00 to 3.00. ESs in social science and education tend to range from 0.00 to 2.00. Normally in meta-analyses, the ES estimate is reported as a delta (Δ) and is often calculated as follows: $\text{Mean}_{\text{experimental group}} - \text{Mean}_{\text{control group}}$ divided by the standard deviation of the control group's scores. There are other ES estimates reported in meta-analyses (see Sink & Stroh, 2006, for an overview of ESs in school counseling research).

CONCLUDING REMARKS

Despite the fact that group counseling efficacy research is generally encouraging, school counselors need to be mindful of the downsides to facilitating school groups. In fact, some studies failed to show student improvement after a group experience, and many are in some way methodologically flawed (Whiston et al., 2011; Whiston & Aricak, 2008; Whiston & Quinby, 2009). For example, Whiston et al.'s meta-analytic review of school counseling interventions indicated that many of the studies utilized quantitative instruments (e.g., surveys, tests, inventories) to measure student outcomes with varying degrees of reliability and validity. Of 117 studies reviewed, less than 39% reported sufficient instrumentation reliability data, and validity concerns were only weakly addressed. Among other issues, many studies did not have adequate controls, large enough sample sizes, or report estimates of practical significance (effect sizes). Consequently, even with the best intentions, preparation, and leadership, groups are not altogether beneficial interventions with students. In fact, there are possible detrimental effects of school-based counseling for children with internalizing (e.g., students with depression and anxiety) and externalizing (e.g., students who fight) behavior problems, as well as those who are grieving, using abusing substances, and in need of substantial social skills training (Nicholson, Foote, & Grigerick, 2009). Schools with challenging environments and limited administrative or teacher support for group counseling may also find them ineffective, especially if they are instituted in a haphazard fashion. For these reasons, the need for quality training in collaboration and group methods with students showing a range of issues is perhaps more pressing now than ever before.

All the same, it is not the lack of evidence that keeps many school counselors from facilitating groups but the pragmatics of developing, implementing, and evaluating small groups. When asked whether they do group counseling, many school counselors we know will respond "Not this year; we just cannot find the time!" As alluded to earlier in the chapter and as you will read about in later ones, the amount of work (e.g., finding a quiet and secure space, coordinating schedules, obtaining permission, pulling students out of class, etc.) involved in setting up a fully operational and effective group can feel like a logistics and bureaucratic tsunami. However, conducting proactive groups that demonstrate student learning, investing time in developing policy changes so that groups are burdensome on the educational enterprise, and collaborating more effectively among faculty, administrators, and counselors can lessen the obstacles (Ripley & Goodnough, 2001).

Other than pragmatic issues, school counselors also report additional concerns about group counseling. For example, there's a "fear factor" involving leadership competency and related ethical issues. Counselors may not feel adequately prepared to conduct effective groups, and the potential risks when working with minors in small groups can be daunting. Confidentiality cannot be assured, possible student psychological harm might occur in the course of a group session, and a leader's ability to deal with troublesome group members can be severely taxed (J. Corey, 2009). These concerns can be lessened by good preservice and in-service group leadership training and by carefully following the professional ethical codes of related to counseling students, including the American Counseling Association's (ACA; 2005, e.g., Section A.8. Group Work) Code of Ethics and ASCA's (2004b, 2010 e.g., Section A.6. Group Work) Ethical Standards for School Counselors. These ethical issues are addressed throughout the later chapters.

Although acknowledging the disadvantages and challenges, there are very good reasons for leading small groups in schools. To reiterate, anecdotal and empirical research supports that groups are a useful way of nurturing student growth and development. In fact, leading school counselor educators Bemak et al. (2005)

> advocate that group counseling in public schools is a more effective intervention in addressing some of the serious social problems facing our youth, particularly at a time when peer relationships, social skills, and social interaction are not considered priorities in an era of high-stakes testing, test results, and academic productivity. In fact, group counseling meets earlier calls for schools to become training grounds for social development and moral development. (p. 381)

However, merely facilitating groups does not make them a valuable responsive service. Effective group counseling leadership requires specialized theoretical and research knowledge and well-honed skills. Counselors must also refine their collaboration and advocacy skills needed to implement groups in schools with many legitimate and competing agendas (Pérusse et al., 2009). Navigating these issues can be very challenging. In the following chapter, the focus shifts from theory and research to quality group processes and procedures.

CHAPTER 2 SUPPLEMENT

USING NARRATIVE COUNSELING IN SCHOOL-BASED GROUPS

An emerging theory in school counseling is the narrative approach. Narrative counseling is built on the premise that stories shape our lives (Freeman, Epston, & Lobovits, 1997; M. White & Epston, 1990; Winslade & Monk, 2007). These stories, which give meaning to students' lives and affect how they interact with others, are constructed and told in relationships. Language, both verbal and nonverbal, organizes events into narratives, which give, ascribe, and hold meaning (M. White & Epston, 1990). A student who is told that she will never be a "math-wiz" may start to believe this script, leaning into it until she no longer applies herself in math classes.

A narrative, or life story, reveals what the student deems important, which affects his or her behavior (Eron & Lund, 1996; Freedman & Combs, 1996; Parry & Doan, 1994; M. White & Epston, 1990; Zimmerman & Dickerson, 1996). A student who talks a lot about baseball may value sports. Healthy stories are dynamic. The student who loves baseball may also like to read and to hang out with friends. Problems occur when stories become static. The student who likes baseball thinks that that is the only thing he is good at and that being a pitcher in the major leagues is the only job he could want.

It is the thin story, the stuck narrative that is the problem. The student is not the problem; the problem is the problem. This is not to excuse bad choices or negative behavior, but to take that behavior outside of the student and alter the action while seeing the strengths within the holistic person. The baseball-loving student is not unmotivated; he just needs to see other strengths and how his skills that make him a good player bode well for him in other areas of life (e.g., the math that helps him figure out his "earned run average" can also be used to help him in science classes).

Stories are not static. A problem-centered story may be transformed to an account of success and hope. Narrative theorists encourage bonding, or joining, with students by hearing their story, using their language, and collaborating with them (Winslade & Monk, 2007). First, the counselor maps the problem. When is the problem the problem? Who is there? How long does it last? How does the student help the problem go away? Next, the counselor helps the student to see the problem as an external entity. Externalization is an approach that encourages objectification and personification of problems. The problem becomes a separate entity. This can be done via language or by giving the problem a name. For example, a narrative counselor would not ask a student if he were sad. Instead, the counselor would ask, "When is sadness inside of you?" Problems can also be externalized giving them a name. For students who are quiet in class, a group leader could ask, "What eats all your words when you are in class?" The student could name the word eater, and the group could help members fight against the word monster taking away the students' voices.

After the problem has been mapped and externalized, the counselor helps students rewrite their stories to have unique outcomes to the situation. This shows that alternatives are possible and that the problem is not all encompassing. Finding unique outcomes is similar to the solution-focused technique of asking about hypothetical solutions. The identification of unique outcomes and the discovery of new meanings around these outcomes assist students to identify their power over the problem and work against it. A richer story is retold to include solutions and hope.

Winslade and Monk (2007) offered an eight-lesson school-based small group in their text (pp. 136–152). Each group member identifies a challenge. Then, the group works to challenge the challenge by offering other members support and feedback. The leader's role is to offer support, help externalize the problems, and investigate the unique outcomes. Each student in this group may choose a different problem. The narrative approach may also be employed when there is an identified goal for the group. For example, when running a group on coping with test anxiety, early sessions may explore what the feeling of test anxiety in each student is (mapping the influence). During the early and middle stages of the group, the group leader will start to use language to externalize the groups' experiences of test anxiety. For example, students may draw pictures of themselves, using red to fill in where they feel the anxiety (mapping the influence). The group leader may then pose an externalizing question such as, "What would you name this red, anxious spot?" After the student gives the problem a name (e.g., "the fiery pit"), the leader begins to help the member to alter the narrative to help identify skills, attributes, and resources that keep the fiery pit from taking over the student's whole body (finding unique outcomes). This will help the group write a thicker narrative with solutions that students create for themselves and learn from other group members.

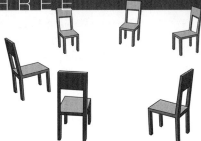

Basics of Group Preparation and Implementation

It felt like I could cooperate with my family. I never really let what was in my mind out before the group. When I got in the group, I knew the people and felt comfortable.

After my dad died, the entire world turned on me. I became a hider, and an escaper. No one knew how I felt … I joined a grief group provided at my school, and quit because I didn't want to talk about my dad with kids I barely knew. For some reason, my name wasn't taken off the list by the next group meeting. I remember getting called in from Math, and sitting through another group meeting. The beat of my heart grew faster as it was almost time to share what reminded me of my dad. When it was my turn; I decided to share how I felt seeing his truck everyday once I came home from school. With a gust of wind, the weight was taken off my shoulders. Something unexplainable happened in that room that day; and I knew I needed to trust the people who were trying to help me. There was nothing to be afraid of. I would definitely recommend this. It really did teach me a lifelong lesson.
—Comments from two ninth-grade Washington State students, commenting on a grief group they attended during the previous year in middle school.

LEADING BY EXAMPLE—WISDOM FROM THE AGES

Two traveling monks reached a town where there was a young woman waiting to step out of her sedan chair. The rains had made deep puddles and she couldn't step across without spoiling her silken robes. She stood there, looking very cross and impatient. She was scolding her attendants. They had no where to place the packages they held for her, so they couldn't help her across the puddle.

The younger monk noticed the woman, said nothing, and walked by. The older monk quickly picked her up and put her on his back, transported her across the water, and put down on the other side. She didn't thank the old monk, she just shoved him out of the way and departed.

As they continued on their way, the young monk was brooding and preoccupied. After several hours, unable to hold his silence, he spoke out. "That woman back there was very selfish and rude, but you picked her up on your back and carried here! Then she didn't even thank you!"

"I set the woman down hours ago," the older monk replied. "Why are *you* still carrying her?" (Story retold by Jon Muth, 2005, n.p.)

* * *

When participating in a well-functioning small group, both students like those quoted in the chapter epigraph and the group facilitators may find the experience a little Zen-like. The timeless parable retold above exemplifies the influence group counselors can softly, yet noticeably exert in guiding members toward personal well-being and social growth. If the group experience is run with skill and care, students will recognize that change is an inevitable process related to effective decision making, problem solving, and goal attainment. Like the Zen master in the preceding tale, leaders model with few words how to relate with less than desirable people and to successfully manage frustrations and emotions. Students may then apply what they have observed to their interactions.

As such, the practical side of group leadership is now explored, building on the introductory material discussed in chapter 1, and the group theory and research reviewed in chapter 2. In particular, the discussion here summarizes and illustrates the four major phases of group work as well as the specific stages of the group implementation phase. The core counseling functions and skills needed to conduct quality, strengths-based groups are also explored.

PHASES OF GROUP DEVELOPMENT AND IMPLEMENTATION

In all likelihood readers have already surmised that counseling, whether conducted individually or in group settings, is a process much like human development, almost taking on a life of its own. Most group counseling texts address the phases of group work and how it unfolds over time (e.g., G. Corey, 2008; M. S. Corey et al., 2010). Not unexpectedly, school-based groups begin with a formation phase, followed by the group implementation, evaluation, and follow-up phases. To ground our school-based group work, sample practical materials are liberally integrated into the text. For additional group resources, numerous publications are available online and in the counseling literature (e.g., DeLucia-Waack, 2006; Greenberg, 2003; Jacobs & Schimmel, 2005; Jacobs et al., 2009; Shechtman, 2007; Shechtman & Gluk, 2005).

Phase 1: Formation

Prior to conducting the group, many logistical and planning issues need to be considered and worked out. Regrettably, because of the amount of preparation required in this phase many well-meaning school counselors get mired in the details, perhaps in time even jettisoning the practice altogether. Sometimes when asking counselors about why they no longer conduct groups, one often is greeted with such shortsighted reasons as: "It's just too much work and effort." "My caseload is so big; I just don't have time for groups." "Our school will never accept taking kids out of their classes." But if you are new to group counseling, have faith in the vital responsive service; once the group starts flowing naturally, students almost always benefit from the experience. Roughly, here is the group formation "to do" list. With administration and teacher support, the school counselor

- conducts a needs assessment by surveying students, families, and faculty to determine the magnitude of the need as well as the feasibility of the group;
- develops an overall focus or group theme and sets group goals;
- selects the most appropriate group design or format (e.g., psychoeducational versus growth group) based on previous research and best practice;
- applies theoretical constructs and reviews the research on the topic to help guide the group experience and activities;
- composes the group by screening/interviewing potential group members, and with written parent/guardian and student consent selects those students who might benefit most from the group experience;
- develops each session's content and activities;
- works through logistical issues (e.g., finding an appropriate space and times to run the group, notifying students, teachers, and, if needed, families, about these details); and,
- obtains additional teacher and administrator "buy in" through the writing and marketing of a short group plan.

If not addressed in earlier chapters, these formative tasks are explained below and practically illustrated in the remaining chapters.

Conduct needs assessment   What are the most pressing areas of concern for students on a year-to-year basis? Do the school staff and family members agree with how students perceive their needs? Let's assume, for instance, that all parties concur that the most urgent student concern is test-taking skills. Before the group is designed and put into practice, the professional school counselor in consultation with the school administrator must think through the implications of conducting a group on this topic. In most cases, innocuous topics related to educational and career development are readily approved by the principal, but when you want to facilitate a group related to a personal/social issue that is perhaps controversial (e.g., sexual issues), the administrator may ask some questions.

As part of the larger data collection process related to implementing the school vision, school improvement plan, and so on, school counselors also conduct highly focused or schoolwide needs assessments. Basically, counselors devise a survey tool that is individualized to their schools, specific grade levels, target populations, and intended uses. There are numerous sample instruments accessible online and in school counseling publications. You are also not limited to paper-and-pencil formats. Counselors may deploy e-surveys to help with the process. Reputable online programs include, for example, SurveyMethods (http://www.surveymethods.com/), SurveyMonkey (http://www.surveymonkey.com/), and Zoomerang (http://www.zoomerang.com/). In any case, questionnaires should always be carefully designed with a clear purpose in mind and developmentally appropriate. For example, the wording of each survey statement should be developmentally appropriate and the possible response options must be understandable. Given the cognitive sophistication required to self-evaluate one's own learning and developmental concerns, needs assessment measures are probably not that valid for children in Grades K–2. Certainly younger children's parents/caregivers can provide their input.

Here are suggestions for writing high-quality surveys and individual statements:

- Keep the questionnaire "short and simple." In total, surveys should require no longer than 20 minutes to administer and for the respondent to complete.
- Scorers should need only 10 minutes to sum up respondents' ratings for each area (domain) assessed.
- Select the developmental domains best representing the school's counseling program (e.g., academic/educational, personal/social, career/vocational, multicultural, moral/character) and write 5 to 10 statements per domain. If you were interested, say, in assessing the character and social issues of your students, the counselor would construct a 10- to 20-statement survey.
- Keep each statement/item brief, unambiguous in meaning, and reflecting only one idea or theme. Here are some examples.
  - *Academic domain*—Student survey
    - Grades 3–4: "School is hard for me."
    - Grades 5–12: "I need help with doing classwork (or homework)."
    - Caregiver version: "My daughter/son would benefit from more help with their classwork (or homework)."
    - Teacher version: "Students need more assistance with their classwork (or homework)."
  - *Personal/social domain*—Student survey
    - Grades 3–4: "Making friends is hard for me."
    - Grades 5–12: "I need help with making friends."
    - Caregiver version: "My daughter/son would benefit from more help with making friends."
    - Teacher version: "Students need more assistance with their friendship skills."
- Make sure each statement can be answered with a simple response or rating. Survey devisers can employ a Likert-type scale, so that respondents circle one number ranging from 1 to 3 or 1 to 5 that best reflects their opinion. Write the response options as:
  - 1 "do not agree," 2 "not sure," and 3 "agree" (for younger respondents), or
  - 1 "really do not agree," 2 "do not agree," 3 "not sure," 4 "agree," and 5 "really agree."
  - For younger children, they need only circle a face representing for example

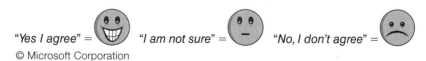

"Yes I agree" =   "I am not sure" =   "No, I don't agree" =

© Microsoft Corporation

- Include brief and uncomplicated directions to the targeted respondent. For example, "Directions:
  Your student attends _____ School. The principal, teachers, and counseling staff would like to know what you think are the *most important learning needs* of your child right now. By filling out this survey and returning it promptly, we can

make plans to *better support your child's learning*. Please take a few minutes to complete this survey and return it to the office by MM/DD."

- Request other demographic information at the beginning or end of survey. For student respondents, ask for their gender and grade level. The name should be optional. The educator survey version should ask for the respondent's school position and grade level. The parent/caregiver survey version might include a question about the respondent's relationship to the student (e.g., mother, father, or other) and child's grade level.
- Make sure you include a confidential statement on the survey such as: "All your responses will be kept confidential and read only by the counseling staff."
- Ensure the surveys have what is called "face validity," meaning that they look professional and relatively interesting. Position the school's name and mascot (logo) on the survey's masthead (top section of the letter). You could also place the school's slogan and its contact information.

Sample abbreviated surveys designed for middle school students, parents/caregivers, and educators (to be administered to, e.g., teachers, administrator, nurse, etc.), respectively, are provided below (see Figures 3.1, 3.2, and 3.3). Notice that the text is slightly modified on each needs assessment survey, depending on the target audience. For elementary or high school levels, minor wording changes will be required. As alluded to earlier, examples of needs assessment surveys are plentiful on the Internet and in relevant school counseling texts. Simply key into your favorite Internet search engine (e.g., Google, Bing) descriptive phrases like "K–12 needs assessment," "elementary school needs assessment," or "high school needs assessment." The results will reveal numerous alternatives available to select from. Should you use a needs assessment questionnaire from a website or elsewhere, to avoid copyright issues make sure to cite the source(s).

In terms of data entry and analysis, Microsoft's Excel program works very well, especially if used with a no-cost, relatively simple add-in software program called EZAnalyze (available at http://www.ezanalyze.com/). According to software designers and in our experience as well, this program extends the functionality of Excel by adding a "point and click" feature for analyzing data, making graphs, and creating new variables. Versions are available for Macs and PCs. With this program, use the simple bar chart function to generate and display the major trends in the data. For example, to enhance comparisons among the school's constituents, select the top five most highly rated needs from the student, parent, and staff data, and then graph them. Figure 3.4 depicts fictional data collected from Wapiti Middle School's (WMS) students, parents, and educators. The higher the scores (i.e., respondents more strongly agreed with the needs assessment survey item) for the three-item questionnaire, the higher the bar appears on the chart. Clearly, each respondent group agreed that getting assistance with homework is the most pressing need. As such, an academic, content-based small group could be devised around this topic.

In terms of soliciting support for the needs assessment and how to collect the data, Ripley and Goodnough (2001) provided some useful school-based ideas. Each year they obtained authorization to carry out the assessment as part of a brief classroom presentation in each language arts class. In collaboration with classroom teachers, a preapproved presentation calendar was circulated to the relevant educators. To maintain

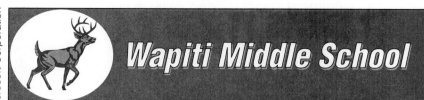

12345 West Stream, Ryne Mt., CN
Student Survey
Your opinions matter! What do you need from our school?
Month, Year

Directions:

The principal, teachers, and counseling department would really like to know about your *most important learning needs*. By answering this voluntary survey and returning it now, they can make plans to *better support your learning*. Please take a few minutes to fill out this survey and return it to the office by the end of today. Your answers will be kept confidential.

Gender: Male or Female   Circle your grade level: 6th 7th 8th

Needs Assessment Statement	Circle one number for each statement				
1. I need more assistance with finishing my homework. (academic skills)	1 strongly disagree	2 disagree	3 not sure	4 agree	5 strongly agree
2. I need more help with making good friends. (social skills)	1 strongly disagree	2 disagree	3 not sure	4 agree	5 strongly agree
3. I need to learn more about jobs. (career skills)	1 strongly disagree	2 disagree	3 not sure	4 agree	5 strongly agree
4. Etc.	1 strongly disagree	2 disagree	3 not sure	4 agree	5 strongly agree
Comments:					

Thank you for your support of MMS. Please return this survey to your teacher or to the counseling office by **the end of today**. If you have questions or want to speak to a school counselor, call (xxx) xxx-xxxx, stop by the counseling office, or write your name here
_____ (You'll be called in.)

FIGURE 3.1 | Sample abbreviated middle school needs assessment survey—student version.

professionalism and the teachers' goodwill and desire to be accommodating, the counselors, in turn, followed carefully the presentation schedule, began on time, and in a timely manner made their presentations.

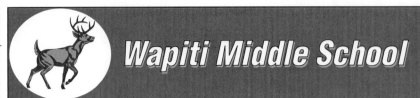

Wapiti Middle School

12345 West Stream, Ryne Mt., CN

Parent/Caregiver Survey

Your opinions matter! What does your student need from our school?
Month, Year

Directions:

Your student attends WMS. The principal, teachers, and counseling department would like to know what you think are the *most important learning needs* of your child. By answering this voluntary survey and returning it promptly, the staff can make plans to *better support your child's learning.* Please take a few minutes to fill out this survey and return it to the office by no later than October 15. All responses will be kept confidential.

Relationship to student: Mother   Father   Other _____ (please specify)

Your child is in: 6th   7th   8th grade (circle one)

Needs Assessment Statement	Circle one number for each statement				
1. My student needs more assistance with their homework completion skills. (academic skills)	**1** *strongly disagree*	**2** *disagree*	**3** *not sure*	**4** *agree*	**5** *strongly agree*
2. My student needs more assistance with their friendship skills. (social skills)	**1** *strongly disagree*	**2** *disagree*	**3** *not sure*	**4** *agree*	**5** *strongly agree*
3. My student needs to learn more about job/career skills. (career skills)	**1** *strongly disagree*	**2** *disagree*	**3** *not sure*	**4** *agree*	**5** *strongly agree*
4. Etc.	**1** *strongly disagree*	**2** *disagree*	**3** *not sure*	**4** *agree*	**5** *strongly agree*

Write your comments here:

Thank you again for your support of MMS. Please return this survey by **October 15** to the office or mail it in using the school envelope. If you have questions or want to speak to a school counselor, call (xxx) xxx-xxxx for an appointment.

FIGURE 3.2 | Sample abbreviated middle school needs assessment survey—parent/caregiver version.

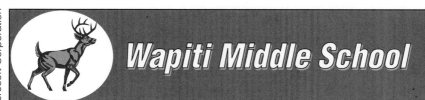

Wapiti Middle School

12345 West Stream, Ryne Mt., CN

Educator Survey

Your opinions matter! What does your student need from our school?
Month, Year

Directions:

The School Counseling Department would like to know what you think are the *most important learning needs* of your students. By completing this optional survey and returning it promptly, the counseling staff can make plans to *better support your students' education*. Please take a few minutes to complete this survey and return it to the office by October 15. All responses will be kept confidential.

Circle your position: Teacher Counselor Psychologist Administrator Other: _____
(please specify)

Needs Assessment Statement	Circle one number for each statement				
1. Students need more assistance with their homework completion skills. (academic skills)	1 *strongly disagree*	2 *disagree*	3 *not sure*	4 *agree*	5 *strongly agree*
2. Students need more assistance with their interpersonal skills. (social skills)	1 *strongly disagree*	2 *disagree*	3 *not sure*	4 *agree*	5 *strongly agree*
3. Students need to learn more about jobs/careers. (career skills)	1 *strongly disagree*	2 *disagree*	3 *not sure*	4 *agree*	5 *strongly agree*
4. Etc.	1 *strongly disagree*	2 *disagree*	3 *not sure*	4 *agree*	5 *strongly agree*

Comments:

Thank you for your support of MMS. Please return this survey to the box in the counseling office by **October 15** at the latest. If you have questions or concerns, please come by the counseling office.

FIGURE 3.3 | Sample abbreviated middle school needs assessment survey—educator version.

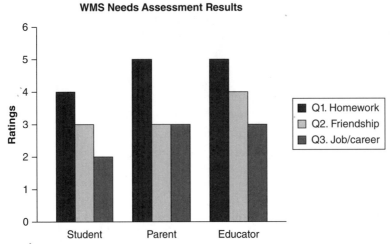

FIGURE 3.4 | Bar chart comparing student, parent, and educator needs assessment results.

Whenever possible include the school principal and the administrative staff in these discussions and schedules, soliciting their support and informing them of the upcoming presentations and data collection procedures. Families may have questions, and the office staff needs to understand when, where, and why students are completing the surveys. If the office staff is suppose to aid in data collection (e.g., collecting and storing the completed questionnaires), make sure they have all the details and materials needed to retain the data in a safe and confidential place. Do not leave any completed surveys out in public view. Sharply put, keep them secure at all times.

Feasibility analysis   Forming a group can be a protracted endeavor, not only because of the needs analysis process but because the feasibility of conducting the group must be considered as well. Feasibility studies are generally instituted by business and engineering professionals to estimate the probability that a planned venture will fulfill its stated objectives. In education, this practice is frequently included in strategic planning (e.g., Kaufman, Herman, & Watters, 2002); however, for our purposes, a feasibility analysis largely involves ascertaining whether the proposed group can and should be launched, and if so, how and when. This is an informal process requiring interdepartmental conversation and later asking other school personnel for their input. School counselors survey the current educational landscape and attempt to process and reply to these sample questions:

- What is the school climate right now? Is it positive and supportive? What is the history of groups in my school? Do I need to invest more time in educating the staff about the value of group counseling?
- Are teachers and families open to this group topic? Will they allow the targeted student members to leave their classroom and miss the lessons?
- Is there a regular, safe, and confidential location to carry out the group?

- Are there any conflicting school activities (e.g., state achievement testing, soccer championship taking place, spelling tournament) that may interfere with the group experience and student attendance?
- Will the administrator support the group leader if there is some negative feedback?
- Will parents/caregivers support this group idea?
- Are there any intangibles (i.e., "red flags") like school district teacher layoffs that might impede the group's success?
- What multicultural and diversity issues need to be considered? Is the proposed group culturally sensitive and relevant? Will students with special needs be included and successful?

Once the counseling staff has worked through the questions, these are usually later discussed in closed-door conversation with the administrator and other relevant colleagues. Sort out your group ideas and rationale before these meetings occur. As a professional collaborator and advocate, remain open-minded, ready to listen, and adaptable to suggestions (Ripley & Goodnough, 2001). To be discussed shortly, develop a group action plan or proposal that is presentable to major decision makers as well.

Create group focus/theme and set general goals   When developing the group, counselors should ask themselves: What am I aiming for? What do I want the group members to learn and practice in their daily lives? If I had to write in a letter home to the students' families explaining what this group is about and what differences parents/caregivers should see in their children's behaviors, what would it say? Situated within theory and best practice, answers to these preliminary questions can provide guidance on selecting the most suitable group format (e.g., psychoeducational, growth group) and "ensure" that the group's proposed major aim(s) and goals are achievable.

The group theme(s) should echo the results of the needs and feasibility assessments. Selecting a topic that is a school counselor's pet interest may be fun and motivating, but not necessarily a meaningful group focus for the participants. Depending on how the items on the needs assessment are written, the most pressing issues for the respondents fall into the three major ASCA (2005, 2008) developmental domains: academic/educational, personal/social, and career/vocational. Supporting the foregoing points, Steen and Kaffenberger (2007) recommended that topics for small counseling groups should be developed "in conjunction with teachers, administrators, and parents. School counselors, in many instances, consult with parents or guardians, school personnel, and other identified parties when developing plans and strategies for promoting student development" (p. 516).

Sample topics fitting for K–12 groups as well as those that are inappropriate are listed in Table 3.1. Most of these are drawn from ASCA (2005) and various school counseling publications. Themes to be avoided are those topics beyond a school counselor's scope of practice and level of competence (ASCA, 2004b, 2010; see also chapter 4). The group areas most likely to generate concern are those related to the remediation of deeper behavioral, psychological, and emotional disorders (see chapter 1 for a longer discussion). Once more, psychotherapeutic groups conducted by private therapists and psychologists are most efficacious for serious and chronic mental health issues. At all times use professional discernment when selecting the group topic. As indicated above, consultation with administrators, other school counselors, and relevant others

TABLE 3.1 | Examples of Suitable and Incompatible Topics for School-Based K–12 Small Groups by Developmental Domain

Developmental Domain	Suitable Group Topics
Educational/Academic	• Cognitive/learning strategies (e.g., memory, attention, planning, organization) • Coping with learning challenges • Educational assets • Help-seeking strategies • Homework completion • How to study at home and in school • Learning in English (e.g., for ELL, ESL students) • Relate school to life experiences • Staying on task and paying attention • Test taking • Tools for educational success (general) • Using the library and Internet for better learning
Personal-Social	• Anger management • Being different • Conflict management • Coping with grief and loss (e.g., family separation, divorce, and bereavement) • Dealing with bullying • Decision making • Developmental assets • Empathy and emotional regulation • Friendship and social skills • Gender-related issues (girl and boy empowerment) • Internet use and etiquette • Peer pressure • Personal/social assets • Relationship building • Resiliency • Responsibility taking • Self-management • Stress management • Self-efficacy and self-concept • Transitions (e.g., new school or grade level, family moving, new sibling, adoption, military deployment)
Career/Vocational	• Academic/educational skills needed for jobs and careers • Career planning • Career/vocational assets • Choosing a career • Discrimination issues • Getting and keeping a job

- Getting along with coworkers
- Goal setting
- Consumer finances
- Planning for the future (postsecondary education and training)
- School-to-work transition
- Values and ethics in the workplace
- Work world

Inappropriate Group Topics

- Chronic depression, anxiety, and diagnosable psychiatric condition
- Coping with family members with serious challenges (e.g., parent with substance abuse issues)
- Emotional, physical, and sexual abuse
- Foster care issues
- Religious issues[1]
- Severe behavior disorders (e.g., self-harm, habitually dishonest, steal, highly aggressive) requiring psychiatric/clinical psychological treatment
- Suicidal tendencies and ideations
- Any topic outside school counselor's level of professional competence

Note: Items drawn from, e.g., ASCA (2005a); Blum and Davis, 2010; Smead (1995); Pyle (2007); Ripley and Goodnough (2001); Stroh and Sink (2002); Steen and Kaffenberger (2007).

(e.g., nurse, school psychologist, district attorney) is strongly encouraged. Make sure the group format is most fitting for the group theme. If the group focus will emphasize personal/social support and sharing among students, a growth group format is probably the most useful.

It may have already become obvious that many group topics, although placed within one developmental domain (see Table 3.1), tend to overlap with others. Most school-based topics can be interwoven into an overall group theme(s); for instance, one high school group addressed both educational and personal/social student needs through its weekly small-group activities (Ripley & Goodnough, 2001).

Finally, because students' concerns and needs are multifaceted, group leaders should avoid becoming so narrowly (and overly) planned that the building blocks (e.g., cooperative learning skills) of educational success are neglected (Steen & Kaffenberger, 2007). The preponderance of group topics in Table 3.1 can be introduced by late elementary school. Create a developmental crosswalk matrix (see ASCA's National Model, 2005a, for details) that includes the core developmental domains, student competencies to be addressed, and grade-level benchmarks indicating when the competency should be "mastered." Using the crosswalk approach, school counselors are more likely to select developmentally appropriate group themes. With the tentative group foci/topics in mind, counselors can draft a short group action plan to share with relevant educators and administration.

---

[1]Spirituality in a generic meaning-making sense (nonreligious) can be touched upon if students raise the issue (see Sink & Devlin, 2011, for clarification and recommendations).

Develop group action plan   This summary document is considered best practice and an efficient way to operationalize the proposed group (e.g., Brigman & Early, 2001; Greenberg, 2003; Smead, 1995). Because teachers want to have their input on most school events affecting their students, a written plan for them to comment on may allay their initial hesitations. Moreover, by communicating to other professionals that you have a well-thought-out group plan, your credibility is enhanced.

More specifically, prior to the group's implementation, relevant administrators, teachers, and other associated educators should have the opportunity to add their input and understand the educational relevance of the group content. Teachers appreciate knowing how their students will benefit from the group experience. Importantly, administrators are skilled at providing information that you may not have already considered (e.g., how different parent groups might to react to your group topic). Once the principal and teachers recognize that the group content, processes, and procedures are well devised, they will generally lend their support. This backing is invaluable when working with parents/caregivers. As you solicit student participants, sometimes parents want to know about the group and its implications for student learning. In our experience, most parents are willing to review a brief document. The plan reinforces in parents' minds that the group experience will assist their child's learning and development. If parents are confident in the group content, they are more likely to give their consent. A short document outlining the group experience also works in your favor with potential student members, who may need to be reassured of the group's value. Finally, the action plan is beneficial to school counselors, for it provides an organizing structure—a group blueprint—to help with pregroup preparations, implementation, and evaluation of the small-group experience. As these plans for different types of experiences are written, they need only be revised for subsequent groups. By collaborating with K–12 building educators and counselors from across the school district, a well-honed collection of group plans are then available for all counselors to utilize.

What basic elements should counselors include in the group action plan? To avoid getting too detailed, only the key points needed to initiate the process are summarized here. For sample plans with varying organizational structures, Capuzzi's (2003) and Greenberg's (2003) practitioner-oriented group texts are suggested resources. Other group plans are included in later chapters.

1. *Cover page and group naming*   The first page includes the proposed group title and contributors' names and contact information. Adding the school name and logo/mascot adds to the plan's upbeat and professional feel. If you can devise an inviting or creative title that forms a "clever" group acronym, so much the better. Obviously, make the titles developmentally appropriate, and avoid unappealing names such as "Study Skills Group," "Conflict Management Group," or "Controlling Your Anger."

   These titles may not be what you would use, but here are some sample group names:

   - "Making Connections" (secondary-level group for new students)
   - "Getting FIT" ("Families in Transition"; secondary-level family transition group)
   - "YEAH!" ("Youth Empowerment and Achievement Help"; any level—generic group)
   - "KIDS Group" ("Kids in Development"; elementary school level—generic group)
   - "Making More Friends" ("MMF" group; elementary school level—social skills group)

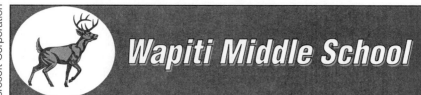

WE GOT GAME!

SMALL-GROUP PLAN

MIDDLE SCHOOL BOYS GROUP TO STRENGTHEN SOCIAL SKILLS

Developed by Hugo Jimenez and Kate Gardner, School Counselors
DATE

SUMMARY: This small-group experience focuses on the strengthening of teenage boys' social and educational skills. The long-term goal is for these students to be more successful in school. Specifically, the group leader will assist students to learn how to get along better in situations that make them frustrated, angry, or upset. The small-group curriculum is based in part on an established program called Student Success Skills.

FIGURE 3.5 | Sample small-group plan cover page.

You can also give the group a nonspecific title and during the first meeting have the participants make up a name. For a sample title page, see Figure 3.5.

2. *Overall theme (group focus)* Above we discussed the question: "What is the major focus of the group?" On the cover page or on the following page, add a summary statement much like this one: "This small-group experience focuses on the strengthening of teenage boys' social and educational skills. The long-term goal is for these students to be more successful in school. Specifically, the group leader will assist students to learn how to get along better in situations that make them frustrated, angry, or upset." Note to plan writers: Attempt to keep the focus positive and hopeful.

3. *Rationale and potential benefits for group members* The reasons for conducting the group experience are closely associated with its major theme(s). In a few statements provide the basic rationale for why, for instance, addressing educational and social skills development is a valuable group focus. If you have some research to support the group focus, this could be included in nontechnical language. Keeping with our "We Got Game" educational and social skills group idea, here is an example of a rationale statement: "Small-group experiences have been shown to improve student behavior and learning. Some of the WMS boys are struggling to maintain focus in the classroom and during nonschool times. In order for the boys to be more successful in school, they need to learn how to effectively manage their reactions to personal and social obstacles. The small-group curriculum is adapted from the well-researched Student Success Skills (SSS; Brigman et al., 2007; Webb & Brigman, 2006; see also http://www.studentsuccessskills.com/materials.htm) curriculum."

Although mostly obvious to the readers of group action plans, do not overlook adding a statement or two reiterating for educators and parents the benefits for students that may result from group participation. As summarized by Berg, Landreth, and Fall (2006), depending on the group type, group counseling (a) provides a safe environment for preventive care and support, (b) assists with student development, (c) encourages self-discovery and improvement, (d) allows for peer support and validation (i.e., students see their peers with similar concerns), and (e) promotes interpersonal awareness and prosocial behavior. Individualize these benefits to each student group member.

4. *Sample objectives*   Each group experience has preplanned but tentative student objectives. These arise both from the group members' observed and stated needs and from the overall group focus. Word these statements in an understandable, relatively unambiguous, and succinct manner. Sometimes educational objectives are stated in performance-based language. Namely, student objectives are framed in such a way that one can actually "measure" changes in student behavior. Essentially, then, as you write objectives, specify the information and/or skills students are to learn and what they will do to demonstrate proficiency. From the SSS curriculum (Webb & Brigman, 2006), here are some sample modified objectives for our fictional "We Got Game" group:
   • Students will be able to identify three personal "anger triggers."
   • Students will identify one "study buddy" to help them when they feel frustrated during classroom assignments.
   • Students will demonstrate three strategies to handle stress during a role-playing activity.

5. *Group content (session topics) and use of mobilizing activities*   A professional group plan includes short descriptors relating to each session's primary theme or focus as well as any related activities used to energize and facilitate intermember discussion and reflection (DeLucia-Waack, 2006). Accordingly, if you are hoping to conduct a 6-week group, the plan will include the same number of topics or themes. For example, based on a synthesis of behavioral theory, social learning theory, and reality therapy, the six topics for our "We Got Game" group might be: (a) getting started and introduction to social and self-management skills; (b) identifying constructive and harmful social behaviors and how they relate to classroom learning; (c) identifying those cues and situations that are social-emotional triggers; (d) trying out new positive social skills; (e) hearing and accepting of social feedback; and (f) consolidating group learning and closing activity. Another example of the group content summarized as weekly topical descriptions (see Table 3.2) was provided by Malott, Paone, Humphreys, and Martinez (2010). Their 8-week intervention group was designed to scaffold the ethnic identity development of adolescents of Mexican heritage.

As mentioned above, groups with children and youth use mobilization strategies often called catalysts or icebreakers. You will notice in Table 3.2 that the descriptions refer to various activities used to address the session's content in an engaging way. Essentially, as DeLucia-Waack (2006) pointed out, there are multiple reasons to use activities. They (a) are good ways for group members to get to know each other, increase self- and other awareness, and reduce within- and between-group member anxiety; (b) provide

TABLE 3.2 | Content of Intervention Small Group With Adolescents of Mexican Origin

Session	Weekly Topic
1	Ice breaker—Alligator river activity
2	Identity exploration—Ethnic-labeling activity
3	Values exploration—Creation of craft representing values
4	History and historical Mexican role models—Creating a representational mask
5	Mexican/Latino identity creative writing
6	Personal history—Sharing a personal story and key family members with a craft
7	Discrimination and barriers to success—Role playing with good/bad scenarios to address peer pressure and racism
8	Closing activity—Identifying one's own and others' strengths, and creating a personal portrait

Note: From Malott et al. (2010).

structure to the session (i.e., students know where the group is heading); (c) promote and focus member active involvement; (d) help students further internalize knowledge and skills as they practice the skills learned in the activity; and (e) facilitate closure and consolidation of learning during the final session. Because these activities are so vital to student participation and promoting group effectiveness, counselors need to ensure there is "meaning attribution." DeLucia-Waack suggested that group members must understand the activity they participated in for it to be meaningful. In processing the activity during the group experience with the students, school counselors can ask such open-ended questions as these: "What was your understanding why we did this group activity together? What value did you find in the activity? How was it significant to you, if at all?" The sophistication of these processing questions must be correlated to the students' grade levels.

Finding sample resources, catalysts, and content is not at all difficult. They are so numerous, one cannot catalog them here. Simply use an Internet search engine and check online booksellers (e.g., Amazon.com or Borders.com). For instance, type in germane descriptive words or terms for the content or icebreaker category you might want to review. Access Google, for instance, through the Internet, and key in the terms "small-group counseling personal/social icebreakers" or "group counseling curriculum," and links to pertinent curricula, lesson plans, therapeutic games, icebreakers, energizers, sample books, and so on are easily found. When implementing any predeveloped ("prepackaged") group action plans, content, activities, or catalysts from Internet or print sources, it is nearly always necessary to scrutinize them for relevancy and quality. Regrettably, the merit and usefulness varies widely from resource to resource. Conscientiously adapt the material to the group's major theme(s) and to the particular needs of group members. For your convenience, sample resources to guide your content and activity development are included in Table 3.3.

TABLE 3.3 | Sample Resources for Small-Group Content, Activities, and Catalysts

Sample Resources (*Title*) for Small-Group Leadership

Websites

Counseling and Guidance Lesson Plans. http://www.fldoe.org/workforce/programs/cd_lesson.asp

Games and Icebreakers: http://www.idealist.org/ioc/learn/curriculum/pdf/Games-and-Icebreakers.pdf

Group Activities, Games, Exercises, and Initiatives: http://wilderdom.com/games/

Icebreakers, Warmups, Energizers, and Deinhibitizers: http://wilderdom.com/games/Icebreakers.html

Lesson Plans Sorted by Title: http://www.schoolcounselor.com/macomb/all-sites.asp

Teambuilders/Energizers/Icebreakers: http://www.drexel.edu/OCA/l/tipsheets/Teambuilders.pdf

Publications

Brigman and Early (2001). *Group counseling for school counselors: A practical guide.* (numerous small-group plans and activities)

Capuzzi (2003). *Approaches to group work: A handbook for practitioners.* (many useful group plans)

Conyne, Crowell, and Newmeyer (2008). *Group techniques: How to use them more purposefully.*

Cooley (2009). *The power of groups: Solution-focused group counseling in schools.*

DeLucia-Waack (2006). *Leading psychoeducational groups: For children and adolescents.*

Erford (2010). *Group work in the schools.*

Fehr (2010). *101 interventions in group therapy.* (some good examples of groups for children and youth)

Harpine (2008). *Group interventions in schools: Promoting mental health for at-risk children and youth.*

Kaduson and Schaefer (2001). *One hundred and one more favorite play therapy techniques.*

Liebmann (2004). *Art therapy for groups: A handbook of themes and exercises.*

Pavlicevic (2003). *Groups in music: Strategies from music therapy.*

Senn (2004). *Small group counseling for small children.*

Smead (2000). *Skills for living: Group counseling activities for young adolescents.*

Winslade and Monk (2007). *Narrative counseling in schools: Powerful & brief.*

Note: For detailed bibliographic information on texts, see the References.

Sessions should vary in their intensity level. They need not always focus on serious verbal exchanges with a therapeutic tone; rather, meetings need to also include a sense of adventure and enjoyment, where students can still act like children. Meetings should reflect an inventive spirit wherein students are allowed to express their humorous sides, relax, and be themselves. Incorporating activities, ideas, insights, and materials from personal journaling, drama and role playing, art therapy, bibliotherapy (bibliocounseling), narrative therapy, and play therapy are invaluable to generate this caring but creative group atmosphere. Moreover, for those group members who are young, less verbal, or prefer sharing themselves through other means, these creative approaches encourage movement and self-expressiveness (Shechtman, 2007). Because this is a rich and valuable area for further exploration, you are again encouraged to review the pertinent resources listed in Table 3.3.

6. *Logistics (practical considerations)*   Perhaps the most detailed part of the plan is thinking through and writing down the "nuts and bolts" of the group experience. This is where you summarize the issues that many teachers and administrators want to know most about. This section is tailored to the type of group you are aiming to facilitate, addressing such questions as: How will this proposed group interfere with the students' academics? When will this group be taking place and for how long? How will teachers be involved? Specific pragmatic issues to consider are overviewed here.

   * *Consent to participate*
     All group plans should include a statement of how students' rights are going to be protected and how informed consent will be obtained. Reread ASCA's (2004b, 2010) and ACA's (2005) ethical guidelines as you formulate this section. Mention that written permission for their students to participate in the group will be gathered from parents/caregivers through, for example, a letter/consent form sent home. On school letterhead, devise the letter/consent form in consultation with the school administrator (see Figure 3.6 for an example). If the student is 18 years or older, parental consent is not legally required, but it is still advised. You will observe that the term *group counseling* is not used on the letter/permission form; rather, the term *group experience* is included. This intentional omission is not meant to deceive parents but to avoid controversy over their understanding of the term *group counseling*. Some parents still believe that group counseling is synonymous with group psychotherapy. The letter also clearly indicates that it originates from the school counseling department, so parents who have questions will know to contact the school.

Assuming each student participant has the cognitive wherewithal to provide his or her written consent, school counselors should obtain this. An "easy to complete" permission form is prepared and reviewed with each potential group member during the pregroup screening/interview (see below for details). Ethical considerations are further discussed in the following chapter, but to reiterate some of them here, before the group commences, students should be familiar with the group's overall theme(s), what type of activities they may be asked to participate in, and what the basic group member expectations are (e.g., actively participate, be positive, come on time, etc.). Finally, students should know that (a) they are volunteers, (b) they have the right to nonparticipation, and (c) their teacher(s) and parents/guardians have agreed to their involvement.

Wapiti Middle School

12345 West Stream, Ryne Mt., CN

Date

Dear Parent/Guardian,

The school counseling department at WMS is pleased to announce that beginning January 15, several educational small group experiences for students will be offered. We are inviting your daughter/son to be involved and need your written permission. Please carefully review this letter and sign it at the bottom in the space provided. Please return this signed copy in the pre-addressed and stamped envelope or to drop it off at the counseling office by no later than January 10.

Your child will also be fully informed about the small group experience. This is a voluntary experience and not required for any class. Students will meet one time a week for approximately 40 minutes and no academic time will be used.

The group experience will address social and educational needs of your child.
Here are some answers to commonly asked questions:

What will my child learn during the small-group experience? Under the guidance of a well-trained school counselor, students will learn about and practice important skills related to school success. Groups give students an opportunity to try out new educational and social skills.

Does my child's teacher know about and approve of this small-group experience? Yes. All teachers have been consulted and given their approval for your son's or daughter's participation in the group.

Can my child leave the group if he or she does not want to attend any more? Yes. This is a volunteer experience that your student will probably really enjoy, but she can always leave the group without any consequences.

Will the counselor or my child tell me what's going on in the group? Most likely your student will give you some general information, but not always. Confidentiality laws will be followed. Student discussions in group settings are generally protected by law; however, if students talk about harming themselves or others or breaking state or federal laws, parents/guardians and appropriate authorities will be consulted.

What if I want to discuss this more? If you have any other questions or concerns about this exciting group opportunity, please don't hesitate to let us know! Feel free to contact the counseling office at (xxx) xxx-xxxx or Ms. Kirkland, school principal at (xxx) xxx-xxxx.

Thank you for your support!

Hugo Jimenez and Kate Gardner

School Counselors, WMS

NOTE: If at all possible, this letter/consent form can be translated and explained. Please contact the counseling department for assistance.

PARENT/GUARDIAN PERMISSION FORM

Dear Counselors:
I give my permission for _____ (write your child's name) to participate in a small group experience conducted by the school counselors during winter semester.

Please print your full name: _____
Sign here:_____ Date: _____
Please return by **January 10** using pre-addressed and stamped envelope or drop it off at the school's counseling office.

Thank you.

FIGURE 3.6 | Sample parent/guardian informed consent document.

- *Group composition issues* There are still various issues to decide before actually launching the group. These should be briefly summarized in your group action plan. Regrettably, definite research does not exist on these topics, so our recommendations here are based largely on expert consensus (Greenberg, 2003; Jacobs et al., 2009; Smead, 1995) and many years of group counseling experience.

Group size Specify in your plan how many group members are going to be served. You may be then wondering, what is the optimal size for small counseling groups? Factors influencing this decision include the students' grade and maturity levels, the group's focus, the potential intergroup dynamics when mixing students with varying personalities and interpersonal skills, the number of parent consent forms returned, and so on. Undoubtedly, with younger children the most advantageous group size is between four and six members; for late elementary (Grades 5 and 6) to high school students, the group size can be increased to around eight members or sometimes even to 10. If you decide to include students with learning and behavioral challenges, the group size may need to be adjusted downward to better accommodate these children's personal/social and learning needs.

School counselors may be tempted to undersize the group, believing they will have more "control" of the group process with fewer participants. This may be true; however, more control is not necessarily the most beneficial goal for effective group counseling. Group members must be allowed the opportunity to manage their own group behaviors. Just like teachers want students to take responsibility for their own learning, why not, ask student to be accountable for their group actions? Obviously, the level of leadership control varies depending on the age of the members, with the youngest requiring the most substantial behavior scaffolding.

Moreover, students, like us, tend to be very active and every now and then cannot attend a meeting. Doing so is generally for various legitimate reasons. Although frustrating for the group counselor's plans, members will skip group due to, for example, unplanned sicknesses, classroom activities that students cannot miss, test makeup days, preplanned vacations, or class field trips. In this situation, if you limit the group to, say, five members, on a particular day one student may be sick and another has to leave school early for a sporting activity. The group leader is then left with three students, making for an awkward and challenging small-group experience. To reiterate, these suggested participant numbers are not fixed; counselors use their professional expertise and consultation skills to optimize the group experience for all participants.

Attracting potential group members Who should be in the group and what are effective ways of attracting group membership? Once school counselors have tallied up the results from the needs assessment discussed above, selected a group topic/theme, and received approval and support from relevant decision makers and teachers, it is time to solicit potential group members. Your group plan should, thus, highlight how you intend to "recruit" students to volunteer for the group experience. In other words, how do you propose to "market" the group? There are many ways to accomplish this, and here are some examples. First, publish a "snappy" announcement in the school newspaper, parent newsletter, and on the school website. Second, to encourage students to consider volunteering for different group counseling opportunities, with permission from the principal post around the school student-friendly, creative, and interesting recruitment or promotional flyers (see Figure 3.7 for an example). Third, make a personal announcement in classrooms and at general assemblies. When possible, take with you one or two students who have enjoyed and benefited from their group experiences to help with promotion. In our experience, students prefer hearing about groups from peers. Finally, although perhaps not widely practiced, Bostick and Anderson (2009) reported that teachers and school counselors identified the neediest children (e.g., students who had the lowest scores on a screening instrument were considered students most in need of small-group counseling) and screened them for group participation. The bottom line for soliciting students for groups? Use multiple methods and creativity.

Participation criteria and pregroup screening/interviewing A summary of your pregroup screening process is another necessary component of the action plan. Some counselors may take liberties with the process, neglecting or minimizing the screening process. Suppose a particular student read a promotional flyer posted on the school wall or heard about the upcoming group and comes to the counseling office to volunteer. Understandably, counselors may assume these keenly interested students are perfect candidates for groups. But as seasoned group counselors know, not every student is appropriate for group counseling. Some students are simply "joiners" ("the group looks fun"), whereas others see the group as an easy way to get out of a class. School counselors cannot be sure of students' suitability for a particular group experience until they screen all possible group members.

Before the face-to-face screening interview takes place, establish some loose group participation criteria. In general, group counselors look for those students who (a) are likely to benefit from the group focus and activities; (b) possess sufficient communication, cognitive, and social skills to participate; (c) express a willingness and ability to engage in the group experience; (d) indicate a readiness to accept and follow the group rules or guidelines; (e) want to learn in cooperation with other group members; (f) commit to attending all group sessions and arriving on time; and (g) will have parental/guardian consent. Supplementary criteria are usually added depending upon the nature of the group.

To facilitate a meaningful and successful group, school counselors need to ascertain whether potential members meet the conditions for group participation (Greenberg, 2003). All ages can be screened, but the process changes depending on the child's level of understanding and maturity. The screening process includes not only speaking with each student in the privacy of the counseling office but also consulting with the potential group member's teacher(s) and other relevant educators as well. With these two sources of information and the counselor's own history with each student, a tentative list of members can be compiled. Attempt to have a few more potential members than you can actually accommodate in the group. School experience suggests that even though all students say they want to participate, normally one or two (or more), for whatever reasons, will not attend.

The actual screening "interview" can be relatively informal. Definitely keep the atmosphere light; establish initial rapport using student-relevant open-ended questions (e.g., "What is your favorite movie? How come?" "Have you heard _____'s

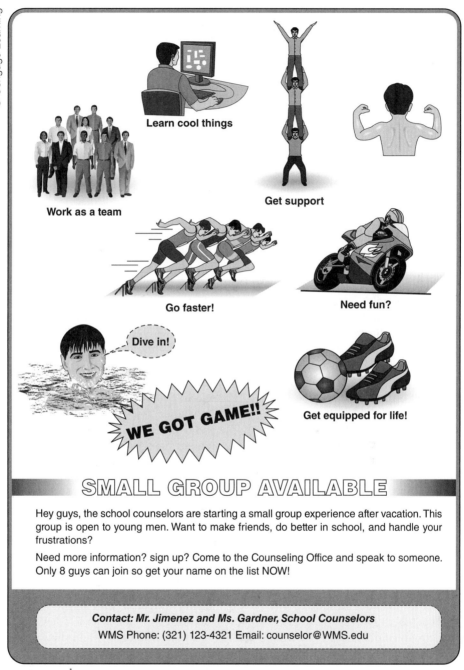

Learn cool things

Work as a team

Get support

Go faster!

Need fun?

Dive in!

WE GOT GAME!!

Get equipped for life!

SMALL GROUP AVAILABLE

Hey guys, the school counselors are starting a small group experience after vacation. This group is open to young men. Want to make friends, do better in school, and handle your frustrations?

Need more information? sign up? Come to the Counseling Office and speak to someone. Only 8 guys can join so get your name on the list NOW!

Contact: Mr. Jimenez and Ms. Gardner, School Counselors
WMS Phone: (321) 123-4321 Email: counselor@WMS.edu

FIGURE 3.7 | "We Got Game" small-group promotional flyer.

[insert name of a popular band] latest CD?"). After this "warm up" dialogue, explain the purpose of the screening meeting (use another more gentle phrase, e.g., "getting to know each other"), overview the group focus and content, and indicate that you will be asking a few questions about the student's interest in group participation. Craft open-ended questions around the group participation criteria listed above. For younger children, the queries need to be simple, requiring perhaps a few words in response. Sometimes a "yes" or "no" from a kindergartener or first-grader will suffice. Moreover, for early elementary-age children, the use of puppets, play, and artwork can facilitate the conversation.

Here are examples of useful screening questions. The first criterion—students will benefit from the group experience—can be explored by asking about the student's interest in the group: "Tell me about your interest in this group." "What about this topic seems cool to you?" "What do you think you might learn in this group?" Criterion 2 (student has reasonably good communication, cognitive, and social skills) is deduced from the screening conversation and your consultation with relevant educational staff. To determine whether a prospective group member will get involved and engage with others (Criterion 3), nonthreatening questions like these can be asked: "How do feel about talking in front of other students that you don't know well?" "How do you best learn? For example, do you sit back and wait for things to happen or do you jump right in?" "How do you feel about sharing stuff that is sort of personal?" To see if the student will follow the group rules (Criterion 4), talk with the relevant educators who have observed this student's classroom and school behavior. Remind the student about the group rules or guidelines (see below for details) and give a few illustrations (e.g., "I will speak for myself." "I will listen to others."). Ask students about their comfort level with rules; for instance, ask the student: "How do like following rules?" "When you break a classroom rule and the teacher gets mad, what do you do?" Questions related to Criterion 5 (cooperation) can be as simple as: "How do you get along with others in your class?" "What do you prefer, working alone or in a group? Say a bit more …" Whether the student will come to all the sessions and be on time (Criterion 6) is a tricky one to get solid answers to. Check with the student's teachers about this issue and ask the student: "We are meeting during lunchtime every week on Thursdays and it's very important that you're on time. What might keep you from not regularly attending or arriving at the start time?" Criterion 7 is self-explanatory; if the student brings back the parent permission slip signed, then you have your answer. Naturally, individualize the questions to the student's level of comprehension.

One effective but optional way for students to set some pregroup personal goals and for you, the school counselor, to assess whether the group will be useful for each member is to conduct a short, postscreening individual meeting with all the selected group members. During this 10- to 15-minute meeting, counselors refer to a few established group guidelines (e.g., "I will do my best to attend all meetings and show up on time." "I will maintain confidentiality." "I will try to participate in all group activities and sharing."). After reading over these guidelines, ask students questions like these: "What would you like to get out of the group?" "Are there specific things you'd like to see happen in the group?" (The school counselor may suggest possible goals and ideas.) For future reference, the counselor writes down the student's thoughts and goal(s). Each group member signs a guidelines form and then takes it home for a parent/caregiver signature, hopefully returning it the next day. Before sending the students back to class, they are each queried about whether they, their teachers, or their parents/caregivers have any concerns. This is also a time when the members can air their questions. Finally, the counselors use this short one-on-one time to remind the students when and where the first group meeting will take place.

Timing issues This aspect of the group plan merely notes when the group is slated to begin, for how many weeks, the duration of each group meeting, and when during the school day. If you plan on varying the group times and days, this can be a logistics nightmare but still workable with much advance scheduling. There is no definitive research precedence for what is the most efficacious number of group meetings, but a general guideline is between six and eight sessions. To solidify learning, counselors may choose to extend the group beyond the allotted number of weeks. Whether to do this or not is based largely on time constraints of busy school counselors and limitations on how many periods students can reasonably be absent from during a semester without negatively affecting their academic performance. The length of each meeting is largely determined by the developmental level of the group members. For younger children, 30 minutes tends to be a workable time frame, whereas for older students, the entire class period is usually required to accomplish session goals. Finally, some counselors will conduct two group meetings per week rather than the customary weekly session. Again, there is no school-based evidence to suggest that this practice of "doubling-up" is more or less effective than running the group only once a week, so it's largely the group leader's choice.

Other considerations for maximizing the benefits of small groups School counselors are also cognizant of additional, yet vital nuances of facilitating groups. The following are not in any particular order of importance, but each should be considered before starting the group experience.

Keeping teachers informed First, most instructors want to stay in the communication loop while their students are participating in group. Thus ongoing counselor-to-educator collaboration is good practice and improves "public relations." Although chapter 4 tackles this topic in more depth, when you dialogue with teachers or other educators about the group experience, maintain confidentiality (i.e., do not divulge students' contributions) unless the major exceptions are revealed (i.e., student expresses desire to harm self or others, or illegal behaviors may be involved). Counselors are free to share general trends. For instance, without giving out any details counselors can provide a status report every now and then, sharing in a noncommittal way about a student's attendance and progress. Here's a sample comment a group leader shared with a curious teacher: "The group's going reasonably well given we've only had two meetings; your two students are contributing to the group. I am pleased see Ricardo and Simone. Thank you again for allowing them to miss your class for a few weeks. Is there anything I can do to help the students catch up?" Always keep the teacher apprised of when the group is beginning, when it's ending, and the times and days of weekly sessions. If the schedule happens to change, send a note to the teachers. Of course you will want keep the parents/caregivers in the communication circle as well.

Including exemplary students as role models Another group issue discussed by group counselors relates to the inclusion of peers as role models (Akos, Hamm, Mack, & Dunaway, 2007). Supported by the views of social learning (observational learning) theory (e.g., Bandura, 1986, 2001) and group counseling research with special populations (e.g., learning disabilities; see Leichtentritt & Shechtman, 2010), this strategy tends to be a useful practice. It allows for students with good personal/social skills to demonstrate prosocial behavior to those who may be deficient in some ways. A serious limitation to this practice is when the regular group members feel as if the "exemplary" students really do not understand where they are or have been. In other words, there is too much social "distance" between the "model" group members and the other members. If you use this practice, and again, this can be an effective method, spend time with the model student preparing him or her for the experience (Akos et al., 2007).

Multicultural and diversity considerations Although fully addressed later in the book, leaders must take into account for the potential subgroup dynamics when planning and facilitating small groups. For instance, research on small groups conducted with adolescents of Mexican origin clearly indicates that counselors must think through developmental issues related to ethnic identity (Malott et al., 2010). You need to consider the between-subgroup (e.g., differences between ethnic and cultural groups; students with learning challenges and those labeled "gifted and talented"; socioeconomic levels) and within-subgroup differences (i.e., disparities within the special education population, a particular ethnicity, etc.). If diversity issues significantly impact how the small group will be conducted, these issues may need to be briefly addressed in your group plan (see e.g., Molina, Brigman, & Rhone, 2003, for a longer discussion).

 To further illustrate this issue further, here's an example of the challenges involved with conducting groups with a diverse set of learners. Despite the fact that the Asian American population is not monolithic in characteristics and behaviors, Asian American children and youth were found generally to experience comparable social-emotional adjustment problems (e.g., loneliness, isolation, rejection, anxiety, low self-confidence; Zhou, Siu, & Xin, 2009). Therefore, on the surface, a small group conducted with students of Asian heritage as members could address these adjustment issues. Sensibly, however, the effective leader does not assume that all Asian student members will experience these social-emotional concerns in a similar fashion. Thus, before leaping to the implementation stage, the school counselor facilitating this group will reflect on the inclusion of each potential group member and he or she might impact the group as a whole as well as with specific members. It is inevitable, for example, that a high school small group comprised of one recent Thai immigrant to the United States, three second-generation Korean American students, a single Japanese exchange student, and two third-generation Vietnamese American students will experience their home and school situations in relatively disparate ways. In short, effective group leaders organize, plan, and conduct the group experience with cultural sensitivity to not only between-subgroup differences but also within-subgroup differences. Readers may want to also peruse DeLucia-Waack and Donigian (2004), among other books, to further understand how to develop and run a culturally responsive small group.

Voluntary versus involuntary membership Briefly stated, voluntary group membership is ethical and most likely more successful than "forced" membership. Administrators may want to use group counseling as a "discipline" tool, requiring students with academic or behavioral problems to either attend a group addressing these issues or receive a stiffer penalty such as detention and in- or out-of-school suspension. Most students will opt for the group experience, not because they are keen to attend but to avoid what they perceive as a harsher punishment. Although used in clinical settings with, for example, incarcerated youth (J. Corey, 2009; Jacobs et al., 2009), avoid involuntary members on the grounds that it is unethical to require students to attend groups against their will. Sharply put, school counseling best practice does not recommend this "participate in group counseling or else" approach to discipline.

Open versus closed groups Your group action plan probably should specify whether students can join the group or not once the experience has begun. For the sake of long-term group cohesion, closed groups are good practice (J. Corey, 2009; Jacobs et al., 2009); however, in a skills-based group format (e.g., psychoeducational group), adding new members within the first couple of meetings may not affect student bonding to any major extent (Smead, 1995). When facilitating a growth group, where students are focused on self-improvement and personal exploration, open groups are especially ill-advised. Ultimately, the decision should come down to student needs, the nature of the group, and professional judgment and experience.

Location of group Work with the facilities "manager" (e.g., the school's administrative assistant, vice principal) about where you can hold the group on a regular basis and include the site in the group plan. Students, rightly so, are self-conscious in groups, schools are hectic places, and private space is at a premium, so addressing the group location question early on in the planning process is crucial. If at all possible, do not settle for a semiprivate space (e.g., the corner of the lunchroom or hallway) where other students or staff can access during the group time. This may mean looking for an empty classroom during the scheduled group time. Asking the school psychologist or nurse whether his or her office may be free during the school week is another good option. If the weather's pleasant, even going outside on the playground may work better than using a high-traffic, nonconfidential location like the school conference room or library.

Development of ground rules As highlighted earlier, all groups have expectations for member behavior. Because a group experience is probably new to most students, Berg et al. (2006) wisely recommended that the leader distribute to the members at the first meeting a suggested list of general guidelines or ground rules to read through; subsequently, each student selects one rule that is perhaps most challenging to follow and explains why. Other group members are then encouraged to provide ideas on how they might follow that particularly difficult guideline. With input and guidance from the facilitator, another method is to leave it up to the students to develop these rules during the initial group meeting. No matter how these group guidelines are developed, sample ones could be included in the action plan.

Rules should follow the ethical standards of professional organizations, such as ASCA (2004b, 2010). When writing these behavioral expectations, use a positive tone,

TABLE 3.4 | Sample Group Guidelines (Rules) With Grade-Level Benchmarks

	Elementary		Secondary	
Group Guidelines (Ground Rules)	**Early**	**Late**	**MS/JH**	**High**
My hands and feet need to stay close to me.	✓			
Pay attention to the group leader.	✓	✓		
Wait my turn to talk.	✓	✓	✓	
Let others share without interrupting.	✓	✓	✓	
Listen carefully to others.	✓	✓	✓	
Be positive to others (no "put downs").	✓	✓	✓	
Ask my questions politely.		✓	✓	
Take part in activities and sharing.		✓	✓	✓
Support others in this group.		✓	✓	✓
Tactfully share my feeling, thoughts, and opinions.		✓	✓	✓
Allow for the feelings, thoughts, and opinions of others.		✓	✓	✓
Maintain confidentiality.		✓	✓	✓
Speak in the "here and now." (Stay present centered.)			✓	✓
Speak for myself.			✓	✓
Take responsibility for my feelings, thoughts, opinions, and behavior.			✓	✓

Note: Checkmarks represent at what grade level a group rule should be stressed. For additional rules, see, for example, Greenberg (2003).

keep them relatively unambiguous (avoid vague rules), limit the number to five or so, and make them developmentally relevant. For younger students, reminding students to monitor their own nonverbal and verbal behaviors is essential; whereas for teenage group members, the focus is more on maintaining confidentiality, owning their voice, and avoiding storytelling and negativity. One way to reinforce group rules is to have the members create an "artistic" poster summarizing the group rules. Leaders then bring it to each group meeting, referring to it as needed. Table 3.4 lists sample group rules or guidelines with very rough developmental benchmarks as to when the rule should be emphasized (also see chapter 5; DeLucia-Waack, 2006; Greenberg, 2003, for additional examples). Although maintaining confidentially is vital at all grade levels, group leadership experience suggests that this issue is far more difficult for younger children to follow than older students. Fortunately, the consequences of breeching confidentially with early elementary-age group members are generally less harmful. However, by late elementary school and certainly by middle school, breaks in confidentially can have dire consequences. Some of the rules that leaders emphasize with younger children need not be stressed with upper-grade-level group members. Older students should have already learned the basics of group behavior. Including such students with highly deficient social skills in a group is probably a mistake. As a caveat though, every group is different, so the rules will need to be individualized to each group experience and theme.

Phase 2: Implementation

Once school counselors have checked off all the group formation tasks mentioned above (e.g., writing the group action plan; identifying potential members; creating the weekly "lessons" and activities; consulting with relevant teachers, administrators, staff, and parents), the actual experience can commence. Prior to moving ahead too quickly, however, readers may recall from an earlier discussion that group dynamics, processes, and procedures (i.e., implementation strategies) are more successful when a learner-centered framework is utilized. Specifically, the research-based recommendations of the American Psychological Association (see Stroh & Sink, 2002) on quality educational reform recommend a learner-centered approach to education. Thus it is advisable that school counselors incorporate a learner-centered approach to group work. Not unlike what M. S. Corey et al. (2010) suggested, the learner-centered group leader is one who provides facilitation, guidance, and support. Members learn through the leader's modeling of appropriate behavior and communication skills (e.g., listening, openness, sharing, empathy, accepting feedback). Group counselors pay close attention to and show respect for students' diverse voices and viewpoints, encouraging social responsibility, and acting as colearners or conavigators. As a facilitator, observe student needs, abilities, and interests. These factors should influence the group's processes, content, and expectations. Again, a learner-centered facilitator mobilizes the group experiences, but its members, as much as possible, are encouraged to share the responsibility for the group's progress (M. S. Corey et al., 2010; Smead, 1995).

In short, the type of group leader we are advocating for here is not one who runs the group like the interpersonal expert, directing students with little preparation or simply relying on a structured or "canned" curriculum; rather, a learner-centered facilitator creates a dynamic group experience using meaningful and real-life activities for students to work through. As developmentally appropriate, the well-thought-out materials and counseling techniques promote student reflection and contributions. Group catalysts are customized to the student needs and strengths.

Stages of groups   Generally speaking when groups are implemented, they loosely evolve in overlapping stagelike fashion. Although there is not enough research documenting how school-based groups evolve over time (Greenberg, 2003), a normal group experience might evolve over three (Jacobs et al., 2009) to five stages (e.g., G. Corey, 2008; M. S. Corey et al., 2010; Gladding, 1994; Tuckman & Jensen, 1977). In an attempt here to blend leading perspectives on the topic, five stages plus the pregroup and postgroup phases are depicted in Figure 3.8 and described below. As a caution, the stages are not so neatly experienced by group members, and unproductive groups may get bogged down,

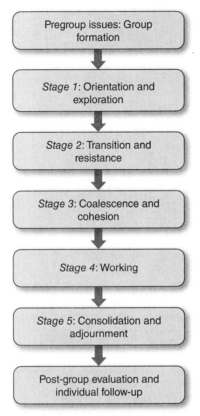

Pregroup issues: Group formation

Stage 1: Orientation and exploration

Stage 2: Transition and resistance

Stage 3: Coalescence and cohesion

Stage 4: Working

Stage 5: Consolidation and adjournment

Post-group evaluation and individual follow-up

FIGURE 3.8 | Provisional stages of small-group development.

for example, in transition (M. S. Corey et al., 2010). Groups proceed with different pacing and may revert to an earlier stage if things shift in an unhealthy direction.

At the outset, the group goes through a formation period (G. Corey, 2008). After the group is organized and planned, it begins in earnest with the "orientation and exploration" stage. As the label suggests, during this period group counselors help students to become better acquainted with one other and more comfortable with group dynamics. Implementation strategies and activities are devised with these outcomes in mind. Counselors need to be aware of potential member anxiety, because for some students, meeting their peers for the first time can be a social challenge. Well chosen 5- to 10-minute icebreakers are deployed early on to foster nascent empathy, mutual respect and trust, sharing (self-disclosure), and probing of members' "below the surface" level thoughts, feelings, and behaviors. More often than not, although members are generally excited and motivated to get going, they will test the leader's skills and group limits, so reinforcement and enforcement of the ground rules need to be judiciously emphasized. To avoid the leadership trap of facilitating with too much leniency (e.g., trying too hard to be non-teacher-like or "cool") or with needless severity (e.g., acting as a disciplinarian), effective modeling is in order. To avoid group members dwelling in "there and then" (storytelling and focusing on what happened in the past), engaging activities are selected to foster goal setting, team building, as well as a "here and now" (present-centeredness) (M. S. Corey et al., 2010). If it seems appropriate, a contracting exercise may be in order, where students create a written agreement for themselves. In brief, the counselor's role at this stage is to facilitate a warm climate of sharing and caring, where members feel safe to speak, desire to reveal more of themselves to their peers, and set individual goals for their group experience.

By the third group session, characteristics of Stage 2 ("transition and resistance") generally emerge. At this point, group leaders must anticipate and plan for student demonstrations of "storming" (Tuckman & Jensen, 1977), where members exhibit a heightened sense of personal anxiety. Some engage in avoidance behaviors, or show signs of uncertainty, resistance, and perhaps even hidden agendas (G. Corey, 2008; M. S. Corey et al., 2010). These overt or covert behaviors are often directed at the leaders themselves or to the group experience as a whole. Potential intergroup conflict may erupt. Corey et al. further portrayed this stage, commenting that it is often marked by group members struggling to define themselves and group norms (i.e., "here's the way things are in this group"). Members start to jockey for position in the group (Gladding, n.p.). Thus leaders will find themselves working through student fears, disagreements, silence, and so on. The importance of using potent and enjoyable team-building exercises cannot be overemphasized. When students are asked to collaborate on an enjoyable task, their energy is redirected away from negativity to achieving a common goal. Providing a small, tangible reward for working effectively together is always appreciated by group members of all ages. Finally, if redirecting and refocusing does not help to turn the group around, you may need to try some gentle confrontation with those difficult and challenging group members.

After students generally progress beyond their fears and need for individuation, they hopefully begin to experience in Stage 3 what Gladding (1994, n.p.) calls "the spirit of we-ness." Specifically, group members at this stage feel more included and positive, and constructive sharing is more common. This "we-ness" phenomenon is referred to as member "coalescence" or "cohesion," for participants experience a sense of diminished intergroup tension and increased psychological closeness. Until the group evolves into a productive team, the leadership role is challenging. Clearly then, the goal at this stage is to create the conditions wherein members also experience "other-ness," where they are far less focused on themselves and reach out to their peers in caring support. Again, as in the earlier stages, the well-timed use of evocative activities can facilitate group flourishing. The counselor links student comments, finding thematic commonalities among member sharing. Given time limitations, school-based groups sometimes get to only this level of intimacy and connectedness. Although this is not a negative, for some learning has taken place, groups can go deeper. This stage naturally blends into the next one.

During the "working" or middle stage (G. Corey, 2008; Jacobs et al., 2009), students show more obvious signs of deeper exploration, personal and social adaptability, collaboration, and assimilation of new perspectives and behaviors. When groups reach this level, interdependence has occurred and members play an important role in mutual support. The comfort level among group members is at its highest. Students are working on their personal goals and attempting to do constructive problem solving. According to some sources, this stage can take up 50% of a group's time (Gladding, 1994) and is the core of the group process (Jacobs et al., 2009). As the group further gels and flows, predictably benefits for students continue to accrue. For example, members learn and incorporate new information, explore more fully session topics and lessons, complete growth- and skill-related tasks, as well as engage in deeper sharing and therapeutic work (Jacobs et al., 2009).

What are the group counselor responsibilities during this working period? Simply stated, they do more of the same. Akin to the previous stage (coalescence and cohesion) and as the situation warrants, counselors mobilize the action toward richer group sharing with challenging and productive activities and exercises. Counselors continue, for example, to direct intergroup traffic and flow, manage student contributions so they remain therapeutic and growth producing, change course if the group requires it, and suggest relevant exercises for students to practice outside the group setting. To "ensure" the health of the working group, Jacobs et al. (2009) indicate that sometimes counselors will even alter the group format, leadership style, and/or structure, as well as make other changes. The point being, group facilitators remain flexible and adaptable to the needs of the members, laying aside their weekly agenda when the situation demands a course revision. Lastly, at least 2 weeks before the end of the group, counselors start reminding students, parents, and their instructors that the group is coming to a close. For the parents and educators, a note or email should suffice. Moreover, students are strongly encouraged to take responsibility for achieving their group goals. By making this announcement and processing it with the students, members start preparing for this eventuality. The counselor subtly communicates that if members want to raise any additional or unfinished issues, time to do so is running short.

During Stage 5, group leadership is aimed at helping members close out their experience by consolidating their learning, working through any "unfinished business" or leftover unresolved issues, and preparing for adjournment. To reduce possible feeling of loss, counselors have already announced to students and their teachers when the last session will occur. The final session then is an occasion where students can "round out" their group experience, express their "goodbyes" to one another, and celebrate the accomplishment of any personal or group goals. Reassurance is provided to the group members, informing them of the availability of ongoing follow-up support after the last meeting. You probably will not need a catalyst for this session, but always be prepared to activate one if the group comes to a standstill. Generally speaking, by adopting a strengths-based approach during the session, students are encouraged to share their positive feelings about their experience. Those students who found the group less productive should be allowed to contribute as well. Ask students to think of ways they can apply their group learning to home and school life. Concrete action plans are useful, particularly if some members need measured reinforcement for maintaining their changed behavior, thoughts, or feelings.

Closing rituals or exercises are sometimes practiced (see Smead, 1995, for examples). These involve students sharing a meaningful activity that yields positive sharing between members. It is important to be creative and culturally relevant (e.g., Brinson, 1995), yet not silly or overly dramatic. Younger students might make a small gift for each member of the group. Older members could write a short poem emphasizing other students' strengths. Perhaps for the final sharing ("go around"), group leaders could also provide constructive feedback about each member's personal accomplishments and contributions to the group experience. You might say something like, "Raphael, you've been an emotional support to several others in this group. When they were hurting, you were there to give them a hug, smile, or a caring word. Thank you for these gifts to us all. My hope for you is that you take your gentle, supportive nature and share it with your friends and family. Your teachers would love to see it as well [counselor smiles]."

At the closing stage some counselors have students evaluate their experience and personal progress. This conversation generally centers on whether members met their group goals, what they are taking away from the experience, and what learning they can use at home or school. Other counselors institute the group evaluation during the individual follow-up meeting with students. More will be said on this issue shortly.

Summary and final thoughts about implementation   Whether each stage is reached in a typical 6- to 8-week school-based group, the research is equivocal. Anecdotal evidence does indicate that only aspects of these stages are commonly reported by student members and school counselors leading small groups. In any case, the point is: By the end of the group experience, healthy and constructive small groups move forward from a low to high level of intermember cohesion and support. It is your role to facilitate this positive and supportive process. To achieve this positive outcome, leaders use group counseling techniques such as modeling, active or reflective listening, open-ended questioning, group problem and decision making, linking, paraphrasing, and blocking/cutting off inappropriate behaviors or sharing. Chapter 5 discusses the prerequisite communication/facilitation skills needed for a successful group experience.

No matter what stage the group has reached, to be an effective leader, key implementation tasks are required. As a reminder, group leaders establish rapport with members, scaffold intergroup sharing, encourage peer support, and assist students as they work toward personal goals. Moreover, effective leaders

- model behaviors that foster mutual caring and a safe learning milieu,
- manage the group's focus and flow with equanimity,
- encourage all members to "own" (take responsibility for) the group experience and engage as fully as possible,
- reinforce and enforce (manage challenging behaviors) the group's ground rules or guidelines,
- refocus the group when members are straying too far from the session's aims,
- mobilize the group to move forward by employing an assortment of connecting activities,
- collect data to evaluate the impact of the group experience on student outcomes, and
- facilitate the group in an ethical and professional manner (e.g., leaders are non-coercive or heavy-handed, avoid dual relationships, use multiple counseling techniques, act with impartiality, etc.).

As a way to wrap up this section, no matter which stage the group is in, school counselors must avoid serious leadership flaws. For example, leaders should avoid counseling students as individuals as opposed to leading the group as a unit. Leaders provide the group compass, directing the process to a relatively clear purpose. Group members who remain clueless for too long tend to disengage and perhaps even disrupt the flow. Finally, the greatest temptation perhaps for school counselors is to be the group's broker, doing most of the psychological work for the members. In other words, if your leadership style makes you the hub and all the action goes through you, group members tend to acquiesce to your influence and do little of their own work.

Phase 3: Evaluation

The research on the effectiveness of group counseling, as summarized in chapter 2, is relatively promising. Nevertheless, school counselors cannot assume that their specific group leadership skills are productive for all members. Rather than simply hoping that counselors' work with students is leading to positive outcomes, the profession now operates from an evidence-based position (Dimmitt, Carey, & Hatch, 2007; Johnson, Johnson, & Downs, 2006; Stone & Dahir, 2011). Specifically, ASCA's (2004b, 2010) ethical standards require ongoing assessment of one's group counseling services, for positive evaluation data can enhance your credibility with the school's educators. In contrast, less than complimentary feedback often helps counselors further refine their group practice. Accordingly, group counselors need to answer two accountability-related questions:

1. In what ways do student members benefit from the group experience?
2. How does this practice add to the value of the school's comprehensive school counseling program?

Simply put, school counselors want to ascertain whether (a) students reach their personal goals and change their behavior as a result of the group experience and (b) this vital responsive service increases the efficacy of overall counseling program. Assessing parent/caregiver and teacher perceptions of student behavioral changes is a bonus.

To respond to the first question, several ways are available to the school counselor. Perhaps the most efficient approach is to utilize student self-report data collected with a pregroup and postgroup evaluation survey. School counseling experts suggest that the profession use action research (Rowell, 2006), emphasizing "hands-on" tools for gathering application-based outcome data. Most likely a survey or questionnaire, written in a developmentally appropriate way, is employed. The instrument should include two relatively brief sections, one with knowledge-based questions and the second with self-perception items. To assess student understanding of group content, the survey items can be written using various response formats. These may include any or all of these options: fill in the blank, true or false, multiple choice, and short answer.

Most of the guidelines for writing needs assessment items discussed above apply here. For instance, items need to be succinctly and clearly worded, and the overall survey must be understandable to your respondents, as well as straightforward to administer and score. As with needs assessments, make sure the surveys look professional and not thrown together at the last minute. Face validity goes a long way to enhance response rates. Sample evaluation tools are plentiful on the Web for no cost. However, constructing your own questionnaire is a better practice given that you can tailor the survey to the group's primary objectives, and it improves the ecological validity (the survey best represents the content and learning environment where the data are to be gathered) of the evaluation process.

Here are sample survey items that could be used by our fictional WMS school counselors who are interested in whether the boys in the group learned (i.e., knowledge-based item category) to appropriately respond to peer pressure. A fill-in-the-blank question may read as follows:

What are three *positive* ways to react to a friend's pushiness? Write one idea on each blank line. (Don't worry about spelling; just get your ideas down.)

1. _____
2. _____
3. _____

In a later chapter another example of a fill-in-the-blank small-group assessment tool ("Hang Time Survey") is provided.

A sample multiple-choice item addressing the same knowledge area could be written similar to this:

- You are at a sleepover and some kids want to watch a movie that you know your parents would not allow you to see at home. What's the *best* way to deal with this situation? Circle one answer only.
  a. Pretend that it's okay and watch the movie anyway.
  b. Get mad and leave the sleepover.
  c. Tell your friends that you cannot watch the movie because your mom is really mean.
  d. Find someone who doesn't want to watch the movie and play a game together.

A true–false question could be devised as follows:

- T F (circle one) It's always better to keep your best friends happy and do what they say.

Finally, here is a sample short-answer question:

- A good friend asks you to do something that you know is not nice. What do you say to your friend? (Don't worry about your spelling!) _____
  _____
  _____

Perception-based questions are fairly simple to construct using Likert-type scaling as discussed above in the needs assessment section. Sample postgroup questions for students to answer could read similar to these:

- How much did you learn about peer pressure in this group? Not much Some A lot
- The group was helpful to me personally? Never Sometimes Most of the time Always

© Microsoft
Corporation

- My group was: "good"   "okay"   "not so good" (This response option would be used with students who may have significant learning challenges or with younger participants.)

Assuming you have quantitative data, determining easy-to-report and -describe methods of representing the information is the next step. The intent here is to clearly

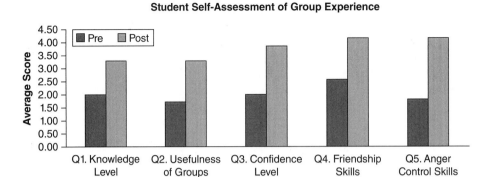

FIGURE 3.9 | Bar graph showing group members' mean score improvement from pre- to post survey.

demonstrate that participants found the group experience beneficial. Figure 3.9 represents pre- and postsurvey data collected from the eight boys in our fictional "We Got Game" group. The survey has five Likert-scaled questions with the response options ranging from 1 = Strongly Disagree, 2 = Disagree, 3 = Not Sure, 4 = Agree, 5 = Strongly Agree. The higher the score, the more strongly the student agreed with the statement. For Item 1 (Q1), for example, it reads as follows: "I know a lot about how to control my anger." The bar graph reveals that on the "pretest" administered by the school counselor during the pregroup interview, all students on average disagreed with the statement. By the end of the group experience, 6 weeks later, the average score improved from approximately 2.0 to 3.25, suggesting that members generally believed they had learned something about the topic. Looking more closely, Figure 3.9 plainly shows that group members' mean scores increased from pre- to postsurvey administration across all five items, suggesting that the "We Got Game" group was a success. Similar data can be graphed for teacher and parent perception. An additional sample high school group counseling evaluation form is included below as part of the chapter's supplemental resources.

Another useful way to assess the value of a small-group experience is to observe students outside the group to determine if they are applying any of the lessons learned to another environment. A short "observation recording sheet" could be devised (see Figure 3.10 for an example). The observers could be the school counselor as well as one or two other school staff members (e.g., the student's teachers, lunchroom staff, nurse, librarian). These "evaluators" monitor the student in, for example, the lunchroom, library, hallways, or classrooms, as well as in other potentially challenging social situations (e.g., at a dance; during a club meeting, pep rally, or sporting event). This form should identify those major behaviors the group is addressing from week to week. If our two WMS counselors were targeting the improvement of the boys' prosocial behavior in the "We Got Game" group, they would create an observation form that has, say, 10 key positive behaviors. These target behaviors could be drawn from the group's objectives.

Observer:

Student initials:		Observation							
Group Objective	Target Behavior	No. and Date			Location				Description
		1	2	3	CR	LR	HW	Other	
1. Students will be able to identify their "anger triggers."	Recognizes situation that triggered anger	Date							
	Did something to calm down	Date							
2. Students will identify one "study buddy" to help them when they feel frustrated during classroom assignments.	Recognizes situation that triggered frustration	Date							
	Seeks out help from study buddy	Date							
3. Objective	Target behavior 1	Date							
	Target behavior 2	Date							

FIGURE 3.10 | Sample observation recording sheet to be used as group evaluation tool.

SMALL-GROUP OBSERVATION RECORDING FORM

Instructions: Please use this short form to record when you see this student performing one of the target behaviors listed below. Please use this form for **2 full weeks,** recording perhaps up to three observations. Please enter in the date for each observation, location (CR = classroom, LR = lunchroom, HW = hallway, Other = [e.g., field, bus stop, etc.]), and a brief description of what you observed (e.g., "walked away," "lowered fists," "went back to desk").

Phase 4: Postgroup Follow-Up

Although not a stage in the sense that the group reassembles as a whole, this is a significant time when, a week or so postgroup, members individually reconnect with the leader to discuss and evaluate their experiences. The counselor and each group member process the experience and assess any learning that took place. Personal goals and behavioral contracts, if developed, are reviewed as well. Students are encouraged to continue their progress and growth and are assured of ongoing counseling support. Should referrals for outside mental health counseling be required, these are provided. In this situation, school counselors' consultation skill set would be used.

CONCLUSION

Not to belabor the point, but the previous discussion must be framed with a sharp eye toward group counseling theory and best practice research. As school counselors plan and organize their groups' central themes and the content of each session, as well as when they conduct the group experience, these two foundational pillars should always guide practice. Group leaders also should carefully reflect on the needs of potential members, attempting to create an experience that will optimally address those concerns. During the formation phase, numerous pragmatic issues and logistical challenges must be assessed and resolved. Clearly, much preliminary work will be done before the students arrive for the first session. Once the group experience begins, counselors are attentive to the signs of group development. They realize that some groups evolve steadily toward the working stage, whereas others may become mired in conflict, reflecting the transition and resistance stage. If all goes well, group members consolidate their learning and apply it to their school and home environments. During the last session or in the follow-up time with the school counselor, evaluation tools are used to ascertain whether the experience was productive for the group members. Hopefully they reached their group and personal goals. Positive member changes might be observed, for instance, by the teachers and significant others as well as reported by students themselves. In chapter 4, we explore more in depth the major ethical and legal issues related to group development and implementation.

CHAPTER 3 SUPPLEMENTAL RESOURCES

The following is a more involved needs assessment tool developed by Chris Wood (2007) & his school counseling students at the Ohio State University.

High School Needs Assessment

This is a survey asking your opinion about your needs and some of the things you are experiencing at _____ High School. There are no right or wrong answers, but we ask that you take this survey seriously and be thoughtful about how you respond to the questions. This survey is confidential and your individual responses will not be shared with your teacher or fellow students. The total results of the survey will be used to assist the school counseling staff to better support you.

Please feel free to ask any questions. Thank you for taking the time to answer this survey! ☺

Age: _____   **I am:** Male Female   **I am in:** __ 9th __ 10th __11th
                                                          __ 12th grade

Ethnicity: (Circle the ethnicity that best describes you; if you are multiethnic, you may circle more than one.)

Asian/Pacific Islander   Native American   African American
White/Non-Hispanic   Hispanic   Other: _____

School district: _____

Content: Personal/Social Audience: Students

Directions: For the following items in this section, **FIRST rank in order** each topic from 1 to 5 (1 = the LEAST serious problem, 5 = the MOST serious problem). **SECOND**, from the choices in parentheses ( ) following each area, **circle the concern that you believe is the "biggest" problem at your high school.**

_____ Peer pressure (cliques, alcohol/drug use, sexual activity, gang involvement)
_____ Conflicts due to differences between students (race/ethnicity, money, religion)
_____ Self-image (body image, depression, extreme academic stress, perfectionism)
_____ Violence (bullying, controlling anger, fights in or out of the classroom)
_____ School unity (making new friends, difficulty fitting in, lack of school spirit)

Directions: For the following items in this section, circle the number that **best** represents your opinion.

I WOULD LIKE TO KNOW MORE ABOUT ...

	Low Priority		High Priority	
How to deal with peer pressure	1	2	3	4
How to get along with students who are different from me	1	2	3	4
How to manage personal stress	1	2	3	4
How to handle conflict at school	1	2	3	4
How to fit in at my new school	1	2	3	4

Directions: Answer to the best of your ability.

Describe any other personal/peer-related issues about which you would like to learn. (This is an opportunity for you to discuss any other problems at your school that were not listed above.)

(You can use the back of this page if you need additional space.)

Content: Career Audience: Students

Directions: Please **rank** the following career-planning activities in order of importance to you using the numbers 1–8.

1 = least important   8 = most important

_____ having the opportunity to job shadow
_____ creating an educational plan
_____ learning where to find information on choosing careers, information about careers, etc.
_____ attending presentations given by professionals in different career fields in my community
_____ practicing interviewing skills
_____ learning to write a resume
_____ researching my career interests by using multimedia sources (Internet, books, newspapers, etc.)
_____ attending a career fair

Directions: Please **circle the number** that demonstrates your confidence level for the following items.

	Not Confident		Very Confident	
I can relate my career interests to my personal skills, abilities, and interests.	1	2	3	4
I know what college majors relate directly to my career interests.	1	2	3	4
I can effectively balance schoolwork and leisure time.	1	2	3	4
I can set achievable goals.	1	2	3	4

Directions: Please answer the question below by **listing as many sources of career information you know**. If you cannot think of any answer, then just write "NONE" in the space provided.

I can find occupational information (information about careers, wages, where to go to school for a certain career, etc.) from the following sources:

_____

_____

Directions: Please complete the following statement.
When it comes to career planning, I need the most help with _____
_____.

Content: Academic Audience: Students

Directions: Please **rank** the following topics using the numbers 1–5 in the order of priority for you.

1 = I need the LEAST help on this topic (highest priority); 5 = I need the MOST help on this topic (lowest priority)

_____ Study Skills (how to prepare for tests or assignments)
_____ Time Management (between school, extracurricular, leisure, family, friends)
_____ Organization (keeping all your academic materials organized and easy to access)
_____ Communicating for Help (how and when to ask for it)
_____ Test Anxiety (calming your nervousness before a test)

Directions: Please circle your answers to the questions according to the scale provided.

	Never		Always	
I am confident about my ability to prepare for a test.	1	2	3	4
Although I have prepared for a test, I feel an over-whelming sense of nervousness just before taking a test.	1	2	3	4
I am overwhelmed by the number of activities I am involved in.	1	2	3	4
I turn in my assignments on time.	1	2	3	4
When I need it, I will ask for help on my assignments.	1	2	3	4
I feel confident about my ability to take charge of my own education and learning.	1	2	3	4

Directions: Please answer the following questions.

Describe how you prepare for a test:

Describe a way you use to manage your time:

SAMPLE GENERIC HIGH SCHOOL GROUP COUNSELING EVALUATION FORM[3]

My Group Counseling Experience

Student Version

The school counselors want your real feelings and comments about your group experience. Your answers will be shared only in the counseling office. **Please circle the number that best reflects your group counseling experience:**

Strongly Disagree	Disagree	Not Sure	Agree	Strongly Agree
1	2	3	4	5

1. The group helped me make progress toward my personal goals.		1 2 3 4 5
2. I learned how to work on my personal challenges.		1 2 3 4 5
3. I can better talk about my thoughts and feelings.		1 2 3 4 5

---

[3]This form would be administered either in the last session or during the postgroup meeting.

4. I am more accepting of others.   1 2 3 4 5
5. The group experience helped me do better in school.   1 2 3 4 5
6. I can better cope with difficult situations.   1 2 3 4 5
7. My relationships with my peers are getting better.   1 2 3 4 5
8. The counselor did a good job leading the group.   1 2 3 4 5
9. Overall, I liked the group experience.   1 2 3 4 5
10. What was the purpose of the group?_____
11. What did you like most about the group experience?

_____
_____
_____

12. What would you change about the group?

_____
_____
_____

13. What other comments would you like to make about the group experience?

_____
_____
_____

How many group meetings did you go to?   Some   Most   All (circle)

Name: _____ (optional)

_____

I am: Female   Male (circle)   I am in Grade: 9   10   11   12 (circle)

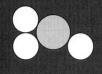

FRAMING—FOLLOWING PROFESSIONAL GUIDELINES FOR SMALL GROUPS

Professional Considerations in Conducting Groups in Schools

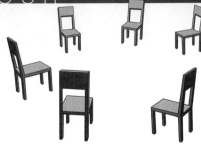

Professional school counselors (PSCs) are educators with graduate-level training in school counseling focused on addressing the personal/social, academic, and career domains of all students through individual, small-group, and schoolwide interventions. They are specifically trained to be group leaders who are able to attend to the various needs of students at all levels through the effective use of group counseling skills and techniques. During their time of professional service, PSCs must keep abreast of best practice considerations and professional, legal, and ethical expectations related to group work.

The ASCA (2005a) National Model calls for a comprehensive school counseling program to include small-group work in K–12 settings (Jacobs & Schimmel, 2005; Newsome & Gladding, 2007). The ASCA (2008a) position statement on group counseling further emphasizes the importance of this school counseling intervention (see Table 4.1). Despite the profession's strong commitment to small-group counseling, at the school level counselors see the value in the practice but its implementation can be spotty. Whether you are working in a school where this is the case, or in one where groups are commonplace, there are professional expectations, laws, and ethical guidelines that should be followed before starting your group as well as during and postintervention. This chapter begins with sample vignettes related to these issues and follows with recommendations, ethical guidelines, and legal mandates to think about when considering starting a small counseling group. Each vignette includes discussion questions that may be considered individually, as a group, or for class discussion.

TABLE 4.1 | ASCA (2008) Position Statement: The Professional School Counselor and Group Counseling

---

American School Counselor Association (ASCA) Position

Group counseling is vital in the delivery of the ASCA National Model to students and should be supported by school districts as part of an effective comprehensive school counseling program.

The Rationale
Group counseling, which involves a number of students working on shared tasks and developing supportive relationships in a group setting, is an efficient, effective, and positive way of dealing with students' academic, career, and personal/social/emotional

developmental issues and situational concerns. By allowing individuals to develop insights into themselves and others, group counseling makes it possible for more students to achieve healthier personal adjustment, cope with the stress of a rapidly changing and complex environment, and learn to communicate and cooperate with others. Research on group counseling suggests that this intervention is rather robust for a variety of academic, career, and personal/social/emotional concerns (Gerrity & DeLucia-Waack, 2007; McGannon et al., 2005; Paisley & Milsom, 2007; Whiston & Sexton, 1998).

The Professional School Counselor's Role
The professional school counselor's training in group facilitation is unique to the school setting. School counselors provide group services to students and parents and may utilize their specialized training to facilitate school staff and administration on relevant professional issues or topics. Group services offered to students and parents are based on school and community needs, which are assessed through survey data. School counselors prioritize group offerings based on analysis of survey data. Group counseling should be offered to all students in a PK–12 setting.

Summary
Group counseling is an efficient and effective way to meet students' developmental and situational needs. Group counseling makes it possible for students to achieve healthier academic and personal adjustment in a rapidly changing culture. Groups are an integral part of a comprehensive school counseling program and should be included and supported by every educational institution. The professional school counselor's training in group facilitation benefits students, parents, school staff, and administration. Group counseling has a positive effect on academic achievement and personal adjustment.

Note: For references, see the ASCA website: http://asca2.timberlakepublishing.com//files/PS_Group% 20Counseling.pdf.

 SAMPLE VIGNETTES

Consent? What Consent?

Ms. Ching is a first-year school counselor at Apple Elementary. She enjoyed running groups during her internship and is very excited about the prospect of starting groups at Apple. After a carefully implemented needs assessment process, it was apparent that bullying prevention groups would be beneficial to the Apple Elementary School population. Ms. Ching was careful to review various bullying prevention curriculum in collaboration with the school principal and choose the one that appeared to be culturally sensitive, developmentally appropriate, and a good fit for the school demographics. Ms. Ching decided to start with the fifth-grade classrooms, and requested referrals from the classroom teachers. As taught during her graduate school internship, she carefully conducted pregroup interviews and selected her group members. Ms. Ching's group started off great and seemed to get better each week! After the third group meeting, however, Ms. Ching's principal notified her that a parent had called and was furious with his child's involvement in the group. Ms. Ching was confused and said that she did not realize parental consent forms were needed. She thought they only used them during her internship because she was a student counselor.

(continued)

SAMPLE VIGNETTES (continued)

Discussion Questions:

- Did Ms. Ching do anything inappropriate by not receiving parental consent for student participation in a small group? Why or why not?
- What might she have done differently, if anything?
- Is this a professional issue? Ethical? Legal?

Not during my class!

Mr. Lopez's principal asks him to lead groups on study skills and test anxiety prior to the upcoming State Assessment of Student Learning (SASL) tests. Being a conscientious professional school counselor, he sought out interesting and exciting curriculum that would draw students to this tough topic. After weeks of preparing, he felt he had an "awesome" curriculum that would not only support students during their preparations but would also be fun and enjoyable. Mr. Lopez spent weeks putting together posters and flyers, and making announcements in various classrooms to encourage group membership. He was disappointed when very few students signed up, so he decided to ask the classroom teachers if they would encourage students to become involved. He was informed by both classroom teachers he approached that they would rather their students not be involved in the group. Mr. Lopez was frustrated and disappointed! He had worked so hard on this group! Come to find out, Mr. Lopez had scheduled the group meetings during key times blocked out for academic course work.

Discussion Questions:

- Did Mr. Lopez do anything inappropriate by not consulting with classroom teachers prior to planning the logistics of his group? Why or why not?
- What might he have done differently, if anything?
- Is this a professional issue? Ethical? Legal?

Scope of practice

Ms. Dorsey decided to lead a girls group at her school to focus on positive body image and self-esteem. Five females self-referred for her group. As Ms. Dorsey conducted her pregroup interviews, it became apparent that the five young ladies were in dire need of support in this area and might need additional counseling as well. Ms. Dorsey received signed consent forms for the "Girl Power" group, which was described as a self-esteem group for girls. At the first group meeting, three of the five girls self-disclosed that they had eating disorders, although Ms. Dorsey suspected the other two might have indicators as well. Ms. Dorsey decided to shift the focus from self-esteem to eating disorders, although she was nervous about it, given her lack of training in this area. She quickly pulled together different curricula that would best meet the more intense needs of this group of girls.

Discussion Questions:

- Did Ms. Dorsey do anything inappropriate by changing the focus of the group? Why or why not?
- What are the concerns related to consent forms? Ms. Dorsey's training related to eating disorders?
- What might she have done differently, if anything?
- Is this a professional issue? Ethical? Legal?

KEY PROFESSIONAL ISSUES TO CONSIDER

There are many issues to think about when facilitating groups in schools. Above all are the ethical and professional expectations and mandates for school counselors. As you may know from your previous legal and ethical course work and training, professional ethics call us to a higher standard than state laws, although these are important to follow as well. One area that many beginning school counselors neglect to consult is individual school and district policy. Many policies have specific language around the types of topics that may be attended to within counseling or referrals that can be made by the school counselor. For example, your district may not allow school staff to discuss the topic of sexuality with students unless the student is the initiator of the conversation, whereas the topic of intimacy is allowed in the curriculum. You may find during pregroup interviews that a student is not appropriate for the group but would benefit from community counseling, or you find that in the course of working with a member in a small group, it becomes apparent that additional counseling would be warranted. In either case, you will want to refer to district policy with regard to referrals, as liability for the financial cost of such recommendations may be the responsibility of the school if initiated by a school staff member. Again, these are just examples of important considerations; the previous instances are not necessarily the norm but are certainly worth considering prior to starting the group work process.

You may discover that your school principal or district has expectations for groups or other school counseling interventions beyond those covered by state law and your ethical guidelines. It would behoove you to familiarize yourself with your district policy and discuss with administrators, classroom teachers, staff, and other school employees considerations and preferences that may be unique to your building or are unspoken practice. Remember, it is often the principals who are called when there is a problem with a group—you will want them on your side. Along these same lines, it is often the classroom teachers who refer students for potential group membership, so these folks are important to have as advocates of group guidance. Last, but certainly not least, it is other school support staff who often have their thumb on the pulse of the school and see and hear students' needs that go unnoticed by others. Let's now turn to a major issue: the legal and ethical regulations covering group work in schools.

Legal Considerations

You might have heard the expression "An ounce of prevention is worth more than a pound of cure." The saying is especially true when thinking about group counseling practice. Although this chapter is not intended to replace a legal and ethical course, we provide a few key points to consider that are referred to as the five Cs of staying out of legal hot water.

Carefully review state laws, as well as the ethical guidelines and district policies regarding group practice. Familiarize yourself with these documents and regulations, and ask questions if there are aspects you do not understand. Three documents in particular that address ethical standards include the *Ethical Standards for School Counselors*

(ASCA, 2004b, 2010), the *American Counseling Association's Code of Ethics* (ACA, 2005), and the *Association of Specialists in Group Work Best Practice Guidelines* (ASGW, 1998). The first is most applicable to group work in the schools; however, ACA and ASGW resources may provide support as well. School handbooks and district policies may include information relevant to school counseling interventions, including group counseling. For example, a district may require parental/guardian permission for participation in any school counseling services aside from general academic or schoolwide interventions. State laws may dictate who may provide counseling-related services in the schools, what topics may be addressed, and training required to conduct group experiences. For example, in Washington, state law (WAC 181-78A-270) requires that school counselors receive specific training in group work. This law emphasizes the importance of school professionals running groups in schools having the specific training to do so.

Even with the completion of a course specific to legal and ethical issues, translating these guidelines to group work can sometimes be tricky. In such cases, consultation (discussed further later) is especially helpful. Stay current regarding state and national trends and legal mandates by maintaining membership in your state counseling organization as well as ASCA, read the organization's newsletters, and visit their websites. Often organizations notify members of legislative changes that impact professional practices such as group work. Additional resources that may be helpful to staying current regarding legal mandates are textbooks, scholarly journal articles, and attending workshops at state and national conferences. School districts may also provide training for school staff related to district policies and local legal mandates. Familiarizing yourself with legal and ethical expectations and staying current on any changes will allow you to be aware of the expectations for professional practice related to group counseling at the district, state, and national level.

Consent Obtain informed written consent of group members and their legal guardians. Students have a right to know what they are getting into, a right to refuse participation, and a right to terminate involvement if they choose. Parents and guardians have a right to know that their students are involved in a small counseling group or to refuse participation. Consent is most effectively obtained by providing parents and guardians a form that indicates that the student has permission to participate in the small-group counseling experience. The form should include the following details:

- Your name and role at the school. Here's an example: "Greetings Sunnyside Elementary Parent or Guardian, my name is Mrs. Edwards and I am the school counselor."
- Basic information regarding the group such as the title, general topics, main goals, or objectives. Example: "In April, I will be facilitating a group of approximately six students to talk about friendship skills. The focus of the group meetings is to provide the opportunity for fourth-grade girls to learn more about friendship, learn ways to make new friends, talk about how to be a good friend, and discuss friendship concerns. Group members will have the opportunity to choose the name for this friendship group."

- Indication that the group is voluntary. Students and parents have the right to decline participation. Example: "Your permission is required for your student to participate in this friendship group. Your student will not be permitted to attend group meetings until this consent form is signed and returned. Attendance and participation is voluntary, but I do ask that if your student agrees to join the group, that she or he attends all group meetings when able."
- Information about the consent form. Example: "I am excited to begin meeting with the girls starting in 2 weeks! If you are in agreement for your student to be a part of this group experience, please sign the form below and return to the school no later than next Monday [include a specific date as sometimes these forms get lost in students' backpacks and lockers—caregivers might receive them days or weeks later than when you first send them out]."
- Your contact information. Example: "If you have any questions regarding the friendship group or school counseling services at Sunnyside Elementary, please contact me at any time. I can be reached at 206-222-2060 or cedwards@sunsideelementary.edu."

Of course, do not expect consent forms to be returned the next day. Plan ahead and allow several weeks for the consent form turnaround. You may need to send out several copies. If you send the forms home with students, check in with them to make sure that the forms did indeed arrive home. Some school counselors find it useful to utilize email or postal services to either send the consent forms or send reminders to parents/guardians that the forms will be coming home with their student. Be aware of language, visual impairment, or literacy challenges that may impact a parent's or guardian's ability to read the consent form. Some school districts offer translation services for school documents that are sent to non-English-language-speaking parents and caregivers. For those parents/guardians with visual impairment or literacy challenges, you might call the student's home to share what is included on the form and ask if there is another adult who might be a support to them with signing the form if they are in agreement with their student's participation in the group experience. In lieu of sending a detailed consent form, some school counselors find it useful to create a generic consent form for all small-group experiences and attach it to a cover letter with group-specific information. Examples of consent documents such as a cover letter and consent form are included in the chapter supplement.

In the quest to expedite the consent process, some school counselors utilize what is often referred to as a passive consent, or they allow for verbal consent for participation. Passive consent is the use of a consent form that informs the parent or guardian of the plans to run the group and indicates that consent will be assumed unless otherwise notified. This is the equivalent of a party invitation that says "regrets only" rather than RSVP, which means "please reply"; it is assumed you will be there unless you let the host know otherwise. There are several problems with utilizing this common practice. First, there is no guarantee that the parent or guardian actually received the consent form or that the form was read or understood. Second, the school counselor has no proof that there was consent if parents or guardians indicate later that they did not consent for their student to be a part of the group experience. The same issue holds true for verbal consent. Although the school counselor would have assurance that the parent or guardian (if they know for certain that is whose voice is on the phone) was informed of the details of the group, once again there is no proof if consent was later denied.

Student consent is also important to acquire. This may be obtained during the pregroup screening (discussed further in the next paragraph) or during the first group meeting. Make the student aware of risks and benefits of participating in the group. For example, some benefits include meeting new people, learning new skills, or learning something new about oneself. One risk is the possibility of confidentiality being broken by another group member. Another risk is related to the emotional challenges that self-awareness attained through group work can initiate or exacerbate. One example of this would be where a student became aware of personal behaviors that were hurtful to others, and the awareness of such behaviors created significant sorrow or stress to the student. Student consent may be obtained through a consent form similar to one utilized for the parental/guardian document or for a less formal process such as participating in a group activity. Group members can give their written consent by creating a poster of group rules together and signing their first name inside a tracing of their hand. The school counselor can assess what means of student consent is most appropriate based on what is developmentally appropriate for the group members and fits with the culture of the school and group topic. Informing potential group members and parents/guardians of the risks and benefits of group counseling participation and obtaining consent demonstrates a regard for counseling ethics and law related to the right to refuse participation. By obtaining written consent, professional school counselors have documentation that parents, guardians, and students were informed and given the option of participation. Doing so also complies with Section A.1.d. of the ASCA Ethical Standards for School Counselors (2004b, 2010), which calls for professional school counselors to be familiar with laws, regulations, and policies in an attempt to inform and protect students.

Conduct Pregroup Screening Utilize the pregroup interview as a time to assess the appropriateness of the student as a group participant. Will the student be a support or hindrance to the group process? Will the student benefit from the group or could the group be a hurtful or an otherwise poor experience for the group member? Ask questions to ascertain fit. Professional school counselors have a legal and ethical responsibility to demonstrate a good faith effort to protect group members from physical, emotional, or psychological harm. ASCA (2004b; see also 2010) Sections A.7.a and A.7.b address the issue of students who are a threat to themselves or others.

The pregroup screening process allows for a brief assessment to identify students who may be negatively impacted by group counseling services or have the potential to harm others during the group counseling experience. It is not uncommon to receive a referral for a student to participate in a small group where the individual who has referred the student (e.g., a teacher, administrator, or parent) feels that the student would be "perfect" for a group. What this sometimes means is that the student would really profit from the material covered during the group experience and may benefit from the peer support of group work. What it does not inevitably mean is that the student is, indeed, "perfect" for group participation. There are situations where a student may benefit from group process but her or his behaviors may have a negative impact on the group as a unit. That person's attendance may be detrimental to individual group members as well. For example, you might run a group to create awareness and appreciation for cultural diversity at your school. A student who is thought to be extremely racist has been referred to the group in hopes of creating awareness of his or her inappropriate bigoted comments and of actions that the student has demonstrated. As the school counselor leading this group, you are aware that there will be ethnically diverse students in the group who are referred due to feelings of being different and feeling out of place in a predominantly white school. Although the student with a history of racist behaviors may benefit from the group experience, the potential harm to other group members outweighs the potential benefit to this one student. In this situation, you might work with the student one-on-one or provide community resources and referrals if available. Similarly, a group member who is referred to a grief group due to a recent death in the family may seem at face value appropriate for group participation. The pregroup interview identifies significant depression, and it becomes clear that this student is in need of therapeutic support above and beyond that which can be provided through school-based group counseling. In this situation, the student is referred to a community counselor in compliance with district policy on appropriate referrals. Supplementary to those discussed in other chapters, here are a few examples of questions that might be asked to make certain that the student would be a good fit with the group you are planning:

- Do you understand what it means to be a group member?
- What do you hope to gain from being a part of the group?
- What do you feel you could offer as a fellow group member?
- What do you understand about the concept of confidentiality (explain to be certain)?
- Do you feel that you could maintain the confidentiality of your fellow group members?
- How could you let others know you care for them and are listening to what they are sharing during group?
- How could you demonstrate that you would be willing to share about yourself during group?
- What are your concerns about being a part of a group?
- Do you have any other questions?

The exact wording and specific questions asked should be developmentally appropriate. From a legal and ethical perspective, it is important that the pregroup screening/interview process allow time for the professional school counselor to get a sense of whether or not the student is a good fit for the group experience. Section A.6.a of the *Ethical Standards for School Counselors* (ASCA, 2004b, 2010) addresses the importance of screening group members in order to avoid physical or psychological harm to group members as a result of group interaction. Group members who are known to be physically violent or verbally abusive should be screened carefully to assess whether or not they are a risk to other group members. If the screening process provides indication that there is a risk, not only is the student inappropriate for group participation but it is important to make the appropriate referrals to child protective services, parents, community agencies, and/or the police as indicated by district policy. In these cases document the outcome (i.e., the decision not to include student in group as well as any other referrals or notifications to others) and follow up with the appropriate agencies, parents, and the student to ensure that student's needs were met. When contacting child protective services, note the name of the caseworker you spoke with and the date and time of the call. Know that although an anonymous referral is an option with child protective services, this does not fulfill your responsibility as a mandated reporter.

Confidentiality This issue must be clearly discussed with group members. Emphasize the significance of members maintaining confidentiality, while at the same time indicate that you, the group leader, cannot guarantee confidentiality when certain topics are discussed (e.g., abuse/neglect, duty to warn/protect, subpoena). Specifically, use developmentally appropriate language to explain that what is said in group should remain in group. Students should understand that you will not inform others of what is said in group unless a member shares information related to child abuse or neglect or self- or other harm. In the event a court order is issued to release information regarding a student's participation in the group, this directive must be honored. Inform members that in these situations, you are legally obliged to share with the appropriate authorities. To ease students' concerns about these issues, inform them that one of your major roles as a group leader is to help keep students safe. Talk about the importance of group being a caring and safe place to share with each other and how group members would feel if personal information was discussed outside of the group context. Some group leaders find it helpful to allow members to decide potential consequences for breaking this confidentiality guideline. For example, if a member tells others about personal information discussed in group, he or she is asked to leave group or apologize to the offended student(s).

In conversations between professional school counselors and parents, guardians, and teachers related to confidentiality, ask group members during the first session what you may share with others while still maintaining their privacy. Let them know that parents, caregivers, and often teachers are curious about the group experience and interested in knowing what you talk about. Ask them what they think about informing interested adults about the topics that are discussed. See if it is appropriate from the students' perspectives whether general topics can be divulged to their significant others. Members need to understand that you will not share personal information or stories divulged in the group. Most likely students are comfortable with this policy. This open conversation can avoid leaving students feeling that their trust was broken when they come home to a parent who innocently comments, "I heard you talked about what it feels like to lose someone you care about." In short, by prefacing that you will discuss only group topics with the parent/caregiver, students will appreciate knowing that whereas you did disclose some nonspecific information about the group, you did not reveal any personal content. Similarly, teachers who have referred students to group or who have approved the student missing class will naturally be interested in how the student is doing. Being proactive with consent facilitates communication with teachers while maintaining confidentiality.

Consultation Talk with your school counseling colleagues regarding concerns about your group. Some readers may have to be creative in what you consider colleagues. Although many individuals only have to yell over a room divider to touch base with a fellow professional school counselor, others may have to reach out within their district, call an instructor or peer from their graduate program, or contact a friend in the counseling profession. When you are unsure if a situation warrants breaking confidentiality or whether a student is appropriate for group counseling, consult with other school counseling professionals.

TABLE 4.2 | The Five Cs of Conducting Small Groups in an Ethical Manner

The Five Cs of Ethical Group Leadership

1. **Carefully** review legal and ethical considerations for group work.
2. **Consent** should be obtained prior to group participation.
3. **Conduct** pregroup interviews.
4. **Confidentiality** should be emphasized.
5. **Consultation** with other professionals can provide support.

Utilizing an ethical decision-making model (see Bradley & Hendricks, 2008; Foster & Black, 2007) may help guide your consultation. There are a number of ethical decision-making models available to you in the counseling literature. Most approaches include some variation of the following steps:

1. Identify the ethical dilemma.

2. Apply the *Ethical Standards for School Counselors* (ASCA, 2004b, 2010).

3. Consult with colleagues.

4. Generate possible courses of action and consider pros and cons.

5. Choose an option.

6. Evaluate your selection.

7. Implement your decision.

An outline of an ethical decision-making model is available in the chapter's supplement. Remember, although it may seem efficient to discuss concerns with a respected teacher in the building or your administrator, these individuals most likely do not share the same code of ethics for professional practice or have training as a counselor.

Consulting with colleagues regarding challenging cases will demonstrate a desire to implement what is best practice among trained professionals. This is often a key issue when improprieties or allegations surface; the obvious question will be asked: Did the counselor follow legal and ethical mandates and act in a manner that is common among his or her profession in similar situations? Consulting will not only provide legal and ethical support but will also enhance your professional growth as a group leader and professional school counselor. We have summarized in Table 4.2 these "five Cs," providing a quick reference. Crespi (2009) provides a nice supplement to this chapter, expanding on the legal and ethical topics specific to group facilitation in the schools.

As with anything in life, there are no guarantees. Although there are recommendations provided earlier in this chapter in reference to staying out of hot water, the reality is that we live in a litigious society and individuals can sue for almost reason. Prevention is key when it comes to avoiding legal or ethical violations. The saying "It's easier to ask for forgiveness than permission" does not apply here; school counselors must be proactive.

POTENTIAL LEGAL ISSUES RELATED TO GROUP COUNSELING

Similar to any counseling intervention provided in the schools, group leaders need to know their rights and limitations. Any state law even remotely addressing school-based group counseling must be followed. Like Washington State, many states specifically require school counselors to receive training in group counseling. Other laws, although not specific to group practice, impact group counselors. For example, New York's Social Services Law 413 identifies school counselors as mandated reporters of child abuse and neglect (Silver & Green, 2001). In cases where a student discloses information that creates suspicion that abuse or neglect has occurred, the professional school counselor has a responsibility to report it to child protective services. Note that the term *suspicion of abuse* is used, not *confirmed abuse*. Many school counselors worry that they need to confirm that the abuse or neglect has occurred or is occurring in order to make a report. The counselor fears that the report, if unsubstantiated, may cause family hardship. Although making a report should be a thoughtful process, keep in mind that school counselors are mandated reporters, not mandated investigators; and, though well-meaning, asking too many questions could do more harm than good. A case that ends up in court may be thrown out if the questioning is perceived to have been handled inappropriately or was done by someone who was not trained in forensic interviewing. Practicing as a professional school counselor requires substantial education and training.

Because training may vary between programs and states, it is important that group counseling is within your *scope of practice* prior to starting group work independently. This technical phrase is used to describe an area or skill in which you have received specific training, experience, and supervision. Although there are many group counseling theories from which to frame your group leadership, it is imperative that your choice of theory and interventions is considered to be common practice in the profession—*tried and true,* as the saying goes. The school is not the appropriate forum for radical, alternative intervention strategies that are on the cutting edge. For example, over the years various counseling techniques have emerged that require extremely loose (or no) boundaries between the counselor and counselee or that call for extensive physical interaction or restraint. For obvious liability reasons, as well as best practice aspirations, such strategies are inappropriate for school-based groups.

School counselors must use common sense and follow closely the professional and practical guidelines learned in their graduate school training. Specifically, as indicated above, small-group counselors should not (a) "wing it" (i.e., facilitate groups without any or little preparation), (b) lead without preservice supervised group training, (c) direct student experiences in areas for which they have no training and are clearly outside the school counseling role (serious mental health issues related to, e.g., eating disorders, psychotic disorders, major depression, self-harm, etc.), and (d) utilize techniques that are obviously inappropriate for school settings (e.g., hypnotism, religion-based meditation, or rebirthing/attachment therapy [not to be confused with attachment theory]). Failing to report abuse, threats to self or other, and poor boundaries are also common infractions. In brief, the above examples of poor group leadership practices may lead to serious legal repercussions (e.g., school district reprimand, parental lawsuit, suspension/termination of certification or licensure). It never hurts to reiterate this advice: When in doubt, always consult with your professional colleagues (e.g., counselors, school psychologist, school principal), the district attorney, and other relevant officials.

TABLE 4.3 | *American School Counselor Association (2004b, 2010)* Ethical Standards for School Counselors *(also see 2010 revision)*

Section Identifier and Topic

Section A.6. Group Work

a. Screen prospective group members and maintain an awareness of participants' needs, appropriate fit and personal goals in relation to the group's intention and focus. The school counselor takes reasonable precautions to protect members from physical and psychological harm resulting from interaction within the group.

b. Recognize that best practice is to notify the parents/guardians of children participating in small groups.

c. Establish clear expectations in the group setting, and clearly state that confidentiality in group counseling cannot be guaranteed. Given the developmental and chronological ages of minors in schools, recognize the tenuous nature of confidentiality for minors renders some topics inappropriate for group work in a school setting.

d. Provide necessary follow up with group members, and document proceedings as appropriate.

e. Develop professional competencies, and maintain appropriate education, training and supervision in group facilitation and any topics specific to the group.

f. Facilitate group work that is brief and solution-focused, working with a variety of academic, career, college and personal/social issues.

Codes of Ethics   As previously mentioned, our professional codes of ethics call school counselors to the highest standard regarding our professional behavior (Remley & Herlihy, 2009). These codes provide specific guidelines for the practice of counseling professionals. The *Ethical Standards for School Counselors* (ASCA, 2004b, 2010) is a publication of the American School Counselor Association and provides direction for school counselors related to professional and ethical practice. Section A.6 of the standards is specific to group work in the schools. Table 4.3 provides the complete excerpt from the ASCA standards. Although this section is specific to group work, it should not be reviewed independent of the complete standards given that there are ethical considerations that are relevant to group work (i.e. diversity, dual relationships, etc.) that are covered in other sections of the standards.

In addition to the ASCA (2004b, 2010) Ethical Standards, counseling professionals in all areas of expertise can seek the advisement of the *American Counseling Association's Code of Ethics* (ACA, 2005). There are two sections of the ACA Code of Ethics that specifically attend to ethical guidelines related to group work. Section A, which focuses on the ethics of the counseling relationship, highlights the importance of screening during the group process as well as the need to protect group participants from physical, emotional, and psychological trauma.

Section B, which attends to the issues of confidentiality, privileged communication, and privacy, emphasizes the importance of confidentiality during group work. As with all

TABLE 4.4 | American Counseling Association's (2005) Code of Ethics—
Sections Pertaining to Group Work

Section Identifier and Topic
Section A The Counseling Relationship
A.8. Group Work A.8.a. Screening A.8.b. Protecting Clients
Section B Confidentiality, Privileged Communication, & Privacy
B.4. Groups and Families B.4.a. Group Work

counseling, trust is the cornerstone. Students need to trust the group leader in order to feel comfortable self-disclosing during group. The group leader must explain the concept of confidentiality as well as the limits of confidentiality as discussed earlier in this chapter. Some students confuse the term *confidentiality* with privileged communication (for an excellent overview of the differences between these two concepts, see the article by Glossoff and Pate [2002] and chapter 5 of Remely & Herlihy, 2009). The latter concept guarantees that a court cannot compel an individual to release information shared in confidence, even when subpoenaed. This right is mostly reserved to the relationship between patients and physicians or clients and attorneys. Rarely, state courts expand the interpretation of this right to other mental health or counseling professionals, so it is imperative to familiarize yourself with your state law as it pertains to school counseling licensure or certification.

Privacy is another right that belongs to the student related to self-disclosure (see chapter 5 of Remely & Herlihy, 2009, for additional information on this topic). Although it is true that our students are often interesting, school counselors request self-disclosure for information that will assist the school counselor to be a support to the student's personal/social, academic, or career success. For example, a student may share that her mother was young when she gave birth to the student. You may wonder just *how* young? It is important to ask yourself, is this relevant to my support of this student or am I just curious? Students have a right to privacy and to know that the information that they choose to self-disclose is for support purposes. Table 4.4 highlights the sections of the ACA (2005) ethical code that addresses small-group practice. In summary, group leaders have a responsibility to carefully screen group members, do their best to ensure that the needs of the group members are compatible with the goals of the group, select group members who will not hinder group progress, and explain the importance of and limitations related to confidentiality within group counseling, and they are encouraged to promote change in group members that improves the quality of their lives (ACA, 2005).

The *Association of Specialists in Group Work Best Practice Guidelines* (ASGW, 1998) is a publication of the Association of Specialists in Group Work (ASGW). The document provides guidelines to supplement the ACA Code of Ethics (ACA, 2005) related to group practice. As with ASCA, ASGW is a division of the American Counseling Association. ASGW is very clear in this document that the intention is not to

TABLE 4.5 | Association for Specialists in Group Work Best Practice Guidelines

Section Identifier and Topic

Section A: Best Practice in Planning

A.1. Professional Context and Regulatory Requirements
A.2. Scope of Practice and Conceptual Framework
A.3. Assessment
A.4. Program Development and Evaluation
A.5. Resources
A.6. Professional Disclosure Statement
A.7. Group and Member Preparation
A.8. Professional Development
A.9. Trends and Technological Changes

Section B: Best Practice in Performing

B.1. Self-Knowledge
B.2. Group Competencies
B.3. Group Plan Adaptation
B.4. Therapeutic Conditions and Dynamics
B.5. Meaning
B.6. Collaboration
B.7. Evaluation
B.8. Diversity
B.9. Ethical Surveillance

Section C: Best Practice in Group Processing

C.1. Processing Schedule
C.2. Reflective Practice
C.3. Evaluation and Follow-Up
C.4. Consultation and Training with Other Organizations

supersede the ACA's ethical code but rather to make clear the expectations specific to group work. The ASGW guidelines focus on three areas of group work: Best Practice in Planning (Section A), Best Practice in Performing (Section B), and Best Practice in Group Processing (Section C) (ASGW, 2007). Table 4.5 identifies the subtopics within each section.

As is intended, the ASGW document complements both the ASCA (2004b, 2010) and ACA (2005) codes of ethics. Combined, these three publications encourage the professional school counselor to carefully attend to the ethical aspects of group work. Specifically, ASGW's guidelines insist that group leaders:

- assess the needs of the population being served when considering the types of and frequency of groups offered;
- screen group members appropriately;
- provide informed consent;
- obtain parent/guardian consent when working with minors;

- define confidentiality and its limits;
- consider their personal values as well as knowledge and ability related to the groups they lead;
- demonstrate cultural sensitivity;
- evaluate the group efficacy;
- remain competent and seek consultation when appropriate;
- be aware of technological trends and the impact on group practice; and
- follow all professional, ethical, and legal expectations related to group counseling practice.

Although screening, consent, confidentiality, and consultation were discussed previously, the areas of group evaluation, technology, and cultural sensitivity require brief elaboration. Evaluating group efficacy allows for accountability and encourages school counselors to use group counseling interventions that work well to address group objectives and student developmental competencies. Group efficacy, or effectiveness, can be accessed through pre- and postgroup interviews, teacher check-ins, or classroom observations.

The use of technology in schools is an ever-changing challenge for small-group work on multiple levels. With recent technological advances in smart phones and their wide usage, even among the very young, group leaders must be savvy in maintaining the focus of group activities and confidentiality. When creating group rules with members, school counselors may find it helpful to create a guideline regarding texting and other cell phone use during group. Be clear that no recordings or photos are permitted. Social networking is common practice for many students as well. Discussions of confidentiality might include specifications related to information shared on sites such as MySpace, Facebook, Twitter, and related sites. As a group leader, know that email and other Internet-related correspondence are not considered confidential. School counselors are wise to limit information shared electronically and may consider including a statement automatically included in all outgoing email messages indicating that the content of emails is not confidential.

Cultural sensitivity is obviously relevant to school counselors when assisting culturally diverse students and when promoting overall cultural awareness in the school. Remaining culturally aware and sensitive is part and parcel of acting multiculturally competent. This issue is examined in more detail next.

MULTICULTURAL COMPETENCIES

Although not specific to group practice, the Association for Multicultural Counseling and Development (AMCD) approved the "Multicultural Counseling Competencies and Standards" (Sue, Arrendondo, & McDavis, 1992). These encourage counseling professionals to improve their multicultural counseling awareness, knowledge, and skills. This publication includes a conceptual framework related to cross-cultural counseling competencies, focusing on the application of (a) counselor awareness of own assumptions, values, and biases; (b) understanding the worldview of the culturally different client; and (c) developing appropriate intervention strategies and techniques. Each of these three characteristics is considered to have three dimensions: (a) beliefs and attitudes, (b) knowledge, and (c) skills (Sue et al., 1992).

Cultural competence is an important professional consideration when running groups in schools. As evidenced in today's schools and touted time and time again in the multicultural literature, we are becoming an increasingly diverse society (Sue & Sue, 2007). Multicultural, racial, and ethnic groups will be the rule rather than the exception. There are unique issues to be cognizant of when working with diverse groups. Further exploration of this topic is provided in chapter 10.

ADVOCACY COMPETENCIES

The ASCA (2005a) National Model calls for school counselors to serve as advocates for all students. The ACA Code of Ethics (ACA, 2005) encourages counselors to "advocate at individual, group, institutional, and societal levels to examine potential barriers and obstacles that inhibit access and/or the growth and development of clients" (p. 5). Moreover, the ASCA *Ethical Standards for School Counselors* (ASCA, 2004b, see also 2010) clearly state that "professional school counselors are advocates, leaders, collaborators and consultants who create opportunities for equity in access and success in educational opportunities" (Preamble, ¶1). The profession's ethical guidelines are thus unambiguous. School counselors are in a pivotal role not only to serve and care for students who are often overlooked or whose needs are often not met, but to go a step further to be an activist and ensure that their academic needs are served by others as well.

This expectation permeates every role of the professional school counselor, including small-group leadership. Although the importance of advocacy for those students who are often underserved or marginalized is vital to consider, advocacy for all students to achieve educational success in K–12 settings must also be part of the school counselor's responsibility. Remember that school counseling interventions are ideally preventive and proactive. Small groups can support this quest to support student achievement by considering the needs of all students when choosing the type of and frequency of groups to lead in your school.

The ACA Advocacy Competencies (Lewis, Arnold, House, & Toporek, 2005) provide a framework for counselors to serve as advocates for individuals and groups. The competencies highlight five domains, which include client/student empowerment, client/student advocacy, community collaboration, systems advocacy, and social political advocacy (see Table 4.6).

SO MANY GUIDELINES TO FOLLOW!

Reviewing the various professional guidelines can be a daunting experience. This chapter has discussed the ASCA National Model (ASCA, 2005a), the ACA Code of Ethics (ACA, 2005), the ASCA Ethical Standards for School Counselors (ASCA, 2004b, 2010), and the ASGW guidelines for group counselors (ASGW, 1989), among others. You might be asking yourself: "Which one do I follow?" The answer is, "all of the above." Although the ASCA guidelines are the most relevant for the professional school counselor, the other ethical codes and guidelines should provide direction for practice as well. In addition, the ASCA National Model, the multicultural competencies (Sue et al., 1992), and the ACA advocacy competencies (Lewis et al., 2005) serve as additional support for best practice.

TABLE 4.6 | ACA Advocacy Competencies

The ACA Advocacy Competencies are focused on advocating with and on behalf our clients, our communities, and the social systems within which we all reside

There are five domains to the ACA Advocacy Competencies:

Client/Student Empowerment
- An advocacy orientation involves not only systems change interventions but also the implementation of empowerment strategies in direct counseling.
- Advocacy-oriented counselors recognize the impact of social, political, economic, and cultural factors on human development.
- They also help their clients and students understand their own lives in context.

Client/Student Advocacy
- When counselors become aware of external factors that act as barriers to an individual's development, they may choose to respond through advocacy.
- The client/student advocate role is especially significant when individuals or vulnerable groups lack access to needed services.

Community Collaboration
- Their ongoing work with people gives counselors a unique awareness of recurring themes. Counselors are often among the first to become aware of specific difficulties in the environment.
- Advocacy-oriented counselors often choose to respond to such challenges by alerting existing organizations that are already working for change and that might have an interest in the issue at hand.
- In these situations, the counselor's primary role is as an ally. Counselors can also be helpful to organizations by making available to them our particular skills: interpersonal relations, communications, training, and research.

Systems Advocacy
- When counselors identify systemic factors that act as barriers to their students' or clients' development, they often wish that they could change the environment and prevent some of the problems that they see every day.
- Regardless of the specific target of change, the processes for altering the status quo have common qualities. Change is a process that requires vision, persistence, leadership, collaboration, systems analysis, and strong data. In many situations, a counselor is the right person to take leadership.

Social/Political Advocacy
- Counselors regularly act as change agents in the systems that affect their own students and clients most directly. This experience often leads toward the recognition that some of the concerns they have addressed affect people in a much larger arena.
- When this happens, counselors use their skills to carry out social/political advocacy.

Note: From Lewis et al. (2005).

Remember that these various guidelines are not intended to serve as an easy guide to tell you what to do in each situation, but rather serve as a framework to pair with professional judgment and collaboration in consideration of the issues in context (Stone, 2005).

As we conclude this chapter, let's revisit the three vignettes presented at the beginning. The first scenario addressed the issue of parent/guardian consent and asked the following questions:

- Did Ms. Ching do anything inappropriate by not receiving parental consent for student participation in a small group? Why or why not?

    Because small-group counseling involves students' personal lives and is outside of the standard school counseling activities provided for all students, it generally requires parent/guardian permission for involvement. Section A.6.b. of the ASCA Ethical Standards for School Counselors (ASCA, 2004b, 2010) addresses the appropriateness of parental/guardian notification. School culture, state laws, and district policy may have clear expectations regarding group participation by students. Although a consent form may not be officially required, as discussed in this chapter it certainly provides support if there was any question regarding informed consent or parental approval for participation. Although it may seem time consuming to track down consent forms, the commitment may pale in comparison to the time it takes to consult with your legal department and testify in court.

- What might she have done differently, if anything?

    In an effort to be proactive with regard to potential parent/guardian concerns or allegations, Ms. Ching may have benefited from providing parents/guardians with a cover letter and consent form requiring a signature prior to group participation. She could have also created some way for the fifth-grade students to demonstrate their consent for participation through an activity or form.

- Is this a professional issue? Ethical? Legal?

    Assuming that there are no state laws or district policy requiring parental consent for group counseling participation, this may be a professional "best practice" issue only, as the ASCA Ethical Standards for School Counselors (ASCA, 2004b, 2010) leave it to the discretion of the professional school counselor after legal and district policy consideration.

    The second vignette addressed the issue of group planning and organization and asked the following questions:

- Did Mr. Lopez do anything inappropriate by not consulting with classroom teachers prior to planning the logistics of his group? Why or why not?

    This issue is addressed in three sections of the ASCA Ethical Standards for School Counselors (ASCA, 2004b, 2010). First, Section A.6.b acknowledges the importance of notifying staff of student participation; and although it does not indicate exactly when to communicate, it is our opinion that consulting with teachers and administration when planning school counseling interventions is a best practice recommendation, promotes future collaboration, and encourages buy-in regarding group counseling interventions by colleagues. Section C.1 addresses the issue of professional relationships and encourages school counselors to establish and maintain professional relationships and demonstrate respect toward colleagues. Demonstrating thoughtfulness regarding class schedules and teacher preferences encourages a positive working relationship between teachers and school counselors.

Section D.1 focuses on the school counselor's responsibility to the school and community. Professional school counselors want to ensure that the group counseling experience does not interfere with student learning. At times it may make sense to permit a student to leave class for group participation. In these situations, the school counselor should collaborate with classroom teachers to discuss the benefits of the group experience weighed against the cost of missed class time.

- What might he have done differently, if anything?

    Mr. Lopez most likely would have achieved greater success with group member referral and participation had he connected with the classroom teachers whose students he was hoping to recruit. Through collaboration, he could identify the best times to schedule his group and which students might be most appropriate (rather than rely solely on self-referral).

- Is this a professional issue? Ethical? Legal?

    It is unlikely that state law would dictate collaboration; however, it is possible that district policy may address this type of issue. As indicated above, there are both ethical and professional considerations.

    The third and final vignette addressed the issue of scope of practice and asked the following questions:

- Did Ms. Dorsey do anything inappropriate by changing the focus of the group? Why or why not?

    Although one might argue that eating disorders are related to body image, for the purpose of school-based counseling groups the focus should be on prevention rather than responsive therapeutic services. The signed consent forms specified that the group focus was primarily on self-esteem. Although it is not uncommon to make minor adjustments to group topics to meet the group needs in the midst of group meetings, this is a significant shift that would warrant additional consent.

- What are the concerns related to consent forms? Ms. Dorsey's training related to eating disorders?

    A parent or guardian who may have been comfortable with their student focusing on "girl power" may be less enthusiastic about a group focused on addressing eating disorders. Ms. Dorsey acknowledged her limited training related to eating disorders. It is unlikely that she could argue that this topic was within her "scope of practice."

- What might she have done differently, if anything?

    When it became apparent that the girls had needs beyond her scope of practice and beyond the role of school counselors, she should have consulted with colleagues to ascertain whether or not it was in their best interest to continue with the current "girl power" group. A referral to a community counselor to address the eating disorder issue was probably in order here. If it was deemed appropriate, the school counselor should request a release of information to the community counselor to inform her or him that the student is involved in her group and consult regularly to ensure that the group involvement does not put the student or others at risk due to the student's work with the community counselor. If eating disorders appear to be a significant issue for the larger school population, it would behoove the school counselor to obtain additional training in the prevention and identification of eating disorders in order to provide additional preventive school counseling services and make community referrals when appropriate.

TABLE 4.7 | Helpful Websites

- ASCA's 13 Ethical Tips for School Counselors:
  http://www.schoolcounselor.org/content.asp?pl=325&sl=136&contentid=166

- Legal and Ethical Link on the American School Counselor Website: This page links you with the ASCA Scene website where you can post your ethics questions to school counselors around the country. You can also check out various discussion forums in the Legal/Ethical category or email the ASCA ethics chair.
  http://www.schoolcounselor.org/content.asp?contentid=136

- Sex Laws: This website provides legal information involving minors and sexual activity specific to confidentiality and related school counselor issues.
  http://www.sexlaws.org

- Websites and Other Resources Regarding Legal & Ethical Issues in Counseling Compiled by Carolyn Stone, Counselor Educator: This link provides a document that includes a significant number of links relevant to school counselors related to legal and ethical issues.
  http://www.counseling.org/resources/pdfs/Legal_and_Ethical_Website_Info.pdf

---

- Is this a professional issue? Ethical? Legal?

    This vignette addresses professional, ethical, and legal issues. It was unprofessional to represent the group as one topic and then switch the focus after permission forms had been returned. Section E.1.a of the ASCA Ethical Standards for School Counselors (ASCA, 2004b, 2010) addresses the issue of professional competence. Ms. Dorsey was clearly providing services outside of her scope of practice and professional competence. This same issue is relevant from a legal perspective as well. Many states address the issue of scope of practice, such as the Ohio Administrative Code, Chapter 4707-15-01, which indicates that scope of practice is determined by education, training, and practice.

Although all of the documents and recommendations discussed in this chapter are intended to provide support for the professional school counselor when conducting small groups in schools, it is important to remember that you are not alone and you are not required to commit them to memory. They are intended to serve as reference materials. Be familiar with them and always have them at arm's reach, but there is no need to be able to recite them. In addition to having these resources, you will want to utilize peer review, supervision, and consultation throughout your practice. As mentioned previously, this chapter is not intended to replace a legal and ethical course. The text from such a course can serve as a reference resource in addition to those texts cited in this chapter, including Remley and Herlihy (2007) and Stone (2005). Although not all information posted online should be considered a trusted source of information, there are websites that provide helpful information to serve as a support to your professional practice. Table 4.7 provides a few sites that school counselors may use as a reference. Keep in mind that all information obtained via the Internet should be verified specific to your state law and ethical guidelines. Small-group practice is an exciting and fun aspect of professional school counseling—enjoy the experience!

CHAPTER 4 SUPPLEMENTS

Supplement 4.1   Here is a sample letter to be sent home asking for parental/guardian consent.

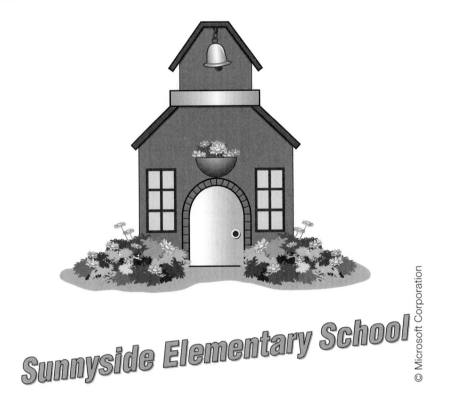

Sunnyside Elementary School

© Microsoft Corporation

March 25, 2011

Dear Parent or Guardian,

Greetings! My name is Mrs. Edwards and I am the school counselor at Sunnyside. In April, I will be facilitating a group of approximately six students to talk about friendship skills. The focus of the group meetings is to provide the opportunity for fourth-grade girls to learn more about friendship, learn ways to make new friends, talk about how to be a good friend, and discuss friendship concerns. Group members will have the opportunity to choose the name for this friendship group.

Your permission is required for your student to participate in this friendship group. Your student will not be permitted to attend group meetings until this consent form is signed and returned. Attendance and participation is voluntary, but I do ask that if your student agrees to join the group, that she attends all group meetings when able. I am excited to begin meeting with the girls starting in 2 weeks! If you are in agreement for your student to be a part of this group experience, please sign the form below and return to the school no later than next Monday, April 4th.

If you have any questions regarding the friendship group or school counseling services at Sunnyside Elementary, please contact me at any time. I can be reached at 206-222-2060 or cedwards@sunsideelementary.edu.

Sincerely,
Mrs. Cher Edwards
School counselor

Supplement 4.2   Below is a sample parental/guardian consent form.

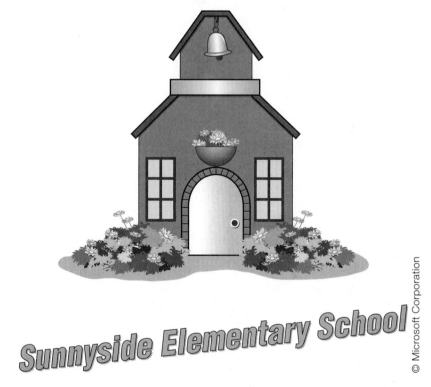

Sunnyside Elementary School

CONSENT FOR SMALL-GROUP COUNSELING PARTICIPATION

I, _____(write name) give permission for my child
_____ (write name) to participate in a counseling group at Sunnyside Elementary School facilitated by the school counselor, Mrs. Edwards. I have received information regarding the group topics and goals of the group.

Signature

Date

Supplement 4.3   Sample ethical decision-making model.

Ethical Decision-Making Model

1. Identify the ethical dilemma.
   - Does something feel "not right"?
   - Would I be okay if my principal knew this was happening?
   - Is this a standard practice for me in my work as a school counselor?
   - Is this a standard practice for other school counselors?
2. Apply the *Ethical Standards for School Counselors* (ASCA, 2004b, 2010).
   - Is there an ethical standard that addresses this issue? If so, what?
   - Are there other ethical codes (e.g., ACA, ASGW) that might inform my work as well?
3. Consult with other professional school counselors.
   - What do my colleagues think when I share the situation with them?
   - What would they do in my situation?
   - Do they agree that I have looked at the appropriate ethical standard?
   - Do they have suggestions for additional resources to help make my decision?
   - Is this a legal matter? Should I contact our district legal support? What is the district policy regarding accessing legal support?
4. Generate a list of potential courses of action.
   - What are options of how to handle this situation?
   - What are the pros/cons of each option?
   - What option do I feel is most congruent with my values and ethical standards?
5. Choose a course of action.
   - Which option do I choose to implement?
   - Do I need to consult with others regarding this decision?
6. Evaluate your choice.
   - How does this choice fit with the *Ethical Standards for School Counselors* (ASCA, 2004b, 2010)?
   - How does this choice fit with the responses from the colleagues that I consulted with?
   - How does this choice fit with my district policies? School culture?
7. Implement your choice.
   - Create an action plan if needed as to how to proceed in a step-by-step manner.
   - Document if appropriate.

Facilitating[1]

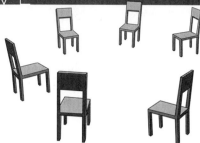

Geneva starts talking about her father's new younger partner in ways that makes Ms. Fearn, the group leader, concerned. Rather than Geneva sharing how her dad's new relationship is affecting her personally in the "here and now," she criticizes her father's choice and blames him for ruining her life. As Geneva goes on a bit longer, the counselor is convinced that this inappropriate storytelling is out of line, breaking not only group guidelines but her father's confidence as well. Ms. Fearn looks directly at Geneva and gently but firmly cuts her off midsentence, saying, "Geneva, let's not talk about your father's choices. He's not here to defend himself. But we'd like to hear how *you feel right now* … Fill in the blank: Right now I am feeling …" Somewhat startled and miffed at being interrupted, Geneva replies, "Ah, um, I am feeling really angry. I've lost my old dad!" The group leader empathizes with her ("It must be very hard to cope with such big changes in your life.") and then draws in the rest of the group, asking them to provide Geneva with some verbal support ("Have any of the rest of you felt like Geneva?"). After this group interchange, Ms. Fearn shifts focus; she asks Geneva to remember back to a time when she's been able to accept big changes in her life.

From this brief scenario, the school counselor facilitated the small group within certain legal and ethical boundaries. Based on her professional skill set and group leadership training, Ms. Fearn knew Geneva's sharing was borderline unethical and certainly inappropriate for a school-based psychoeducational group. As a result, Ms. Fearn used "cutting off," a group facilitation strategy to block and redirect the sharing of the group member.

Facilitating is the process where the group leader engages with students as individuals and, more importantly, with the group as a whole. It is tempting for group leaders who have learned individual counseling skills to manage a group by providing individual intervention while other group members look on as an audience (Jacobs & Schimmel, 2005). However, successful group leaders involve the whole group as their clients. These leaders continually think, "How does this particular student's sharing fit within the group's goals?" and "What interpersonal issues are group members trying to work out with one another?" For leaders who have more experience within individualistic societies, it can be a huge paradigm shift to think of the group itself as the client.

---

[1]With practitioner contribution from Anna Anderson, Laura Bermes, Lorie Bettelyoun, Erin Collier-Bailey, Jennifer Flajole, Michele Ngo, Jacob Olsen, and Sarah Weir

However, with practice, supervision, and strong facilitation skills, group leaders mini-mize the voices of each individual student and start to hear the story of a group as a whole. Although there are going to be times when one student talks (it would be mass chaos if all the students try to share at once!), an effective group leader learns to find themes within all the group members' narratives. For example, instead of simply reflect-ing back what one student says, a group facilitator will paraphrase the similarities and differences of what several students say. This is a complex and important task. Thus the primary aim of this chapter is to explore the skills necessary to facilitate a cohesive and working group.

Once students have been assessed for current issues, a group has been designed to address an issue, and participants who may benefit from the group selected, many group leaders stop and ask, "What do I *do* when I'm sitting with the students in the sessions?" Facilitating a school-based group is a challenging task. Capable group lead-ers use their inherent interpersonal skills such as natural empathy, genuineness, and caring to connect with students (described below). Additionally, more advanced com-munication, such as paraphrasing, reflecting, and summarizing, gets the participants to engage and talk, keep the group productive, and help draw each session to a close (G. Corey, 2008; M. S. Corey et al., 2010; Greenberg, 2003). Following the section on personal characteristics for a group leader, we expound on how these counseling skills (Egan, 2007), which are similar to the techniques that counselors employ in individual counseling, may be fostered within a group context. Solid group communi-cation skills can help build cohesion among members, promote a deeper understand-ing of the students' problems, help students see their strengths and areas of growth more clearly, and help students create new solutions for their problems—all within a group context.

STRENGTH-BASED APPROACH TO GROUP FACILITATION

The ASCA (2005a) National Model calls for school-based groups to be preventa-tive and strength based. Several authors have written about building resiliency and strengths in school counseling (e.g., Akos & Galassi, 2008; Bosworth & Walz, 2005; Eppler, 2008; Galassi & Akos, 2007). There are several ways for school-based small-group leaders to take a strengths-based approach when using group theories and tech-niques to facilitate groups. First, it is important to reframe presenting problems into strengths. In the examples below, an anger group is framed as being able to control actions. A group for young women who have been identified as being at risk for early sexual behavior has been named an empowerment group for females. Next, it is vital to assess both strengths and areas of growth when conducting a pregroup interview. What are students already doing well? (See the Solution-Based Counseling Theory section in chapter 2 and Sklare, 2005, for details on using solution-focused questions.) When designing activities, it is essential to focus not only on what students can do to intervene in their problems but also on what they can do to prevent the same or simi-lar problems from reoccurring. Additionally, when facilitating sessions, group leaders should point out the group's strengths: When are the students being considerate of others? What activities worked well for the group? How is the group showing cohesion? Leaders should be overt in pointing out these strengths to individuals and to the group as a whole.

For example, Eppler (2008) explored using a strengths-based, small-group counseling approach with students who suffered the death of a parent. While setting up the group, a review of the literature will highlight grieving students' emotions of loneliness, fear, anger, and sadness. When a group leader take a strengths-based approach, she or he will find it is important to balance the deficits of grief (e.g., hard emotions) with protective factors such as building positive relationships with remaining caregivers, connecting with caring adults at school, and building a self-concept that balances grief with transcending loss. To help group members bolster resiliency, group leaders may design small-group activities like drawing a favorite memory from before the death. Students may explore both the sadness of the loss and the ability to remember their loved one. Moreover, group members could work on a mural that illustrates their strengths. Members could draw activities they do that help them cope with grief. Additionally, the group could share other ways of dealing with grief with the other group members.

PERSONAL CHARACTERISTICS OF AN EFFECTIVE GROUP LEADER

Although many group counselors are concerned with what they should "do" during a group meeting, it is important for professional school counselors to focus on who they are in a group session. Leading effective groups in the school balances activities and an open group process. M. S. Corey et al. (2010) listed characteristics of an effective group counselor. We have condensed and adapted these traits to fit professional group counselors working in a school.

Courage

A group counselor in the schools must be courageous, as shown through the ability to make and admit mistakes, confront students in a compassionate way, stay with students through difficult processes, take actions on hunches, and draw from the counselor's own life experiences in order to help students (M. S. Corey et al., 2010). These courageous acts can help professional school counselors facilitate groups in several ways. School counselors must be willing to design and implement groups that meet the needs of the students they serve. Within district guidelines, counselors should intervene with all students, including those who struggle with issues of harming themselves, who are considering (or who are) sexually active at a young age, and those dealing with other "at-risk" issues (McWhirter, McWhirter, McWhirter, & McWhirter, 2007). In order to confront these challenging issues, the professional school counselor must have the courage to address what she or he believes about them. This awareness may lead to the counselor taking risks in session by challenging students' attitudes and beliefs about themselves and others. Here's an example of how this might be accomplished.

VIGNETTE

Courage in a Middle School Group

A school counselor at a middle school was asked to lead a group for female students who had been referred to the counseling office by parents or caregivers who were concerned that their daughters were dating and at risk for early sexual activity. As the counselor was newer to the field, she was concerned about how to facilitate a group on a sensitive subject. The professional school counselor decided to lead an "empowerment group for young women." Sessions for this group included talking about what challenges young women faced when dating, how to set boundaries in a relationship, and helping young women to feel strong when faced with pressures from friends and boyfriends. The leader realized that in order to lead this group, she would need courage to have compassion for young women struggling to make big decisions, to block conversations if they became "too gossipy," and to connect with the students who were much younger than herself.

"Courage" Reflection

- How do you show the courage to be vulnerable? In past work with students, how have you admitted your mistakes in a professional way? Would you do the same if you were to make a mistake in a group session? What would you do differently?
- Reflect on "staying with the students through difficult times." What may make this a challenge? How have you seen other counseling professionals maintain their skills and relationship when tough times arise?
- Having courage in group counseling often means taking actions on your hunches. What does this look like for you? How can you "check in" on your hunches to see if they are aligned with best practice?
- It takes courage to disclose what you are thinking about the group members and the group process. How would you use self-disclosure? How will you identify when you are disclosing too much or too little?

Willingness to Model

Students notice what the group leader does and says in and out of the group session. A group leader can promote a healthy group interaction by modeling openness, showing a caring concern for the group members, and taking appropriate risks. For example, when leading the empowerment group for girls, the school counselor modeled respect for the girls and their time by starting and ending the group on time, letting each member have a say in the sessions, preparing thought-provoking questions, and letting the girls make many of the decisions related to the group. In order to role-model empowerment in the group itself, the counselor let the girls decide on group rules; for instance, she asked the girls how it would feel most comfortable for them to be "blocked" if the conversation got offtrack (e.g., by being interrupted, holding up a "timeout sign" by making a "T" with hands, asking for the empowerment ball that gave the group members the floor to talk, etc.). Also, the leader was willing to model openness in the group conversations. She commented during the group that it was often hard to talk about some of the difficult issues that the students faced when dating, and she stated that she did not always have the answers. This willingness to model her vulnerability opened up the space for honest conversation among group members.

"Willingness to Model" Reflection

- How do you see yourself as a model in the group?
- What are the strengths you would want to model to group members?
- What tools will you use to help set appropriate boundaries? How will you verbally and nonverbally communicate these boundaries to the group members?

Openness, Genuineness, Caring, and Being Present

It is a fine balance between being emotionally available for the group and not over-extending yourself so you feel overwhelmed by struggles that group members face. Openness, genuineness, caring, and being present are defined by being who you are and being willing to share the emotions, from joy to pain, of each of the group members. Being present suggests that the group leader is living in the moment, not only thinking of the session's plan or a prescribed agenda but also being open to experiencing what the group members are sharing. It is important for the professional school counselor to reflect on both the verbal and nonverbal statements of the members. What is the mood of the session? What emotions are the members experiencing in the session?

Having a presence is often difficult as it may be easy to hide behind a façade of professionalism. Many new counselors may not have had firsthand experience with many of the issues that students face. Sometimes, it may be easier to stick to an agenda filled with activities rather than really process what the group members are saying. Although having a plan with activities is important, it is also important to be open to the emotional process of the group.

"Openness, Genuineness, Caring, and Presence" Reflection

- When are times that you have felt most "real" around others? How can you use this in group sessions?
- How will you know if you are presenting a façade instead of being fully genuine and present?
- What skills will you use to show your openness to others' ideas and your true caring about the students you serve?

Nondefensiveness in Coping with Criticism and Willingness to Seek New Experiences

Students can be blunt with their feedback. It is important to be aware of one's own anxiety when receiving criticism and use that information to help the group process. It may seem easier to brush off a hard word about the group. For example, a student may protest, "I hate these activities, they are dumb." We may want to say to ourselves that the student does not understand the importance of the activities or is too "blocked" (resistant?) to make use of the information. However, when dealing with criticism nondefensively, be open to the possibility that the students are telling you something important. Maybe they are not ready for the work the counselor has assigned, but they may be willing to share their own ideas that will help them get the most from the group. Dealing with the criticism in a constructive manner—such as asking, "What do you not like about the assignment?" or "What would the group do instead?"—may help the members build skills to talk about situations they do not agree with. Also, the members may need feedback from their peers about how they come across when they complain. After hearing that a group member did not like a task, a nondefensive group leader may ask the group, "Are there other activities that you like that would help us reach our goal? Okay, I'm open to your ideas; tell me a little bit about them." After a new plan is established, the group leader could reflect on the process by sharing, "Sometimes it is hard to receive negative feedback. Is it hard for others in the group? How is it most helpful for someone to tell you that they don't like what you are doing?"

"Nondefensiveness and Openness" Reflection

- How do you handle criticism?
- What is it like for you if you have to change your plan in the spur of the moment?
- How can you be open to the feedback that group members provide?
- Sometimes counselors tell themselves that the group is going well so they do not need feedback. How can you assess if you are doing a good job or if you are closed to constructive criticism? (See Bostick & Anderson, 2009, and other chapters in this text for additional information on assessing group outcomes.)

Sense of Humor

Working with children and adolescents can be challenging and complex; it can also be very enjoyable. Leading groups in the schools requires professional school counselors to be flexible and to use their sense of humor. Counselors do not have to be comedians, but it is important to be open to the joy and laughter in the group. Some professional school counselors fear that they will not be respected if they were to laugh when something humorous happens in a group. That may be the case in some instances. However, the opposite is also true. Students respect and appreciate when they see their counselors as real people with a wide range of emotions.

"Sense of Humor" Reflection

- What type of humor do you use (dry, action oriented, witty)?
- How might students perceive your sense of humor?
- Envision yourself appropriately using humor with a group of students. What does this look like?

The above traits of an effective group leader (adapted from M. S. Corey et al., 2010) are essential personal characteristics of a group leader. There are also communication skills that help a group form, stay on task, and bring the group members together. These are considered next.

GETTING THE GROUP MEMBERS INVOLVED

Building a solid, working group starts even before the first group session. Ethical codes call for professional school counselors to meet one-on-one with potential group members to see if the student would benefit from participating in a group. As discussed in chapter 3, these pregroup interviews serve not only to assess group readiness but also to help set expectations for being involved in the group. The group leader should use the pregroup assessment to clarify what happens during group counseling (see Table 5.1 for examples). Many students may never have been exposed to (or even heard of) group counseling. The rules of a group may be drastically different from what they experience day to day in their classroom setting. For example, the group leader may not expect group members to raise hands before speaking. A student who is used to following the classroom rule of waiting to be called on to speak may not understand that it is appropriate to speak in turn within a group session. Although many of the group expectations and rules will be set and discussed when the group meets together as a whole for the first time, the group leader may use the pregroup interview to set basic ground rules for participating in the group.

In order to get the participants engaged and talking in a group, it is important for the group as a whole to feel a sense of cohesion and have a group identity. Some professional school counselors have tried creative innovations to help group members bond. One practicing counselor had students fill out an "application" to suggest that this was an important place to process issues and work on goals. The application supplemented the pregroup interview by asking why they were interested in the group topic and what they could contribute to the group. For younger students, the group leader helped the group decide on a "mascot." The group came up with the "persevering pandas." The leader used a small, stuffed panda for the group members to hold when they had the floor to talk. This helped remind the students that each person had a turn to talk and it was against the group rules to speak up if the student was not holding the panda.

For the group to arrive at the working stage, members need to build cohesion (G. Corey, 2008; Greenberg, 2003). One professional school counselor did this by having the students focus on their similarities and differences. For an elementary school group, the leader had the group members trace their hand on a sheet of paper. The students drew in the details of their hands. Next, the group leader led a discussion regarding how the students' hands looked different and what similarities they had in common. Group cohesion does not mean that all members are exactly alike, only that the members feel a sense of "connectiveness" that builds trust within the group.

Empowering the members so they feel like they are an integral part of the group is key to building a group that works well together. One way to do this is to let the group members help name the group. Instead of naming the group an "anger management" group (which could have led both the members and others in the school community to identify the students as "angry kids"), the group called themselves the "I CAN Kids," which stood for "I Control Anger Now Kids." Group members should also be empowered to help establish the group rules and consequences. One group leader had the students make a "constitution" of the group rules. The rules were written on a large sheet

TABLE 5.1 | Pregroup Interview Questions That Build Group Cohesion

Elementary	Middle School	High School
• I'm Ms. Christie. I'm here to help students learn how to solve problems. There will be six second-grade students, probably most of whom you know already. We'll have lots of fun while we learn by doing games, fun activities, and sharing stories with each other. Does this sound like something you'd like to join? • Part of being in a group is that everyone shares their own stories, thoughts, and ideas and is willing to talk in the group. How does this sound? • In order for everyone to feel comfortable talking in our group, it's very important that none of us tell other people things that are shared in the group. For example, if someone told us they got in a fight with someone else, we couldn't go tell our friends about it later. Even I won't be telling other people what anyone says during our group time unless someone is unsafe. Does this sound like something you can do? • You don't have to come to our group meetings every week, but in order for everyone to get the most out of it, it'd be great if you came every week and were on time. Is this something you could try?	• Hi! I'm Ms. Christie and I'm going to lead a group about building healthy friendships. Are you interested in joining our group? • In a group, everybody is expected to talk and share their experiences. Is this something you would be willing to do? • A member of the group is expected to try to help other members of the group. Would you be willing to help others who are in the group? • The group will meet six times and you must try to attend all of the meetings. Is this something you would be willing to do? • There are rules in a group that everyone is expected to follow. I will recommend some of these rules and others will be developed by the group. Do you think you'll be able to follow the rules of the group? • We have about 5 minutes; tell me about the kinds of friends that you have. • I have a letter that explains what we have talked about. I will need it signed by your [caregiver] before you can be a part of the group. Will you bring it back signed by Tuesday?	• Hi! I'm Ms. Christie. What is your name? What is something you know about me? • I'm starting a group on [topic]. What are you first thoughts about [topic]? • In a group, group members are expected to share their experiences. Is this something you think you could do? • Everything that you hear in this group must stay private and you must promise not to share anything that you hear in this group outside of the group. Do you think you can keep what is shared in the group private? • Part of the group is being a good listener, and to help other members of the group, do you think you can do this? • The group is going to meet seven times, once a week during class hours. It is expected that you participate in these group meetings. Of course things come up, like being sick, but can you try your hardest to make all group meetings? • As a group we will come up with group rules. Can you help with this process and participate in the group rules we set?

- In order for a group to work well, we need to be able to create and follow rules for everyone to follow during group time. Next week we'll all be creating rules together as a group. How are you at following rules usually?
- The last thing I need to tell you about is this letter I am sending home with you. It basically says everything we've talked about so your [parents/guardians] know what you will be doing in our group. In order for you to be in the group, I need your [mom/dad/caregiver] to read this letter and sign it saying it's okay for you to be in the group. Do you think they will let you be a part of our group? I need you to bring this letter back to school and give it to your teacher by Tuesday. Okay?

- You will be asked to leave class; will you talk to your teacher about this and make up any missing work?
- I have a letter for your [caregiver] that needs to be signed so you can join our group. Will you bring it back to me signed by Tuesday?

---

of paper that was hung up in the counseling room before each group session began. As part of the opening activity of each session, a student would read the "laws" of the group. Sample developmentally appropriate ground rules are presented in Table 5.2.

COMMUNICATION SKILLS FOR GROUP FACILITATION

As mentioned earlier, at least a handful of major communication/facilitation skills are essential to learn before school counselors begin the group experience. These skills are needed to mobilize the action and facilitate the group process. The aim is to create a safe and caring place where students can be open with their peers about their feelings, thoughts, and behaviors. The following skills are summarized below and are also illustrated below within the context of a particular group meeting.

There are several counseling techniques that are useful for both individual and group counseling. M. S. Corey et al. (2010) and Greenberg (2003) listed communication skills that are helpful in facilitating and deepening a group's conversation. These skills are listed below and are defined in terms of using them in a group setting. A table

TABLE 5.2 | Sample Ground Rules for School-Based Groups

Elementary	Middle	High School
What we say stays in this room. It is okay to talk to your caregivers about what you say. But what others say is private. I will keep everything in this room unless someone is unsafe.	What is confidentiality? When do we keep things private? Is it the same as a secret?	What is confidentiality?
What happens if someone tells a friend what someone else said in our group?	What happens if someone breaks one of our rules?	Do I have to talk in group?
What is good listening?	How can we support each other?	How can everyone be a good group member?
Do we interrupt?	What do you think will make a productive group?	What would be disruptive to the group? How can we prevent that?
What can we do if someone speaks before we are finished?	What other rules should we have for our group?	What other rules should we have for our group?
What other rules belong on our list?		
What should be the name of our group?		

of examples and a brief case example follows in order to illustrate how a professional school counselor could use these techniques:

- **Reflecting:** Counselors convey the essence of what the students have said without repeating exactly what they have said. There can be reflection related to both the content and feeling of what the student expresses. The goal for the group leader is to reflect emotions and statements of individual students so they feel validated. And, it is important not to focus only on one-on-one reflections; leaders must also reflect the messages of the group overall. For example, a group leader might respond to a student that she looked upset when she wasn't called on in class. Furthermore, the leader would want to reflect the Gestalt of the group by stating, "I hear that several group members felt left out when they weren't called on in class."
- **Clarifying:** Pulling out a central issue in the students' stories is one way you can keep the group conversation going. Group leaders should listen for both individual members' stories and the central themes among all the members' stories. Clarifying can be used with linking (below) to show how one student's story fits with another

student's experience. For example, the professional school counselor could say, "I hear you saying it is really scary to talk in front of a class. Other members have talked about what freaks them out in class. Let's keep talking about what you have done to feel a bit calmer."

- **Summarizing:** Counselors draw out the most important themes after students have offered good deal of information. The group facilitator can summarize after a student tells a detailed story and/or after several students have shared. The counselor typically closes a group session by summarizing what was learned.
- **Empathizing:** Reflecting feelings to the students in a caring and compassionate way indicates that counselors appreciate what the members are going through. Students should feel understood and validated, and know that other group members understand their thoughts and feelings. However, group leaders should be cautious about not making assumptions that peers may automatically know how students feel in a situation. Furthermore, it is important to normalize that other students struggle with similar issues without minimizing the individual's and group's experiences of dealing with a presenting problem.
- **Questioning:** Without interrogation, the counselor asks thought-provoking (or feeling-eliciting) questions to help the group members think about themselves. Open questions, or questions that cannot be answered with a "yes" or "no" response, are preferred. Sometimes closed-ended questions, or questions that have a yes–no answer, are necessary to clarify or make a point.
- **Linking:** Relating multiple points of view to each other is called linking. This technique also concerns finding the theme within several members' statements.
- **Confronting:** Compassionate challenging assists group members to think deeper or observe their own behavior. One way to confront is to notice the differences between a student's verbal and nonverbal behavior, "I see that you are smiling, but you are telling me about a sad time. What is it like for you to tell the group about your mom leaving?"
- **Supporting:** The counselor supports group members by reflecting a thought that validates, normalizes, and/or affirms students. One caution is not to support too soon. Group leaders may want to jump in and offer encouragement, but it is important for students to express themselves fully. It is also a good idea to help other group members offer support in order to build bonding and cohesion.
- **Blocking/Cutting Off:** When leaders cut off members, they are blocking disruptive or nonproductive behavior. This can be done either verbally or nonverbally. For example, the group could decide that if a student is rambling on, a group leader may show the "T" sign in order to block the talker, allowing other students time to speak.
- **Suggesting:** When you suggest, you are helping students generate additional ideas. Remember effective leaders are not generally advice givers.
- **Drawing Out:** This strategy motivates students to add supplemental information about what they and others have shared. Also, the skill relates to helping students generate further ideas, solutions, or thoughts.

Additional examples of each of these facilitation skills are provided in Table 5.3.

TABLE 5.3 | Facilitation Skills and Sample Leader Verbalizations

Facilitation Skills	Sample Leader Comments
Reflecting	I hear you saying that it is hard to concentrate when you feel stressed. Let's hear other group members talk about what it is like to pay attention in class. 　　When the group talks about having trouble concentrating in class, I sense heaviness in the room. Let's talk about how it feels to feel stuck when you are in class.
Clarifying	I hear some group members saying that it is easy to work with their teachers, whereas I hear others tell us it is harder to ask a teacher for support. I'm curious—when it is easier to seek out help?
Summarizing	We are drawing near the end of the session today. I want to think about what we have discussed. One thing I learned is that there are several ways to cope when we feel anxious. For example, walking away from the situation and focusing on breathing for a few minutes have helped several of the group members.
Empathizing	You are trying so hard to make friends, balance working and school work, and being there for the family. It must be really challenging and rewarding for all of you to be involved in so many areas.
Questioning	I would like for the group to talk about a time when you were able to feel a little bit better when you were under pressure. What did you do to help relieve some of your anxiety?
Linking • Between Group *Members* • Between Group *Sessions*	• I heard Dev saying that she sometimes takes really deep breaths when she feels anxious. I heard Sal say that he tries to talk about what he is thinking. Let's talk about more ways you have been able to feel a little bit more calm. • Last group session we discussed what we could do in the moment when we felt stressed. I would like for us to talk about what we can do to prevent so much stress from building up in our lives.
Confronting	Sal, I notice that when Dev starts talking about her math project you start to look away, fidget, and sometimes talk to the person next to you. 　　I notice that when we start practicing new ways to control our stress that the group starts talking and gets off-track. What makes it difficult to stay focused? What could we do to keep on track?
Supporting	I notice so many things going well in our group. You have been good listeners and you have offered advice to other group members.
Blocking	Dev, I notice that you have answered three questions in a row. I would like the opportunity for everyone to speak. I'm going to pass the speaking ball to Sal.

| Suggesting | I like how everyone has given input. One thing that I haven't heard that has worked with other students is to try … |
| Drawing Out | Sal, you said that it is hard to concentrate. Tell the group a little bit more about that … Group, what questions do you have for Sal? |

Below is an example of how a professional school counselor (PSC) who is leading a strengths-based homework skills group would employ these skills within a group session.

Scenario: Sample Conversation When Leading a Strengths-Based Homework Skills Group

PSC: Hi, I would like to thank everyone for coming today [supporting]. I remember that we have been working on finding our strengths when it comes to studying and homework. Let's take some time this morning for each of you to share what is one thing that you did well this past week when it came to studying [questioning].

JESSE: I turned off the television when I pulled out my homework.

DEV: Got a lot of my work done when I was sitting at my table. I was alone in the room so I couldn't hear my brother play around.

ARI: Yeah, I didn't listen to my music when I was working.

PSC: You all made a quiet place to do your work [linking]. Cool! How do you think this helped you study [drawing out; open question]?

ARI: I don't know; I just had to get stuff done. I usually like to listen to music when I work.

PSC: Well, something quieter worked this time, and you are telling us that sometimes background noise may be OK [clarifying]?

JESSE: Yeah. I hate it when my parents say that I have to sit there and be still and not do anything but study.

DEV: Seriously, sometimes it is impossible to find a place where there isn't a ton of stuff going on.

PSC: That's right [supporting]. So, what happens when you can't find that "perfect" place to study but you still need to get stuff done [drawing out; open question]?

JESSE: Sometimes you just can't get things done.

PSC: Wait a sec, we're focusing on what worked well this week. Let's focus on that for just a little longer [blocking]. Ari, what do you do when it is really noisy, but you still get your work done [open question]?

ARI: Well, I try to create my own noise. If my brother is playing, I put some music on, but just not the really loud stuff.

DEV: No way, I hate listening to music without any words.

PSC: So, Seri, what could you listen to if you didn't want to be distracted but you wanted some "white noise" in the background [confronting]?

DEV: No, I just wouldn't listen to anything. I couldn't do it.

PSC: It is hard not to get to listen to your favorite music [empathy]. So, what do you do instead [drawing out; open question]?

GROUP: {Silence}

PSC: One thing I like to do is play music I know really well. I find I don't really have to listen to it, but it keeps me from noticing everything else around me [suggesting]. What do you think of that idea?

ARI: Yeah.

DEV: {Silence}

JESSE: I don't know, sometimes the music I know well is my favorite so I want to listen.

PSC: Good point [supporting]. I'm thinking that the noise in the room is only one part of what helps us to get our work done [self-disclosure; summarizing; linking]. What else did you try this week that worked [open question; drawing out]?

The group leader must use the counseling communication skills discussed above (e.g., reflecting, empathy, and clarifying) so each member feels heard. Additionally, in order to maintain focus on the group as a whole unit, techniques such as linking and summarizing help the group see what they have in common and their different ideas. Focus on the similarities of the group to normalize and universalize each member's experience. Members need to share their unique ideas and suggestions in order for the group to generate ideas that other group members may not have thought of on their own.

COMMUNICATION PRACTICE

Watch a reality television show where there is a strong group dynamic (e.g., *Real World*, *Survivor*). Write down statements that you could use to show the above communication skills. For example, what empathy could you express? What links do you see in the participants' stories? How would you summarize what the group members said in an episode?

Next, form a small group of four or five people. Identify a leader. Spend 15 minutes talking about "what I did today." The leader's task is to use as many of the communications skills listed above as possible.

- What techniques do you notice that you use most?
- What techniques do not come as naturally?
- Have group members offer feedback about the techniques they noticed. What did the leader do well? What could have the leader picked up on that she or he missed?

USING THEORY TO FACILITATE GROUPS

Active communication is an important way to facilitate conversation in the group. As you discovered in chapter 3 when discussing the foundations of group work, the leader should infuse counseling theory into the group process (Day, 2007). Counseling theory "directs" the session by helping group leaders conceptualize what is essential and by offering interventions to move the group toward its overall goal. For example, a solution-focused brief counselor (SFBC) like Ms. Fearn in our opening vignette will block conversation that emphasizes the origin of the students' problems (Sklare, 2005; also see chapter 3). Instead, the SFBC will draw out the members' stories of success. The leader may ask about times when the problem was a little bit better or what the students would be doing if a miracle occurred and the problem was no longer an issue.

Counseling theory should also be integrated into the proposal and to each group session. The theory guides the counselor's view of the students, what is necessary to help students change, and interventions that may be helpful for members to reach their goals. For example, when choosing activities a professional school counselor may ask, "Does this fit with my theory's philosophy?" or "How does this activity help me reach my theory's larger goal?" Within the session, the counselor should use the concepts embedded in the theory in his or her language. For example, if a counselor approaching the group from a cognitive-behavioral therapy (CBT) model hears the students talking about how everything is going wrong and nothing will work, the counselor could challenge the catastrophic and "all-or-nothing" thinking by saying, "Wow, I hear some big ideas here. You are saying *nothing* can help. That sounds like some open and closed thinking to me. I'm wondering if we were just a little bit open, what options we could come up with together?"

By relying on the theory to help guide the conversation, the group leader is able to focus on the process of what is being said (in the example, how the thinking affects the inert behavior), instead of focusing only on the content (that the students don't think anything can happen). If the counselor is focused on process-level interventions, it helps the group avoid just putting a bandage on the symptom and instead get to the core of the problems. Plus, it helps augment the proposal by helping the counselor find direction in each session.

In summary, we have explored the personal and counseling characteristics that help facilitate group communication and aid process toward the group's goals. Group leaders need to blend intrinsic and cultivated skills such as caring, compassion, and courage. Solid group-leading skills also are evident when the leader sees beyond the individual students and considers the group as a whole. Now that you have a good sense of what facilitation/communication skill set is needed to be an effective group leader, and you practiced these skills, it is time to conduct the first group counseling session.

FACILITATING THE FIRST SESSION

After a topic is chosen, group members are selected, and a semistructured proposal has been developed, you are ready for your first session. As you will recall from chapter 3, make sure you set up the logistics of finding a quiet and private space with enough room for all members of the group (Greenberg, 2003). Depending on the developmental level and the culture of the school, some school counselors believe that it is a good idea to send a reminder note whereas others rely on the students to remember the time and place of the meeting. Counselors may want to walk around to the classrooms and "pick up" students or may want to meet in the counseling space. If you are leading a lunchtime group, some counselors have found it helpful to collaborate with teachers and lunch staff so the group members may leave class a minute early and get to the lunchroom before the crowd so they do not have to wait in a long line.

Most students in secondary schools will probably require a reminder note sent to their classroom teachers. It is also professional to provide teachers with a reminder note at the beginning of each week identifying which students will be leaving their classes on which days and at what times. Ask the teachers how the students should return to class and how they should make up any missing assignments. Be proactive and anticipate glitches in the process.

One of the major anxieties that many new group leaders face is wondering if the members will have anything to say. First, group leaders ought to be aware of their concerns related to the group sessions. What is the worst that could happen? How would a group leader know he or she is off-track? Getting these thoughts out in the open may help alleviate some anxiety related to the group.

Starting the group off on a fun and creative path is usually a good idea. Many professional school counselors employ icebreakers to help members of the group get to know each other and the leader (M. S. Corey et al., 2010; Greenberg, 2003). These icebreakers or catalysts can be any fun activity that the group leader either finds or creates. Some leaders have adapted a "bingo" game so students have to find other students who fit a description listed on the bingo grid. After the students mingle and have other students sign their sheet, the group could gather and talk about what they learned about each other. For example, the group leader could help a student explore how many students were born in the same state in which he or she now lives, how many have brown eyes, and how many like math better than reading. Sample catalysts or icebreakers are included in Table 5.4.

For the younger students, it is enjoyable to have the members work together and say one or two things that they like. Next, their partner will have to draw a picture of the person. Then, each partner introduces the other to the whole group using the picture and saying something that their partner really likes. Because younger students are used to drawing themselves, this is a good way for them to help connect with each other.

An example of a catalyst or icebreaker for older students is to have group members stand in a circle with an arm in the air. A student will be given a ball and told to say the name of someone else in the circle. They will then toss the ball to the person they named. The person who catches the ball will lower their arm. This continues until everyone has caught the ball (signified by no one having their arm in the air). Next, this process is repeated, with students throwing the ball in the same order. Students are encouraged to continue doing this as fast as they can. When they are ready for an additional challenge, more balls are added.

Icebreaker Reflection

- What team games have you played that you feel would work well for elementary students, middle school students, and/or high school students?

After the icebreaker, draw the group together in order for the group leader to explain the expectations for the group. The group leader uses this time to remind the

TABLE 5.4 | Sample Catalysts and Icebreaker Activities for K–12 Groups

Elementary School	Middle/Junior High School	High School
	Title	
"Best/Worst"	"Unique"	"Two Truths and a Lie"
What was the best thing about school this week? What was the worst? What do we have in common? What is different?	Go around the room and have each person share something that makes him or her different from anyone in the group, such as "I've never left the state I was born in" or "I am one of 10 kids." Students give input on each other to determine if the fact is unique or shared.	Have each person make three statements about him- or herself: two true statements and one lie. For example, "I've never broken a bone. I have five sisters. I was born in Yugoslavia." The group tries to guess which statement is not accurate.

students of the rules of confidentiality that were shared in the pregroup interview. Subsequently, the group can decide together what would happen if confidentiality were to be breached. For all grade levels, the group members should provide input on the rules regarding what happens if a member shares about the group conversation to outside students, teachers, and/or staff. Not only does the counselor need to highlight the "don'ts" of breaking the privacy of the group; it is imperative that the leader focus on the positive of keeping the conversations in the group so that the members can trust one another.

Another expectation that the group leader should cover in the first session is that participation is voluntary and that it is important that each student share his or her thoughts and views with the others. Students should be told that they have the right to "pass" on answering any question, although it is important the group hear all points of view (M. S. Corey et al., 2010; Greenberg, 2003). However, the leader should note that even though "passing" is appropriate, each group member is expected to talk about him- or herself and to support other members of the group. A school counselor leading groups could ask what the students think would help create a "safe space" where everyone would feel comfortable sharing. The leader could also ask how other members could help a student who did not feel like talking. There are other ethical issues to consider when starting a group. A quick review of chapter 4 might be your next step.

First Session Reflections

- What are key components of the first session that you would want to cover?
- How would you do this with different levels of students?
- How can you empower students to establish rules and consequences in the group?

Keeping the Group Productive

There are many techniques that a professional school counselor can use to keep the group productive. Although icebreakers are typically used in the first session, it is a good idea to add fun and creative activities to each session in order to connect the students with the leader and with each other (DeRosier, 2002; Drews, Carey, & Schaefer, 2001; Elliot, 1994; D. S. Sweeney & Homeyer, 1999). Art, clay sculpture, games, and puppets are all good tools to help keep the group creative. Additionally, each group session should have a balance of activities and open discussion. If the students are talking productively, it is important for the leader to be flexible and postpone a planned activity. If the group is not as communicative in a session, it is a good idea to have several hands-on interventions (e.g., worksheets, watching a movie clip, etc.). Balancing the proposed plan and going with the flow of the group is an artistic balance. Once a few members become distracted, it may be a good idea to move on to the next activity. Or, the leader could have an alternate activity (e.g., free color time) that some students do while the other students finish a task. It is important to keep the group flowing. Even if all group members have not expressed all their thoughts, it may be a good idea to move on. Counselors can always pick back up on a conversation when the group is more focused.

As mentioned above, the "go around" group facilitation skill is one way to encourage student sharing. One practicing school counselor opened each group by having the students describe one high and one low related to the group's topic. By asking the students to briefly update the others since the last session, the group was able to support and rejoice with the progress that members had made. Students reported that they liked getting an update from the others at the beginning of the group. In a go-around, the students are asked to answer a question (e.g., "What is one thing that you did well since last session?") in the order that they are seated in the circle. The leader could ask for a volunteer to go first and then state, "We will take turns going clockwise [using a nonverbal gesture to suggest the rotation]." Although the students are answering one after the other, the group leader still fosters a group dynamic by linking the students' answers, helping the students find the themes in their answers.

In order for the leader to assist the group to remain productive, the counselor should be familiar with the best practice research regarding the group's topic. Akos and Milsom (2007) edited a special issue of the *Journal for Specialists in Group Work* that offers concrete ideas and suggestions for leading groups in K–12 settings. When reviewing this and other peer-reviewed journal sources, a leader can ask: What has worked in other groups? What are some issues that students with the presenting problem may face? What are key interventions that are proven effective? Knowing about the topic helps the leader normalize the students' issues, helps promote effective intervention, and helps the leader guide each of the sessions.

Another important skill for group members to employ in order to keep group members talking is the use of nonverbal communication. Remember to lean forward, make appropriate eye contact, avoid fidgeting behavior, and use gestures to animate your verbal comments (Egan, 2007). Jacobs and Schimmel (2005) noted the importance of using effective eye movement. They suggested looking around while students are talking to see the different reactions. Leaders should explain that they want to get a sense of everyone's reactions, so he or she may not look directly at the speaker. The leader could also encourage the group members to talk to each other instead of directing their comments only toward the counselor.

Students need to see that what is discussed in the group relates to their own situations. One way to do this is for the leader to offer real-life examples when leading group exercises. During role plays, brainstorming sessions, and other interventions, it is a good idea to use scenarios that the students can relate to. Moreover, it is important that the professional school counselor use appropriate self-disclosure so the students can relate to the leader as a real person (M. S. Corey et al., 2010). This may be done in two ways. First is the traditional use of self-disclosure where the counselor offers an example of a problem or solution from her or his own life story. The counselor may say, "When I was upset with a friend, I counted to 15 before I spoke." Another form of self-disclosure is for the counselor to offer his or her own perspective of what is going on in the group; doing this helps to focus the group by using the here and now regarding group process. For example, a counselor could state, "I'm aware that the group feels pretty serious right now. I like that you are talking about how you feel, and I am thinking that it may be a good idea to switch to an activity before we get too serious. What do you think about pausing this conversation while we continue to work together as a group? We can come back to it when we can be really productive." Pay attention to when students' developmental level affects how much information they can process (Crain, 2005). Rich discussions as well as less serious interactions should be interspersed so that students can let the information they have just shared and learned sink in.

Drawing the Group to a Close

Using counseling skills and advanced communication skills will help the professional school counselor facilitate a strong group dynamic. Time may seem temporal while the group is being productive, but the leader must keep a subtle eye on the clock. Students need time to transition out of the group and back to class. It is a good idea to give a 5-minute warning before the end of each session. This leaves time for group members to share final thoughts and for the group leader to summarize some of what the groups has shared and suggested. Remind students of their plan of action for the next week. Take note of individual and group strengths. To an individual, a counselor may say, "Seri, I really liked how you were a good listener today." To the group as a whole, the counselor could indicate that "I really liked how you all worked together to paint the posters that remind us what we can do if we feel angry."

As the sessions start to draw to a close, the group leader should remind the group regarding the number of many sessions left (e.g., two or three sessions). The leader can focus on the positives by stating that the group has been helpful and that she or he looks forward to working together for a few more sessions. As you can imagine, transitions are hard for students (Turner, 2007), and the thought of a group ending can be difficult for the group members. Some students begin to distance or act out when they realize that the group is coming to an end. To normalize without minimizing these behaviors, counselors observe the behaviors without judging. A leader may state, "I noticed that after we talked about how the group is ending that some haven't been talking as much as you did the past few sessions; I would like to talk about what it feels like for the group to end." Even if the students cannot verbalize their fears or concerns, try to bring them out in the open. It may also help the counselor think about the students' misbehavior if the leader understands the hardship of the group ending.

During the final session (e.g., sixth or eighth), reflect on what took place in the group (M. S. Corey et al., 2010). What do the students remember from previous sessions? What have they learned? How do they think that being in the group is going to help them in future situations? Spend a good part of the final group session processing the termination. Have a time of celebration to honor the accomplishments in the group.

Some leaders have planned a small party for the last session where the group celebrates with healthy snacks, takes a picture of the group for each member to keep, and facilitates a fun game or creative activity.

OTHER KEY ISSUES TO CONSIDER
When Groups Are Unproductive—What to Do

Even when the professional school counselor employs solid counseling skills and uses counseling theory effectively, the group can be unproductive. To avoid pitfalls when leading a group, we offer these recommendations (also see Supplement 5.1). Jacobs and Schimmel (2005) cautioned against:

- having too much "fluff,"
- asking vague questions,
- using activities that are too long, and
- doing individual counseling within a group.

    Because groups are time limited, make sure you:

- start on time,
- build rapport without erring on the side of just playing games, and
- design interventions that are developmentally appropriate and keep the students' attention.

    However, leaders need to focus on creating an appropriate relationship with the students. The group leader must be seen as approachable and caring. Sometimes, having less structure can help students to warm a new situation. Counselors should also attend to the cultural needs of all students. Some collectivist cultures value having an open time to establish relationships instead of jumping into the thick of the session (Marshall, 2002).

    There are other techniques that group leaders may employ to help resolve group issues:

- **Using the Leader's Strengths.** Group leaders should think about their own experiences and strengths when self-assessing their group leadership skills (see Supplement 5.2). If a leader has previous teaching experience, she or he may be drawn to more of the educational aspects of a group. Honor these skills (e.g., being able to write specific and concrete goals and objectives for group sessions) while at the same time cultivate an aptitude toward understanding groups as a process. For example, the directions may be clear when giving the group a task, but what are the roles group members are taking? Is one student playing the clown to distract the group from really working? How do other group members react to this student? It may be necessary to curtail the activity and refocus on the social/emotional aspects of the group. On the other hand, if a leader comes with a strong interpersonal or mental health background, this facilitator may be less comfortable with setting a plan for a group and desire to keep the group more "free-flowing." Again, respect your strengths, while still adding to your skill set (e.g., those leaders with a solid background in leading less structured groups should supplement their groups with planned activities that support the group's educational focus).

- **Understanding Context.** Even when counselors avoid pitfalls and balance activity and group discussion, there are some sessions that just go haywire. Understand where the students have been just before group. If they have been sitting in a classroom for a while, it may be a good idea to let them have 2 or 3 minutes of "free talk time" just before the group begins. If they have just come from gym or recess, it could be a good time to start with a structured activity.
- **Assigning the Behavior.** If the group is excessively talkative, it may be wise to let the group stop and have free-choice time for a few minutes or to break up into pairs to try a role play or other creative activity. One practitioner found it helpful to "assign" the negative behavior. The school counselor asked the group to spend 3 minutes talking, interrupting, and making noise. Afterward, the group talked about how it felt both good and bad to be disruptive. The leader focused the conversation on when it is acceptable to have chaos and when it works well to have some rule. The group leader needs to realize students are like adults; some days they are "on" and others they are not. In other words, students, like leaders, will have more productive days and days that they are less energetic.
- **Addressing Behavior by Linking to Rules.** Of course, not all group members may be on the same page each group session. There may be times when some group members are really working hard and others are goofing off. The leader needs to address a member's negative behavior before it taints the group's process and progress. There was a middle school group where several girls were making faces at one of the more quiet girls in the group behind her back. The group leader did not want to embarrass either the shy girl or shame the girls who were acting inappropriately. Instead, the group leader stated, "I see that some of the members are having a hard time paying attention. I remember that one of our group rules is to respect each other. What are some of the ways the group shows respect?" After all the group members answered, the leader helped the group explore the teasing behavior. She subsequently interjected, "One thing that is hard for me to watch is when one student is picked on. What would each of you feel if you were to be teased?" The leader facilitated a go-around in order to help build empathy. If the negative behavior were to continue, the leader should talk to the students who are teasing and remind them of the rules while setting limits for what would happen if the teasing continued. During this time it is important to notice and verbally comment on positive behavior such as when the group members are looking at the student who is speaking and when participants are listening quietly.
- **Letting the Group Work It Out.** There are times where there may be some disagreements between or among members of the group. At times, it may be important for the leader to step back and let the group work it out among themselves. The leader might say, "I see that we have gotten off track here; I'm wondering how the group is going to work together this afternoon." If the group members are not able to solve their problems, it may be important for the leader to be more overt with an intervention. For example, the professional school counselor could state, "I see that many of you have differences. It can be really hard to talk with others who don't agree with you. I would like to know how teams come together to reach a goal if they don't agree on some of the little details."
- **Returning to Rapport.** There may be groups or group sessions where a few students (or just one student) are either too shy to talk or openly "resistant" to sharing

with the group. Although these students seem to be opposites, the intervention for helping students open up is the same regardless of whether they are shy or verbally expressing their unwillingness to participate. For both types of student, the professional school counselor needs to establish a strong rapport with the student. It may be useful to do a postsession check-in with the student to ask her or his opinion or advice. The student's concerns about the group need to be expressed and validated. Additionally, it is critical that the leader keep in mind that the student's behavior most likely makes sense in context. For example, the shy student may have been teased by some classmates and now does not want to open up to others. The "resistant" student may feel like he or she will only get more of the same advice that other staff have given. It is the leader's job to understand the concerns and make the group a safe place for all members to share. Inform the disconnected student that "it is okay if you need to be a listener for a session or two. We will take the group slowly and I'll check in with you to see if you are ready to share. My hope is that you will find the group useful. What would it be like if you were to connect with the group? What would you be doing?"

- **Understanding Culture.** In addition to understanding each student's background, counselors should know the school's culture in order to understand the group members' behavior. If the school tends to have many programs or events on Friday, that may not be the best day to have group sessions. Students may be more hesitant to join a group if they think they are missing out on other desirable activities such as club meeting, recess, free time, or their favorite subject.
- **Leader's Self-Reflection.** No matter how much knowledge of the students and their school culture a professional school counselor has, there will be times when the group just does not seem to flow. Remember, take a step back and observe what you are bringing to the group. Take a short self-inventory: Are you stressed or harried? What have you tried to do to get the group talking and working? What has worked well? There are times when counselors would like to intervene once and have this quickly work with all the students. However, the concerns and issues that many students bring to the school have taken years to build up. It may be unlikely that one intervention will work. Several tries may be needed of either the same or different intervention for the counselor to notice any change. For example, a leader may have to use the solution-focused technique of finding the exemption several times before the student starts to see when the positive may work (Sklare, 2005). During this time, continue to focus on the positive, look for small changes, and be willing to try and try again. As Glasser (1965) says in *Realty Therapy*, don't give up change. Group counselors in schools should have high yet reasonable expectations for their groups and the group members. Believe that all students can grow, but also be realistic about how fast that change may occur.

Facilitation Reflection:

- What skills will you bring to the group counseling process?
- What do you see as "reasonable and high expectations"?
- What are some of the roadblocks you may face when you facilitate a group?

SUMMARY

In this chapter, we have reviewed how to facilitate effective and working groups. First, it is important to use your own strengths and personality when leading a group. Cultivate your compassion, sense of humor, openness, and caring with the students you serve. Students may learn as much by you modeling empathic behavior than by any activity that teaches empathy. During supervision and training, K–12 small-group leaders should try out innovative interventions and lead groups steeped in evidenced-based curriculum. Additionally, acquire advanced counseling skills to use within a group setting. You may already be skilled in one-on-one communication skills such as active listening and paraphrasing, but how can use these skills when a group of students is your "client"? It is key to deploy these skills in the first session as well as in the subsequent ones to set the tone and trajectory of the group experience and to keep the group working and productive. As you grow in your facilitation skills, you will learn the balance between leading free-flowing sharing and how many activities to have waiting in the wings. You will be able to balance talkative students and students who sit quietly, passing on answering each question. You will be able to summarize the sessions, bringing the group to a close. And most significantly, you will be able to connect with the students and the group as a whole. Your job is to facilitate the group in a helpful way so that group members meet the goals and group objectives.

CHAPTER 5 SUPPLEMENTS

Below is a list of ways to maintain a productive group experience and reduce problem behaviors.

Supplement 5.1 Suggestions for Keeping Group Productive

Reinforce Group Rules

Remind students to be supportive/positive with their peers.
- Speak for themselves.
- Listen without interrupting.
- Allow others to speak.
- Maintain confidentiality.

Giving Directions

- Use a signal (e.g., tugging on one's ear) to get the attention of students before issuing directions.
- Look at students when you speak to them.
- Wait to give directions until all members are paying attention.
- Issue plain, simple instructions.
- Provide only one direction at a time.
- For younger children, use small steps to task completion.
- If need be, write down directions on a poster or a white board.
- Model for students what you're directing them to do.
- Pair up group members (or use triads) so they help each other out.
- Provide time for clarifying questions.
- Use "wait time" (wait 5 seconds before moving on).
- Use positive reinforcement.
- When students don't attend, try using extended eye contact, a gentle touch, a reminder comment, peer pressure, and so on.

Refocusing/De-escalation

- Be aware of students' "fuses" that may lead to acting up.
- Mediate swiftly when the group is being disrupted.
- Use a gentle voice when refocusing/guiding students.
- Gently use the student's name who is misbehaving and tell him or her what he or she ought to be doing.
- Use kinesthetic activities to keep things loose and moving (e.g., games, artwork, role playing).
- Have students do small tasks to refocus energy (e.g., passing out paper, role playing, writing things on board).
- Ask peers to give the disrupting student feedback on his or her behavior.

Group Behavior Management

- Do proactive activities that promote a positive group climate (e.g., team building).
- Unmistakably clarify expectations and energize students with positive reinforcement (create clear, regular schedule and expectations).

- Support positive behavior (reinforcement).
- Use creativity and engaging activities.
- Keep group flowing by eliminating downtime.
- Be organized and ready to go.
- Plan and inform students of group ground rules and consequences for misconduct.
- Be consistent with modeling and interventions.
- Show how and expect students to take responsibility for themselves.
- Help students use "I" statements.
- Validate and empathize with student feelings.
- Remain calm; avoid getting "into it" with students; review the group's and your expectations.
- Separate students if there are continued problems.
- Allow for students to make choices (e.g., "You have a choice. You may ___ or ___).
- Use de-escalating comments (e.g., "I can see you are ticked off. Please use your words to share your feelings." "Yelling at Keisha; how is that helpful?" "Take 2 minutes to think about what you want to say; I'll come back to you.").
- Use "what" questions rather than "why" questions (e.g., "What are you feeling right now?" "What should you have been doing, right now?" "What might you do differently?").
- Follow a structured process when working through a challenging situation: Actively listen, ask open and clarifying questions, and paraphrase what was said.
- Avoid getting defensive with students.
- Retain your sense of humor.
- Steer clear of critical comments.
- Maintain confidentiality.
- Involve the teacher and school psychologist, if need be (assuming confidentiality needs to be broken).

Consequences If Behavior Problems Persist

- Impose a temporary loss of group privilege.
- Impose a time of silence.
- Correct inappropriate action.
- Note serious misbehaviors in a notebook.
- Have the student reflect on the misbehavior through journaling.
- Remove the student from the group (discuss with teachers and make sure parent/caregiver is notified).
- Use a behavior contract (for assistance, see http://www.schoolpsychologistfiles.com/interventions/index.html).

The following is a checklist to self-assess your personal characteristics and counseling techniques used to facilitate groups.

Supplement 5.2   Informal Group Leadership Self-Assessment Checklist

Group Leadership Attribute or Skill	I do this well	I have some skills in this area	I need to cultivate this skill
Group Counselor Attributes			
Courage to make and admit mistakes			
Openness, genuineness, caring, and being present			
Nondefensiveness			
Try out new experiences			
Use of humor			
Others			
Group Leadership Skills			
Modeling			
Reflecting			
Clarifying			
Summarizing			
Empathizing and supporting			
Questioning			
Linking between group members between group sessions			
Confronting			
Blocking/cutting off			
Suggesting			
Drawing out			
Using icebreakers			
Balancing using activities with building group process			
Using a strengths-based approach			
Conceptualizing group as a whole (not just as individuals)			
Others?			

Internet Resources

- The consummate source for group resources and activities is the American School Counselor Association's online store (http://www.schoolcounselor.org/store_category.asp?id=62). They have curricula and activity-based books for use in K–12 small-group counseling.
- A good site for icebreakers, activities, and small-group activities is: http://wilderdom.com/games/
- This web page offers activities and worksheets for child and adolescent growth and current event awareness: http://www.teachablemoment.org/middle/crisis.html

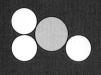

CONDUCTING GROUPS IN SCHOOLS

Groups for Elementary School Students[1]

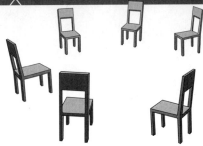

VIGNETTE

Elementary School Group Counseling Vignette—Friendship and Social Skills

It was Ms. Wise's first year as a professional school counselor. She was dividing her time between two elementary schools. With two buildings of students, she wanted to run a few groups to serve as many students as possible during her limited time in each school. Ms. Wise perceived that friendship and social skills were an area of growth for middle elementary school boys. To confirm her intuition, she developed a 10-minute survey as a needs assessment. The results revealed that, indeed, there was a need for boys to build and maintain friendships. Only 25% of the students who responded said "hi" to someone other than their best buddy on the playground, 40% said that they were good at working with others in small learning centers, and 10% of the boys indicated they used "I" statements to solve a problem with their classmates. Ms. Wise talked to the principals and staff to get buy-in and to determine the feasibility of conducting the groups in each building. While doing so, the counselor collaborated with the special education teacher, learning that several boys with educational and emotional differences may be good candidates for the group.

Ms. Wise developed an action plan for the group. Her goals were to teach positive communication skills while helping students identify their friendship strengths. After brainstorming icebreakers and catalysts for the group, Ms. Wise chose several children's literature books with the theme of friendship to use at the beginning of each session as a focusing activity. Ms. Wise planned to have three students from the special needs class and three students from the mainstream class get their lunch, bring it to the group room, and begin eating while she read from the book. The counselor also prepared several reflection questions about the story and characters: Who were friends in the book? How did they use good listening skills? What worked when they were solving a problem with a friend?

Along with leading bibliocounseling and other structured activities, Ms. Wise paid close attention to the group dynamics. Ms. Wise noticed that the group began to coalesce when the boys started to mingle together instead of sitting beside their

---

[1]Contributions to this chapter were also provided by school counseling practitioners Michele Ngo and Laura Lynch.

classmates. To encourage the boys to integrate, Ms. Wise would occasionally assign seats. She also had the boys wear name tags, and she encouraged them to call each other by first names. Ms. Wise was aware that sometimes the boys with developmental or emotional differences might need a little extra time to think about a question. Ms. Wise used her blocking skills to balance which student would answer a question first. One technique that worked for the group was for the counselor to assign the order in which students would answer questions.

By the end of the group, the boys were seen interacting with one another in and out of the group. Two teachers reported that they had overheard the boys using conflict resolution skills when there were quarrels during breakout learning groups in the classroom. Additionally, the boys themselves reported that they had more friends and liked being a friend more than before the group.

Many of the leadership skills needed to conduct this fictional elementary-level boys group were covered in previous chapters (see chapter 3 for logistics and chapter 5 for tips on facilitation). However, each group experience needs to be individualized to its group members and focus. Groups facilitated at varying developmental levels look and feel different. Ms. Wise's proposed group is no exception. As preparation to reading further, reflect on these questions: What makes elementary school groups unique, and what skills are important for school counselors who run groups in the elementary school setting?

This chapter takes a practical look at group leadership at the elementary school level, exploring the basic characteristics of such groups as well as the prerequisite skills needed to run effective children's groups. By way of illustration, a detailed example of a third-grade conflict management group is considered.

CHARACTERISTICS OF ELEMENTARY SCHOOL SMALL GROUPS

Groups facilitated at the elementary school level are energetic, dynamic, and enjoyable. Children in this age range are developing social and personal skills, and small groups are helpful to expand their emerging repertoire. Group work also provides a good way for younger students to connect in a caring and safe milieu (Hoag & Burlingame, 1997). It is important for professional school counselors to run groups for all elementary school students—even the kindergarteners—to meet ASCA's (2005a) National Model recommendation to serve every student in the school (see Gerrity & DeLucia-Waack, 2007, and Paisley & Milsom, 2007, regarding the effectiveness of groups in schools).

As a responsive service, group work fits well with a comprehensive school counseling program model, for they can be preventive or used as an intervention to address a specific concern (see chapter 2 for appropriate school-based group counseling topics). Elementary group examples include those that focus on student resilience and self-worth (Khattab & Jones, 2007), personal wellness (Villalba, 2007), and support for third- to fifth-grade students with incarcerated parents (Lopez & Bhat, 2007). Furthermore, Bostick and Anderson (2009) illustrated the effectiveness of using small groups with third-grade students with social skill deficits.

Moreover, groups at the younger levels tend to be short-term, structured, and engaging (M. S. Corey et al. 2010; Gilbert, 2003; Hoag & Burlingame, 1997; Jacobs & Schimmel, 2005). They are also less conversation oriented or verbally demanding than one might find in groups conducted with older participants. Thus having a range of potential games, worksheets, and other hands-on interventions when leading groups for younger students is essential.

One practicing counselor told the authors that she prepares two activities for each group session. She has one she thinks will be successful and a backup in case the original one is too short or the students do not relate to it. What's more, similar worksheets or exercises can be used to reinforce classroom learning. In a kindergarten group, this counselor started by having the students work on a "friendship pizza." The students were given a piece of paper with a circle drawn in the middle. The group leader and members discussed what went into making their favorite pizza. For younger students, the leader had some precut shapes that looked like pizza toppings. For older students, the counselor had the students draw and cut their favorite ingredients. Next, the group leader talked about what went into having a good friendship. Again, the students were given a piece of paper with a circle drawn in the middle. This time, the students were asked what friendship skills went into the "friendship pizza." For the earlier grades, there were words or pictures the students could choose from (e.g., being friendly or a picture of an ear with good listener written on it). Older children were able to draw and write their own "toppings." These two activities built on each other and afforded the leader the opportunity to link with students in various ways (e.g., modeling behavior when the leader built her own pizza, and building rapport by learning what type of pizza each student liked).

To be adequately prepared to facilitate these exercises, leaders must develop a sound action plan or proposal (see chapter 3 for further details) that includes the goals, rationale, and procedures to be used (such as the activity above), as well as provides an outline of each group session (M. S. Corey et al., 2010; Greenberg, 2003; Jacobs & Schimmel, 2005). The core components of the group are similar regardless of the level of students. However, there are particulars for the elementary school counselor. When developing the plan, the learning objectives of the group must meet state and district guidelines for the younger students. Most states have grade-level competencies; the group plan should align with supporting students to meet these proficiencies. Additionally, elementary school students may need more direct explanations regarding the procedures. Younger students may not have participated in tasks similar to ones older students could do without much explanation. Moreover, elementary school students are probably not as attuned to nonverbal cues and require concrete and specific directions. Older students generally grasp that a stern look is a blocking technique, whereas younger students may need to be verbally coached or have a "talking ball" (i.e., the ball that gives the holder permission to speak) taken from them at the end of their turn.

Although having a specific plan is crucial, the most important skill for an elementary school group leader is to be flexible. Even with the best laid plan, there will be days when the sessions do not end up looking much like what you proposed. Sometimes the members will cooperate and participate in the planned activity. Other times, a group leader may plan a specific discussion, but all the students want to talk about is what happened on the playground. Flexibility also comes in handy when you begin to see the uniqueness of each group. Although you may use the same curriculum again and again, each group will take on a style of its own. An activity that took only 10 minutes in one group may stretch out to nearly a full session in another group setting. Keep in mind that you will often deviate from your plan. It is better to have more activities planned than you may use. But keep recalling that the goal is not to "power through" the activities, but rather to meet the needs of the group by building a strong dynamic that includes sharing, linking, supporting, and bonding.

Even with the challenges of finding good exercises and modeling for them how to be active students, elementary groups are a rewarding experience. Group counseling is important because it normalizes many of the changes and problems that students encounter (Yalom, 1995). For example, students may not realize that some of their peers also live with changing families. One elementary school counselor designed a group for students whose families were adding a new member. The practitioner was able to help the students process the transition of losing the old family constitution while celebrating the positives of adding a new person into the family dynamic. Students were able to talk about what it was like to add a new sibling, caregiver, or grandparent to the family. Because there were mixes of family types (e.g., blended families, multigenerational families, nuclear families), the group was positive and preventive in nature. The group members were able to learn from one another about what worked when families changed. Furthermore, members were able to see that they were not alone in their joys and concerns related to having a "new" family.

Elementary school–based groups can also be a place where students can create friends and learn from one other. The size and duration of the group depends on many factors, including the grade of the students and their cognitive-development levels (M. S. Corey et al., 2010; Greenberg, 2003). Because elementary school groups tend to be preventive and problem-solving oriented, a time-tested guideline is to have six or seven sessions. It generally is a good idea to assemble students by grade levels, combining two consecutive grades at the most (Gilbert, 2003). For younger students, you may have both boys and girls in a group; for older elementary students, it may be necessary to have single-gender groups. One group leader found that with fourth- and fifth-graders, she did more blocking of "budding romances" than facilitating discussion when she included both boys and girls into her small groups. However, you will want to consider the context of the school you work in. Is there a history of blended groups? What has worked well? What are the cultural norms? Are there best practice suggestions regarding the topic or curriculum related to including students of different ages and genders?

VIGNETTE

Elementary School Group Counseling Vignette—Bullying

Mr. Ricardo, an elementary school counselor, learned from his needs assessment that there was a problem with bullying in his elementary school. Collaborating with the fourth- and fifth-grade teachers, the counselor discovered that the problem of "mean girls" was surfacing among some of the female students. After three large-group guidance lessons

(continued)

VIGNETTE (*continued*)

that educated the students on bullying prevention, Mr. Ricardo decided to do some follow-up work with six girls whose teacher had identified as high need for relational aggression intervention (see Bernes, Bernes, & Bardick, 2011, for additional information on this issue). Mr. Ricardo decided that this would be a closed, all-girl group that would meet for seven sessions. He chose to lead the group solo, with the caveat that the health teacher, a female, could join the group if the members requested it. Mr. Ricardo adapted the *Salvaging Sisterhood* (J. V. Taylor, 2005) curriculum, using exercises from the workbook along with ones he created to meet the needs of his school culture. Although other students, both girls and boys, were at risk for bullying behaviors, having an all-girls group allowed the young women to explore their friendship issues in a safe and structured environment.

SAMPLE GROUP TOPICS

As all the mental health statistics indicate (see Sink, 2011, for a summary), young students face many issues today. There is a need for a myriad of groups at the elementary school level. Group topics may include:

- friendship and social skills
- conflict management
- grief and loss groups
- changing families
- study skills
- early career exploration
- cross-cultural adaptation
- test anxiety
- transition to middle school

Inappropriate topics would include dealing with domestic violence in the home, chronic mental health issues, and others that are better served with intense therapy (e.g., conduct disorders, eating disorders, sexual issues).

REQUIRED LEADERSHIP SKILLS

Not only must you select the appropriate group format and topic(s) to best meet the needs of the group members, requisite leadership skills must be adroitly practiced. The major ones are overviewed below. While reading through this section, you might want to do some self-assessment, asking yourself, "Do I practice this skill in my daily life and what might this look like while running a group with 6-year-olds versus 11-year-olds?"

Flexibility

As stated above, a critical skill for an elementary school counselor is to be flexible. In a related way and discussed further below, professional school counselors who lead elementary groups must be creative. There are many enjoyable activities that small groups can do together. As described below, play- and art-involved counseling techniques are a constructive way for the group to have fun and to work on their goals. There are several pertinent resources on the ASCA website (http://www.schoolcounselor.org). Additionally, various publications and guides offer creative interventions when working with younger children in groups (e.g., DeRosier, 2002; Drews et al., 2001; Elliot, 1994; Eron & Lund, 1996; Gil, 1994; Smead, 1995; D. S. Sweeney & Homeyer, 1999; J. V. Taylor, 2005; see also the website http://www.researchpress.com/school-categories.asp).

Group Management

Elementary group leaders need to demonstrate effective management skills. Both time and behavior management help keep the group active and productive. Regarding time management, be direct with younger students, letting them know how many minutes they have to work on an activity, how much time remains in the session, and how many sessions are left in the group. Demonstrate well-honed behavior management skills. For instance, effective group leaders reward positive behavior when they see it happening, and they may set up a token economy, a form of behavior modification (e.g., K. A. Meyer, 1999; Sherrod, Getch, & Ziomek-Daigle, 2009), to encourage good listening skills and other productive group interactions. School counselors must be aware of their students' attention span (Gilbert, 2003). For younger students, be careful to not to draw out activities too long as children may not have the skills to sit or think for a long period of time.

Equitable Treatment

It is essential to treat all students equally. Professional school counselors should be aware if they are allowing one student to dominate the conversation or another student to remain quiet. Students should have the ability to "pass" instead of answering the question, but make clear that input from all students is valued and encouraged. Finding the strengths (or developmental assets) of all members of a group is a useful way to let members know that they are valued. For example, at the end of the session, students may be allowed to choose a colored star sticker as a reward for on-task behavior. The group facilitator should comment on a specific and concrete action that the student receiving the sticker demonstrated during the small group.

Adaptability

School counselors cope with many different changes occurring in the children and in the school, so being adaptable will be a real plus. For example, transitioning in and out of groups can be challenging for some students, so it is incumbent upon leaders to help children move in and out of the group with as much ease as possible. Counselors must consider what the students have been doing right before the group session. Students who were sitting in class may need about 5 minutes of "free" or "wiggle" time to open up the group, whereas students who have come in from recess may be ready to start a more structured activity. Again, flexibility as part of adaptability is the key when leading groups.

Creativity and Play Counseling Skills

Elementary schools are colorful and creative places. In their family lives, classrooms, and friendships, younger students communicate through play and stories. Group leaders must incorporate both play and creativity into the group sessions. Theory, research, and specific techniques from the play therapy literature (Drews et al., 2001; Gil, 1994; Hughes, 2009; Kaduson & Schaefer, 2001; Landreth, 2002) are helpful when engaging group members in meaningful and fun interactions. So, what materials are necessary for group play? Play resources include children's literature books, puppets, art supplies, lined paper for making storybooks, stuffed animals, board games, videos, a dollhouse, and possibly even a sand tray. Play materials should be fun and safe (e.g., Kaduson & Schaefer, 2001). Counselors should consider cultural differences when choosing materials for play. For example, for many Native Americans owls are a symbol of death and may evoke feelings of anxiety. A counselor who brings out "the wise owl" may not receive the anticipated reaction if a student has different associations with that puppet. It is beyond the scope of this chapter to describe the details of play therapy, but a snapshot is offered below (see Landreth, 2002, for details).

Play represents the attempt of children to organize their experiences (Drews & Schaefer, 2010). Children may "work out" personal and social issues by telling fictional stories using puppets, dolls, or inanimate objects (trains, blocks, etc.). Play may be one of the few times in children's lives when they feel more in control of their world and thus more secure to express their thoughts and feelings. Additionally, play helps group leaders connect to group members by building relationships through fun activities (art work, storytelling, reading a children's literature story, etc.). In a group, having time for play may be less directive than other exercises, but it still gives valuable information. For example, a leader may ask the students to each draw something they like to do with their family. The children have the chance to be creative, and the group can build rapport by processing the similarities and differences of the drawings. Or, the group can work together to draw a mural of a caring school. Again, the students have the chance to be artistic while the group leader can notice who is taking the lead, who is quieter during the activity, who works with whom, and so on. These observations can help the group leader process the group's dynamics (e.g., if the members are collaborating as a cohesive team and if the students are in the working stage) while simultaneously focusing on the content expressed in the artwork (e.g., the factors of a caring school such as clear rules, caring adults, having books for learning).

As opposed to more structured activities (e.g., doing a puzzle together), one major benefit of play for younger children is that it tends to require less cognitive focus and energy and provides opportunities for heightened emotional expression (Drews & Schaefer, 2010). There is an emphasis in many groups on learning specific skills and information, but there should also be time for students to become more aware of themselves as individuals and as community members. Group leaders can encourage play with specific toys or in particular ways that are likely to induce feelings and behaviors related to the group topic. For example, if the group's goal is to help students learn more about social interactions, puppets/stuffed animals could be put in the middle of the group's circle. The children could choose a favorite animal and play what it is like for that animal to make friends with other animals in the circle.

The use of stories can be very helpful in small-group work (Eppler, Olsen, & Hidano, 2009). Stories can be a work of fiction or poetry, written by the group (e.g., short story or graphic novel), a video/film, or a story told by the group leader that parallels the conflict or situation that the students face. Because reading and writing are part of the students' typical classroom environment, creating and telling stories are good ways for leaders to draw a parallel between group content and classroom learning. Additionally, school administrators and teachers appreciate when group time attempts to meet educational goals such as bolstering reading and writing learning outcomes. Narratives that the group leader and members create and use toward the group's counseling goals may link students to each other and the academic environment of the school.

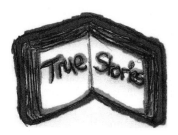

Cultural and Developmental Awareness Skills

The range of students' developmental and cultural backgrounds within an elementary environment is broad. Even at first glance, a first-grader looks small compared to a student who is ready to transition to junior high. It is imperative that group leaders are aware of and knowledgeable about the many developmental, cultural, gender, and other differences among students. First, it is a good idea to have a knowledge and awareness of students' backgrounds (see chapter 10 in this text for additional information on multicultural counseling). Because no student or group of students will align with a textbook case of "culture," counselors should be open and curious when working with all students. Even though two students are in the same grade, are the same age, and come from the same cultural background, they are not the same. Each child is unique, and group leaders who are curious about her or his students will ask questions that show an awareness of developmental ability and culture. Curiosity often is formed in questions: What is life like in your family? How do you see others in your community solving that problem? How are we, as group members, the same and how are we different? Both similarities and differences need to be honored.

Some recommendations for group leaders regarding developmental and cultural sensitivity are that many students may benefit from the group's confidentiality. If students have felt marginalized because of their differences, they may be hesitant to share if they fear shame. Emphasizing that what is said in the group is private may help create a safe atmosphere where students feel safe. For example, some children of New Americans may fear that their caregiver could be sent back to his or her country of origin. Leaders need to speak to the fact that what students share will not jeopardize immigration status because what is said is confidential.

Additionally, group leaders need to proceed slowly when building relationships with the students. Often, students who have developmental differences or are from the non-dominant culture may need time to build trust and respect for both the group leader and other group members. Well-intentioned leaders, whether from a similar or different heritage than that of their students, may want to rush into the working stage, but students may need time to experience the cohesion of the group. Moving slowly also may help the members of the group be able to process information that is presented differently than how they hear it in class and/or in a different language than is spoken at home.

Working With Challenging Students

When collaborating with teachers, administrators, and staff, you may be referred to some of the more challenging students. These are the students who may excessively fidget, not pay attention, and not be prompt. Of the upmost importance is to think about these students' strengths. Even if it is one small thing, what does the student do well? How has she tried to connect with others? What did he do that made someone feel a bit more comfortable? Build a trusting, caring bond with the student. Difficult students may feel as if adults only get them in trouble. Group leaders should define their role as someone who supports, encourages, and guides students into making healthy choices. You may have to return to the facilitation skills found in chapter 5 (e.g., reflecting; being empathic; challenging faulty or unhealthy thinking/behavior while guiding students to take responsibility, share with others, and allow others to have a voice in the group). What's more, for younger students you may have to set up a token economy (see behavioral theory in chapter 2) to encourage participation by reinforcing positive behavior.

LOGISTICAL ISSUES

Making small groups work in elementary schools is a balancing act. Often school counselors are caught off guard when they have to resolve a myriad of conflicting interests and concerns in the school. In particular, elementary schools can be complicated places to navigate when running groups, for school counselors must attend to the varying strictures of school policy and procedures as well as to staff and caregiver concerns. Here are some skills to help you work though major logistical issues.

Collaboration

Effective group leadership requires strong collaboration skills (ASCA, 2005). In particular, school counselors must carefully partner with parents/caregivers, teachers, and other educators who will refer to and support students in the group. One way to connect with these significant others is to send to each one a brief note informing them of the upcoming group experience. Here is an example of such a note a practicing school counselor emailed to the teachers in her school:

> Hello wonderful teachers! I will begin a conflict resolution group in the next 2 weeks. I would like to take a strength-based approach to dealing with anger! We will learn and practice some communication skills (such as "I" statements) and

we will have a chance to develop a plan for constructive ways to cope when angry. At this point, I'm thinking that Wednesday during lunch may be a good time, but I'm open to suggestions! The groups will be 45 minutes long and will be a total of 8 weeks. Would you PLEASE suggest a few students you think would benefit from the group? Also, will you suggest alternate times if Wednesday at lunch doesn't work for your schedule? If I don't hear from you in a week, I'll stop by your classroom for a brief chat. My goal is to support you and the students with these difficult issues! Thanks ☺

Primary components of this letter should include the following: Inform the teachers of the topic (e.g., conflict resolution), of the proposed student outcomes, and that you use a strengths-based approach to the group process (e.g., the group will be solution focused and aim for positive responses). Moreover, the communication should suggest a group start date while at the same time asking for their feedback, stating the parameters of the group (e.g., time of day and number of weeks the group will meet), and soliciting potential student referrals. Allow for both written and verbal feedback. By stating that you will take the responsibility to connect with the teachers, it may open the door for you to obtain both referrals and additional background information on the students. As you may already know, at the elementary school level teachers spend most of the day with a particular set of students, making them excellent resources for learning about the students in the group. We have found that if the initial email does not suggest that a personal contact will follow the letter, it is harder to gain the support of teachers or others who may refer potential group members.

Another way to attract students is to advertise the group. You may be able to alert students in the morning announcements or you might post flyers in the hallway. Hopefully you can make signs that are easy to read, creative, and amusing. Many no-cost, editable templates are available (e.g., see Figure 6.1) and can be found on Microsoft's web page (http://office.microsoft.com/en-us/templates/). Students should be able to leave a confidential note for the school counselor if they are interested in the group. In the announcement in Figure 6.1, notice the group name is "catchy" and that FISH stands for "Friends Involved in Support and Help."

Group Membership

After connecting with teachers, staff, administration, and students, group members will need to be selected. You may have more referrals for the group than you can accommodate. For elementary school, groups work best when there are five to seven group members. If there are fewer students, it is hard to share multiple ideas, and if there are more, it is likely that the group may be too "active" to be productive.

Conduct a pregroup interview with each student as a way of selecting the most appropriate group members (M. S. Corey et al., 2010; Greenberg, 2003). In other words, this individual time with the students allows the group facilitator to connect with them and to assess if they would be suitable for the group. During the "interview," the counselor looks for those subjective characteristics that will balance out a group. For example, if one member is shy, adding another member who is more outgoing could be beneficial. The students who express concerns about the rules may find a better fit in

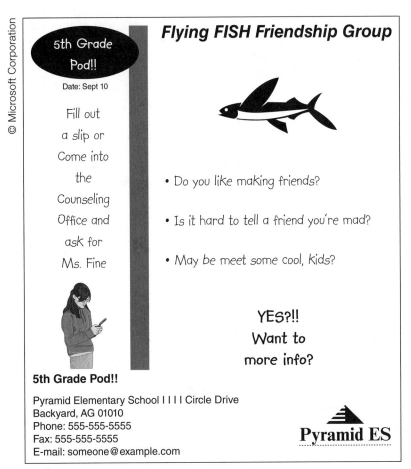

© Microsoft Corporation

5th Grade Pod!!

Date: Sept 10

Fill out
a slip or
Come into
the
Counseling
Office and
ask for
Ms. Fine

5th Grade Pod!!

Pyramid Elementary School I I I I Circle Drive
Backyard, AG 01010
Phone: 555-555-5555
Fax: 555-555-5555
E-mail: someone@example.com

Flying FISH Friendship Group

• Do you like making friends?

• Is it hard to tell a friend you're mad?

• May be meet some cool, Kids?

YES?!!
Want to
more info?

Pyramid ES

FIGURE 6.1 | Elementary-level small-group announcement.

other services provided by the school (e.g., individual counseling, referrals, etc.). There is no "perfect" way to select members who will gel and form a dynamic group; however, pregroup interviews can help a leader choose the students who may benefit most from the intervention and build a strong group process. Table 6.1 provides sample pregroup interview questions for students in late elementary school grades. These questions naturally will need to be adjusted for younger children.

After the student expresses interest in being a group member, engage his or her caregivers in the process. Various state and district laws govern the amount of input caregivers have when their students are involved in school-based small groups. Professional school counselors are called on to collaborate with guardians and other significant adults (ASCA, 2005). Family and key adults in the child's life can be resources as a counselor plans and leads a group. Inviting others into the process of developing a group can help the leader consider diverse viewpoints as he or she plans activities and conversations to have with the students. One way to build a bridge with caregivers is to call them and to initially share some of their student's strengths. After goodwill is established, address the issue of parental/caregiver consent for the daughter or son to participate in the group experience. Following this personal contact, send home a permission letter to be signed. Figure 6.2 is an example of a permission letter for elementary school students.

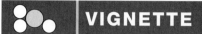

VIGNETTE

Elementary School Group Counseling Vignette—"I Can Kids": An Anger Management Group for Third-Grade Students

When working in an urban elementary school, Michele, a professional school counselor, found that student anger outbursts were a concern of students, teachers, and staff. She saw that many of the third-grade students were unable to express or handle their anger in a constructive manner. The counselor was interested in teaching alternative methods to deal with anger that would help these students become more successful in school while giving them skills to establish lasting friendships with others. Thus she designed "I Can Kids" to help third-grade students build positive anger-coping and communication skills in a small-group setting. She consulted with teachers to gather referrals, led pregroup interviews, and collected signed permission forms. The following description outlines the procedures and sessions, including the first session, early stages (Sessions 2 and 3), middle stages (Sessions 4 and 5), and the later sessions (Sessions 6 and 7). The intent of this overview is to provide group leaders a glimpse into the process of facilitating groups at the elementary school level. Although the illustration is for an anger management group, the process described could be applied to almost any group topic.

Group Goals

The central aims for this group included:

- establishing rapport with the students;
- providing a safe environment to explore their ideas, feelings, values, attitudes, and hopes;
- promoting awareness that anger is normal;
- raising children's understanding of why certain behaviors are unacceptable;
- teaching children strategies to choose from when they are angry; and
- encouraging honest expression and exploration of anger and its consequences.

Group Procedures

There were seven group meetings lasting approximately 45 minutes each. During each session, the general format included:

- welcoming the members;
- reviewing group rules by having members read and explain one rule;
- briefly summarizing the preceding session and emphasizing any concepts taught;
- group discussion;
- activity or several activities;
- round of sharing; and
- a closing activity.

TABLE 6.1 | Sample Pregroup Interview Questions (Upper Elementary Age)

Pregroup Interview Questions (Upper Elementary Age)

- Hi! My name is Ms. Kennedy, and I'm planning to get together some kids to talk about what they can do when they are mad. What do you think about being in this group?

- In this group, I would like everyone to share. Is this something you would be willing to do?

- Everything that you hear in the group is private and you must promise not to share what you hear from a group member with anyone outside the group. You could tell the people you live with what you said, but you should not tell them what another group member says. Would you have a problem with this?

- A member of a group is expected to try to help the other members of the group. Would you be willing to help others who are in the group?

- The group will meet seven times and I would like you to come to all the meetings on time. Is this something you would be willing to do?

- If you are a member of the group, you may have to miss some classes. Of course you would be excused from class by your teacher, but you will be expected to make up any work you miss and turn in all of your assignments. Would you agree to do all of your homework and make up any work that you miss?

- In order to be in the group, your guardians have to allow you to be in the group. You would have to take a permission slip home and ask them to sign it. Do you think this would be a problem?

- What questions do you have?

Group Evaluation Procedure

A pre- and postgroup questionnaire assessed students' progress (see Figure 6.3). Informal assessments included the group leader's observations of members' behaviors and openness to share in the sessions. Collecting data from the groups aligns with ASCA's (2005b) directive for professional school counselors to provide data-driven services to students. It also encourages school counselors to reflect on what works with the students they serve and provides talking points so counselors can share with administrators on the effectiveness of their interventions. For elementary students, keep the surveys simple. For younger students, counselors may have to read questions aloud and help student fill in their answers. A useful way to introduce the evaluation survey to group members is by saying that "this is not a test and there are no right or wrong answers." The counselor may tell the elementary students that "the best answer is the one that you think fits *you* the best!"

Content of Group Meetings

Here the sessions are briefly described.

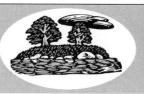

Courage Creek Elementary School

Date

(Address)
(Phone)

Dear Parent/Guardian:

Your permission is requested for [name of student] to participate in a school-based group experience on [Group Topic] conducted by [School Counselor] at [Name of School].

The small group will run seven weeks, meeting on Wednesdays for approximately 45 minutes during lunch and noon break/recess time. The group includes five other students. The group is entitled [Name] and will include discussion about [Goals].

Your student will have the opportunity to learn about themselves and others. Each student will be encouraged to participate; however, this is a voluntary group and the student may choose to not to participate or drop from the group at any time. I would like for each student to attend all the group meetings, however. I will be available if a student needs to meet with me between sessions. [Name of student]'s teacher has been notified of this group and approves of him or her attending.

Because counseling is based upon a trusting relationship between school counselor and student, the group leader will keep the information shared by group members confidential except in certain situations in which there are ethical or legal responsibilities to break confidentiality. Examples are:

1. If the student reveals information about hurting himself/herself or another person.

2. If the student reveals information about child abuse or neglect.

Thank you very much for your cooperation. You can always contact me with any questions or concerns. I can be reached by phone (number) or email (address).

Warm regards,

Kris Kounselor

Elementary School Counselor

If you agree that your student can participate, please sign and date:

_____

Return to the counseling office by: [DATE]

GO BISONS!!

FIGURE 6.2 | Sample parent/caregiver permission letter (consent for daughter/son to participate in small group).

Session 1   For the first session, Michele welcomed the group members. She *introduced* herself by saying, "Hi, I'm Ms. Kennedy and I'm glad we can spend some time together. I'm excited to get to know you. One of the things I like to do outside of school is play

Sample Elementary School Group Evaluation Survey

Name _____ Date _____

Instructions: Read each sentence. Put a circle around the number that shows how you feel right now. Help yourself by being honest.

	1 = Almost Never	2 = Sometimes	3 = Almost Always
1. My anger gets me in trouble.	1	2	3
2. Sometimes I think I am angry all the time.	1	2	3
3. There are some ways to be angry that are OK.	1	2	3
4. I can relax whenever I want.	1	2	3
5. I never feel just a little angry, I only feel a lot angry.	1	2	3
6. Sometimes I get so mad I don't know what to do.	1	2	3
7. I know how to avoid fights.	1	2	3
8. I can deal with bullies/people that tease me.	1	2	3
9. I have my temper under control.	1	2	3
10. I now can say things to someone without getting upset.	1	2	3

(Note to group leaders: Administer this form pre- and postgroup experience to all children. If useful, share aggregated data with teachers.)

FIGURE 6.3 | Sample pre- and postgroup evaluation survey.

basketball, softball, and soccer. I would like to know from each of you what is a game you like to play ...." This icebreaker helped build rapport in the group and was a fun way to get the group started.

After the students said their names and the games they liked, the counselor reminded them of the *group's purpose.* She explained that getting angry is normal and that students can choose healthy ways to deal with anger. Then she described some of the activities that they would be doing during the sessions (e.g., talk with each other, role-play, games, and worksheets). Michele informed the students that during each session they could earn tokens for positive behavior, and if a student had five tokens, he or she could pick out a pencil. The students began with three tokens during this first session, and the only rule was that if a student touched the tokens during the session, the student would lose them. During the next few sessions, the students started with two, one, and then zero tokens.

Next, the leader collaborated with the students to establish and write down *the group rules.* They talked about confidentiality, rules, and consequences. Michele stated what she believed helped make groups work (e.g., taking turns talking, not sharing outside the group, etc.) and asked specific questions regarding the group rules. For example, she asked, "What should happen when a rule is broken?" The members noted that if one student is mean to another during the group, this student should have to apologize. Michele asked another probing question: "What would happen if a group member broke confidentiality?" The group decided to see how much of the trust was broken if that happened. If the group was really hurt, then the person who broke confidentiality could be asked to leave the group. Michele and the students wrote the rules on poster board so they could read them during the opening of each session.

To close the initial session, group discussion was facilitated where the leader used her counseling skills such as paraphrasing, empathy, clarifying, and warmth. She asked the members to reflect on questions such as these: "What was it like for you to be in group today? Who else felt that way?" After linking the common themes shared by members, the leader thanked them for coming and participating and reminded them of their next meeting.

Early Stage: Sessions 2 and 3   For the second and third sessions, the leader again welcomed the members to the group by thanking them for attending. The group rules were revisited by having a group member read over the rules with another member, briefly explaining what each meant in his or her own words. After the rules were refreshed, the leader asked the students what they remembered from the previous session(s). A group facilitation technique called a "go-around," where each student had a chance to answer what they remembered from the last session, was conducted. In an attempt to build group rapport, identify feelings, and relate to one another, there were questions and comments from members regarding what had happened during the week. Although Michele had prepared several activities, she spent time in these early sessions helping to facilitate conversation. Because she was working with elementary students, she promoted conversation by having a range of developmentally appropriate, hands-on activities from which to choose. Some of these activities included:

- **Body outline (adapted from Hitchcox, 2005):** Students were given a sheet of paper with an outline of a body. On it, they were instructed to color in parts of their body where they feel anger. This activity highlighted awareness of the students' anger feelings. Also, students were asked to share where they felt anger, and the group explored the similarities and differences in their responses. After some of the group members shared, the leader inquired, "Does anyone notice someplace new that they could feel an angry feeling?" The counselor modeled how to share using self-disclosure by giving the example of clenching her jaw and saying that her mouth felt tight when angry.
- **Worry balloons:** The group was shown a balloon, indicating that sometimes being worried is like putting a breath of air into the balloon. Modeling, the leader told the group that she worried about doing well in her upcoming soccer game, and then took a big breath and blew it into the balloon. A small balloon was distributed to each of the group members. She asked them to take turns and say something that worried them. After each member shared, he or she would put a breath into the balloon. The leader then asked, "What do you think might happen when the balloon gets really full?" The group shared that they thought it could explode. Michele agreed, stating that "sometimes we get angry after a lot of worry or other emotions build up inside us." The leader also linked together the students' answers and allowed each student to take a turn. She blocked a verbose student who wanted to talk after each group member shared. The group discussed what they could do to help release some of the air out before the balloon popped. Possible solutions were explored.

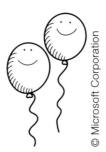

© Microsoft Corporation

During the early stages of the group, the leader noticed who sat next to whom. She noticed that two students sitting adjacent to each other often chatted when others were sharing. In Session 3, Michele requested the group members to sit next to someone whom they had not sat next to before. Also, the leader was aware of her need to block a student who attempted to answer all the questions first. The leader affirmed that the vocal student was a good participant and redirected by being curious about what everyone was thinking. She asked that a student who had not shared yet take the first turn when answering the next question.

In order to close the early-stage sessions, Michele asked, "What is one thing that you either learned or remember about today's talk?" She thanked the students for coming. The students counted their own tokens and were given a pencil if they had earned five chips. At the beginning stages of the group, the students tended to be competitive about the chips. The leader discussed how other members might feel if they were teased about not getting chips. In later stages of the group, the members had built empathy and, often, would help each other earn chips or congratulate each other when they received at least five chips.

Middle Stage: Sessions 4 and 5   As the group was forming and Michele was getting to know the group members, she realized that the students had very diverse ways of coping with anger. The leader's awareness of these differences led her to offer a variety of disparate examples when talking about how anger feels and what happens when people become angry. She empowered the group to provide examples that were specific to them and helped them focus on their strengths when coping with anger. The group dynamic was established by the leader normalizing different anger experiences and helping the members learn from each other new ways to act when they felt angry.

Students at the elementary age require more direction when dealing with transitions within the session. Thus when Michele introduced an activity, she asked the members what they thought that they needed to be doing in order to complete the task. She clarified their understanding by joking about good and bad behavior. For instance, the leader asked if the participants should be jumping on the walls when they were working in a pair. Also, she would give small and specific instructions, such as requesting one student to read two sentences from the worksheet.

During these latter stages, the group should form a unified identity. The leader reminded them at the beginning of each session of the rules and norms, as well as pointed out their strengths and how much progress she had seen in the group and its members. Michele also reminded the group of their individual and group goals. With assistance from the leader, students supported each other by telling the group that they did not have to raise their hand if they had something that related to what someone else was saying. The leader encouraged members to further support each other, increasing the members' empathy and validation of one another. For example, each time a student would keep on topic, Michele would give that student a token.

To open the middle-stage sessions, the counselor would ask the students what they remembered from the last session, encouraging them to share what they had tried in between sessions and what had worked. Michele focused on the student's honesty instead of rewarding "good" behavior. Members were informed that it was "okay" to say that they tried something and it did not work or that they had forgotten to try a new skill. Michele facilitated as much discussion as possible, while also having activities to supplement the time.

Activities for the middle stage of the group included:

- **Anger options:** Students brainstormed what made them angry. For instance, one student was fuming when her sister went into her room and played with her toys. Michele asked all the students to close their eyes and imagine their own situations and think about how their body would feel (e.g., what their face would look like). After putting themselves in the situation, the students were asked to think about one way to deal with the situation that would help the anger without hurting anyone. Students explained their answers by stating they played basketball, drew a picture, wrote a story, or held a stuffed animal. Michele used her group communication skills to link the students' answers. She asked the group, "How are you feeling now about the angry scene you imagined?" and "What was it like for you to allow yourself to work your anger out without hurting anyone?" Additionally, the leader prompted the group to think about how they could use the ideas after leaving the group session.
- **Anger survey:** The counselor distributed a worksheet (Bierma, 2005; see supplement) and asked the group to answer all the questions honestly. After the group individually filled out their forms, she brought the group back as a whole to discuss some of the questions.
- **Small-group role play:** Choosing whom they would work with, the students formed groups of two (dyads). The leader passed around a hat, and one student from each group selected a role play written on a slip of paper hidden in the hat. The following are example questions: "What would you do if you went to get the new toy your friend gave you and someone's taken it from your desk?" "What would you do if you were wearing your new sweatshirt and someone spills their orange juice on it at lunchtime?" "What would you do if you did the dishes last night and now your guardian is saying it's your turn tonight, and your sister's grinning and you know that she knows it's her turn?"

After the group role-played, they shared about their experiences, and the counselor highlighted what worked to solve the problems, underscoring what the students said in the role play that helped express their feelings. Michele linked the answers by asking if other group members felt the same way. Students were directed to tell each other about similar feelings as the group learned new ways to release anger.

For the closing activity, Michele prompted the students to state something new they learned in the group that day. She prepared the following questions to facilitate discussion if the more general question did not get the students talking: "What did you learn about helpful and hurtful ways to deal with anger?" and "How do you feel about yourself when you use better ways to deal with anger and don't end up getting in trouble or hurting other people?"

The members were thanked for their attendance and participation using these words: "I am happy you all chose to be in the group. We had a good session today. I was pleased to see everyone participated." The students were further reminded of the next session's meeting time.

Later Stage: Sessions 6 and 7   As the sessions drew to an end, the leader noticed that some of the students were reverting to "old" behaviors of acting out their anger. Michele collaborated with the teacher and other significant adults in the students' lives to see if the behavior was changing in other environments or if the students were acting out mainly in group sessions. Michele normalized the group's feelings by stating that she knew it was hard to think about the group ending. Starting in the third or fourth session, the students were reminded they were meeting for only a few more times. By the fifth session, the group had a countdown to the last group. The students were empowered by informing them that they were in control of their actions; it was not just the group that helped them control their anger. Also, as needed, a plan to deal with anger for after the group quit meeting was designed, and it was helpful for the members to write their plan down for remembering after the group ended. At the end, a group discussion was held on what the students thought about the group drawing to a close.

The other issue that the leader was aware of during the late stage of the group was her own expectations regarding the group members' progress. She noted that some of the members did not seem to be applying the skills they were learning in group outside of the sessions. Michele fostered a discussion related to what made it hard to apply the coping management and asked the students what they thought she could do to help them. All suggestions were affirmed, while appropriate boundaries were maintained. This was done by reassuring them that she wanted to help them find the strength inside to help themselves. In addition, Michele was transparent in an appropriate way by stating that she was frustrated when she heard that some students in the school had struck or yelled at a peer. She asked the group what suggestions they could give these student to cope with the anger. Although Michele ended up referring some of the students in the group for additional support services, to avoid shaming or embarrassing them she redirected (via displacement) the conversation toward students in general.

To begin the last sessions, the leader informed the students about the plan for the day and described that session's reward (e.g., taking a group photo at the end of Session 7). Michele also fostered discussion by asking, "What have you used outside of group that has helped you not make bad choices when angry?" Activities for the later sessions included:

- **Hang Time:** Michele passed out a workbook (Sink & Zuber, 2005; see supplement) and divided the group into dyads to fill out the pages. After about 10 minutes, Michele brought the group back together and they discussed various answers.

My Group Experience

Please circle the answer that best fits each question, like this:

Never	(Sometimes)	Every time

		Never	Sometimes	Every time
1.	Our group was fun to be at...	Never	Sometimes	Every time
2.	I learned something at group...	Never	Sometimes	Every time
3.	I felt like I could trust Michele...	Never	Sometimes	Every time
4.	I could talk about my feelings in group...	Never	Sometimes	Every time
5.	What we learned about handling anger will help me...	Never	Sometimes	Every time
6.	I felt like I could trust the people in group...	Never	Sometimes	Every time
7.	The thing I liked best about this group was...			

_____

_____

8. The thing I did not like about this group was...

_____

_____

FIGURE 6.4 | Pre- and postgroup evaluation survey.

- **Group Questions and Answers:** The leader had prepared questions listed on note cards. Examples included: "What would you say to the lunch monitor if she accused you of taking someone's cookies when you didn't do it?" "How would you ask your guardian if your friend asked you to spend the night after you were mean to your guardian that day?" "How would you ask a classmate to play with their new soccer ball after you told them they could not play with your jump rope?" After showing the students each card and asking students to read the question, Michele led a discussion about how the members would handle each situation.

The later-stage closing activities involved requesting each student to make a statement concerning something new he or she had learned in the group that day. Michele asked, "How can you deal with people who tease you?" "What does it feel like when you are not able to defend yourself with the right words?" "Does anyone else feel the same way?"

During the final session, the leader had the students fill out an evaluation (see Figure 6.4). Subsequently, the pretest and posttest assessment data were aggregated and shared with administration, teachers, staff, and caregivers (via a newsletter). Michele also used the data plus her own reflection on the group to prepare for her next conflict management group.

To recap, although the group experience required hard work for both the group leader and the members, this elementary school group was well conceived and engaging. Clearly, this type of experience shows how valuable a strengths-based group can be for younger students to establish solid relationships while learning more about themselves and others.

Reflection Questions

The following are some reflection questions for you to consider as you begin to work in the schools. Think about running a group at an elementary school.

- What strengths do you have that will help you facilitate the group at this level? What limitations are you worried about or feel you may need to work on?
- Elementary school groups require a great many focused activities to keep the group moving and engaging. What resources are available to help you guide the group sessions?
- Collaboration within elementary schools is important, and it is hard to balance how much to share and how much to keep private. Here are two scenarios to consider:
  1. Imagine having a conversation with a teacher of one of your elementary school group students. How can you balance sharing information about the group without breaking confidentiality?
  2. Elementary school parents may want to know about their children's progress in the group. How can you use the parents as a resource without going beyond the limits of confidentiality?
- Elementary school students like to share with friends. What would you do if your group members keep talking about the group outside the group?

CONCLUSION

If conducted properly and with adequate foresight and planning, elementary school small groups are effective ways to advance student developmental outcomes. Research cited in this chapter and in previous ones documents their importance to students and to comprehensive school counseling programs similar to ASCA's (2005a) National Model. As a Response to Intervention approach as well, professional school counselors have initial access to students who may otherwise go without any mental health services. Even as groups conducted at the elementary level are not designed to remediate deeper emotional and psychological disorders, they can be one of the first lines of prevention and remediation of potential long-term problems as well as augment the education of struggling learners. Psychoeducational and other content-driven groups are thus helpful to students who may need support with the precursor skills underlying academic competencies. Although logistically, elementary level groups present challenges to implement, in short, they are a vital service to accomplishing the educational mission of schools. Finally, you will find these groups quite enjoyable to facilitate, often seeing the immediate imprint on the students' psychosocial and educational well-being. Students are also largely appreciative of their experience, building some goodwill with the students themselves and potentially with teachers, staff, and the students' family.

CHAPTER 6 SUPPLEMENT

PUBLICATIONS:

- Bostick and Anderson (2009) illustrated the effectiveness of using small groups with third-grade students with social skill deficits.
- Khattab and Jones (2007) outlined an elementary girls group that highlights resilience and self-worth.
- Lopez and Bhat (2007) detailed leading a support group for third- to fifth-grade students with incarcerated parents.
- Seligman, Reivich, Jaycox, and Gillham.
- Villalba (2007) incorporated wellness into elementary school group work.

ONLINE RESOURCES:

- The America School Counselor Association has helpful books, tips, and programs for elementary school counselors: http://www.schoolcounselor.org/store_category.asp?id=46
- The National Center for Youth Issues has elementary-focused resources for anger, grief, tattling, and character education, among others: http://catalog.ncyi.org/
- The Penn Resiliency Project (http://www.ppc.sas.upenn.edu/prpsum.htm) is a group intervention for late elementary students that teaches "cognitive-behavioral and social problem-solving skills and is based in part on cognitive-behavioral theories of depression by Aaron Beck, Albert Ellis, and Martin Seligman." Although treating depression is beyond the scope of practice for school counselors, the outlines and techniques of this program may be helpful to practitioners when forming resiliency-based groups.
- Student Success Skills (http://www.studentsuccessskills.com/) is "an evidenced-based model that helps students develop key cognitive, social, and self-management skills."
- Research Press (http://www.researchpress.com/school-categories.asp) offers an excellent selection of books, games, videos, and activities for school counselors.
- Zenger Media has resources and curriculum for leading groups with younger students (e.g., career awareness, building caring schools, remarriage): http://www.zengermedia.com/c/k6guidance.html?s@ZOzsd72ZSZ.Fk

Sample Evaluation Tools

Anger Survey (Bierma, 2005)

1. How angry would you get if …   1 = not angry   2 = a little angry   3 = very angry

	1	2	3
a) Your parent punished you for something you didn't do …	1	2	3
b) Your parent punished you for something you did do …	1	2	3
c) Someone hit you in the eye with a stick by accident …	1	2	3
d) Someone hit you with a stick on purpose …	1	2	3
e) You saw someone be mean to your friend …	1	2	3

    f) You saw someone be mean to a stranger …   1   2   3
    g) A 1-year-old broke a favorite toy of yours …   1   2   3
    h) A 10-year-old broke a favorite toy of yours … 1   2   3
    i) Your best friend doesn't invite you to a party … 1   2   3
    j) A good friend doesn't invite you to a party …   1   2   3

2. How do you usually show you are angry?

    a) Scream and yell
    b) Sulk and pout
    c) Don't show I'm angry
    d) Other _____

3. How do you usually get over being angry?

    a) by talking about it
    b) by spending quiet time by myself
    c) by doing something physical, like running
    d) Other _____

Hang Time Survey© (Sink & Zuber, 2005)

What is each of these kids feeling? Write **one feeling word** in the box next to each picture.

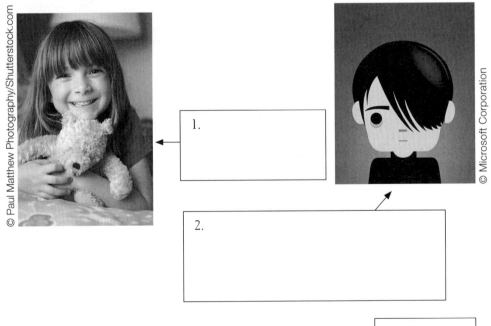

1.

2.

Go to next page ➡

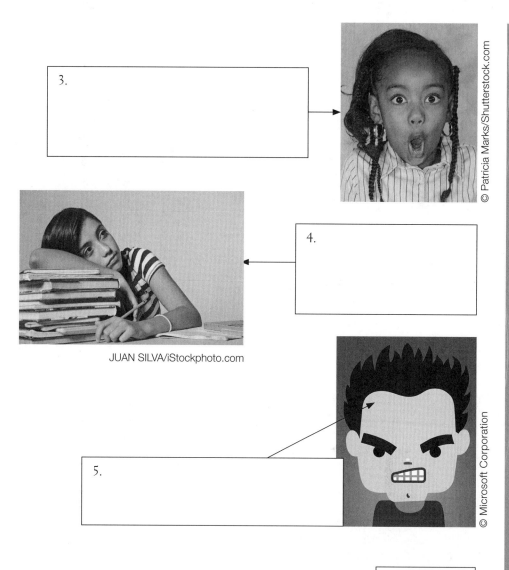

3.

4.

5.

JUAN SILVA/iStockphoto.com

© Patricia Marks/Shutterstock.com

© Microsoft Corporation

Go to next page →

Circle only the pictures of kids who are getting along well with each other.

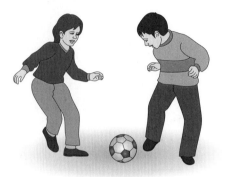
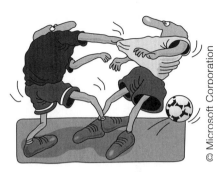

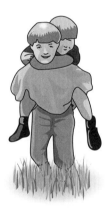

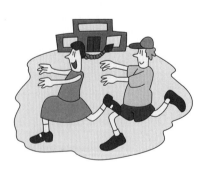
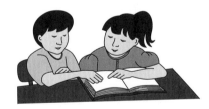

Go to next page ➡

Are these kids handling their anger well?

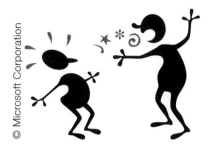

© Microsoft Corporation

Circle one answer:

Yes   No   Maybe

Why did you say yes, no, or maybe?

_____

_____

_____

Which of the following are good ways to help feel better when you're mad?
Circle **all** the best ways!

Hit someone

Calm down

Ask for help

Walk away

Yell at someone

Take a deep breath

**Go to
next page** ➜

☆ What are some of your personal strengths?

1. _____

2. _____

3. _____

4. _____

5. _____

☆ On a good day, what three feelings might you have?

1. _____

2. _____

3. _____

☆ What are three ways to show you care about someone?

1. _____

2. _____

3. _____

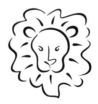

_____

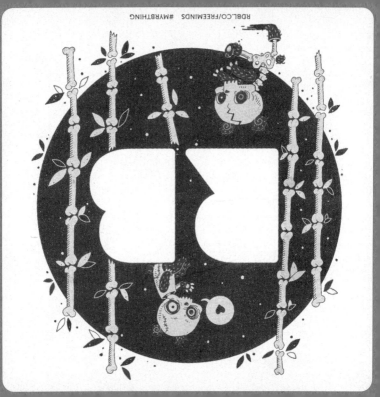

Groups for Middle School and Junior High School Students

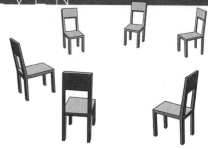

INTRODUCTION

The middle and junior high school years are often filled with emotion and drama. So much is going on physically, emotionally, and psychologically for early teens. It is no surprise that conducting groups for this age group can be quite an adventure. Aronson (2004) discussed the challenges of young adolescent group work, likening early teens to the mischievous protagonist in Sendak's (1963) classic book *Where the Wild Things Are*. Life can be a whirlwind of feelings, thoughts, and shifting values; the world is simultaneously experienced as curious, confusing, frightening, and wondrous. Probably the most constant element of these early teenage years is change.

This chapter begins with a brief discussion of the developmental issues germane to this age group. Next, guidance is provided as to how to successfully negotiate the logistical and practical considerations involved in running groups in middle/junior high schools. Best practice recommendations, potential group topics, and counseling skills particularly relevant to supporting early adolescents are covered. Before concluding, a concrete example of a middle school friendship group is summarized, including specific group topics and activities in the discussion.

DEVELOPMENTAL ISSUES

Middle and junior high school students are ideal candidates for groups that address a variety of pertinent developmental topics. Early adolescents need support as they anticipate career decisions, transition issues, social challenges, and academic hurdles. Professional school counselors who plan on conducting groups for adolescents should therefore review applicable developmental theories and research (see chapter 2 for an introduction). For example, you may recall from previous readings that multiple psychological theorists have addressed this perplexing developmental stage, characterizing it as a time when students struggle with what Erikson (1968) called "identity versus role confusion." Essentially, because adolescents are generally unsure of themselves, they spend time attempting to make sense of their experiences and worlds through self-questioning and reflection. Although perhaps not always openly voiced, early teens wrestle with such existential questions as, "Who am I and who will I become?" Obviously then, transitional issues are the primary theme for adolescents, and they should serve as

187

Anxiety of new school →elem to middle   middle →high

the major foci for group work. For example, groups might address the anxiety students experience as they consider moving from elementary to middle/junior high school and subsequently from middle/junior high to high school. Logistical issues such as navigating a new building, different lunchtimes, locker use, as well as changing classrooms and schedules can be intimidating. Moreover, social issues, including meeting new friends, concerns about bullies, fitting in, having new teachers, and trying out for sports, can be frightening.

Associated developmental tasks to consider when assisting this age group usually involve gender identification and role clarification, friendship/social skills acquisition, morality and personal values refinement, and the increased recognition of the opinions of others (i.e., becoming more "other centered"; Havinghurst, 1952, 1972; Power et al., 1989). For example, observant educators will notice adolescent changes in moral reasoning as many young teens are emerging from an egocentric view of right and wrong ("What will happen to me if I mess up?") to a wider, more socially cognizant perspective ("How will my behavior impact society?"). This population is also experiencing other challenges such as identity formation, developing self-esteem and autonomy, and learning about intimacy (Aronson, 2004). Familiarizing oneself with models of racial and cultural identity (e.g., Aldarondo, 2001; Jefferson, 2002; Kwon, 2001; Rowe & Atkinson, 1995; also see chapter 10) and spiritual formation (e.g., Kwon, 2001; Sink & Devlin, in press; Sweeney & Witmer, 1991) is essential to curriculum planning and the use of relevant group counseling techniques.

Individuals at this age often describe themselves as feeling lonely (Drucker, 2003). Students worry that they are alone in dealing with their experiences, whether they are related to issues of self-esteem, familial challenges, academics, or the like. Sharing in small groups helps to "normalize" what students are currently experiencing; that is, teens often discover the "universalizing aspect of group [work]" (Aronson, 2004, p. 174), where the interaction provides some reassurance that what an individual group member is working through is often shared by peers. As Akos et al. (2007) further explained, *universality* is a primary therapeutic factor in group work with early adolescents, whereby students learn by listening to others who are experiencing similar issues that they are not alone, nor unique in their feelings of hurt and pain, and can learn from others as to how to deal with the issue at hand. Groups also provide the opportunity to learn from each other (i.e., to appropriately socialize and to imitate) through the influence of peer modeling (Akos et al., 2007; Brigman & Earley Goodman, 2008).

With the increased pressure for school counselor accountability, efficacy issues related to group work with adolescents need to be addressed. Empirical support for school-based, small-group efficacy is well documented in the literature (see chapter 2; also Borders & Drury, 1992; Whiston & Quinby, 2009, for specific group topics and populations). Similar findings exist specific to middle/junior high school–age youth identifying the benefits of group counseling interventions for issues related to classroom behavior concerns (Myrick & Dixon, 1985), academics (Greene & Ollendick, 1993), and transition issues (Greene & Ollendick, 1993; Walsh-Bowers, 1992). Akos's (2003) study, for instance, revealed that 93% of fifth-grade students participating in "transition to middle school" groups reported a decrease in their concerns related to the transition process, and 100% reported that the group helped prepare them for middle school.

Group bene RT

To summarize, although further research is needed to fully understand students as they move in and out of this life stage, clear trends in adolescent development are now widely acknowledged (e.g., Blakemore, 2010; Crosnoe & Cavanagh, 2010; Doremus-Fitzwater, Varlinskaya, & Spear, 2010; Klimstra, Hale, Raaijmakers, Branje, & Meeus, 2010; Poulin & Chan, in press). Specifically, research conducted with adolescents documents significant changes in behavior (e.g., increased risk taking), cognitive skills (e.g., less concrete thinking), emotional regulation, familial roles, social understanding and expressions (e.g., friendships and peer groups), physiology (e.g., onset of puberty and brain functioning), morality, and spirituality (e.g., refining personal values and religious questioning).

Young adolescents are, therefore, ripe for small-group discussions and activities related to, for example, diversity, social justice, bullying, friendship, educational success, and behavioral concerns (Akos et al., 2007). This age group is also developmentally appropriate for more intentional career exploration, for they are extending their concept of self to include the world of work, where they begin to investigate various career options and related skills (Brown & Brooks, 2002). With this background knowledge in mind, small-group facilitation with early teens looks somewhat different from elementary school group work (see chapter 6). In this next section, we address the most important areas to consider as you plan, implement, and evaluate groups for middle school/junior high school students.

MIDDLE/JUNIOR HIGH SCHOOL GROUPS IN PRACTICE

Sample Group Topics

✳ Needs survey

As discussed above, most early adolescent groups cover topics that address developmental issues as well normal school and life concerns (e.g., transition, friendship, family, academic issues). Given the broad range of topics appropriate for this age group, you will need to focus on only the most needed ones. Usually school counselors conduct a needs assessment at least at the start of every other school year to ascertain which topics are most pressing as viewed by students, educators, and parents/guardians. Survey results are cross-tabulated to see where respondent perceptions overlap, and counselors tend to devise groups around the high-priority needs.

Furthermore, congruent with the National Model (ASCA, 2005a, 2005b), responsive services should be data driven (DeVoss & Andrews, 2006). Therefore, although recommendations can be made for the types of issues that many students experience at this level, it is pertinent to thoroughly assess the needs of the students at your school to accurately identify what concerns are specific to your population. The demographics and culture of your school will guide your group work as well. Some school populations are more prone to test anxiety and stress management based on community values of excelling academically whereas others may have a significant need for substance abuse and pregnancy prevention education for group work. Many school counselors find themselves in a rut of running the same groups each year due to comfort level and, in some cases, unwillingness to try new topics. It is crucial that school counselors

TABLE 7.1 | Sample Group Topics by ASCA's (2005a) Developmental Domain Appropriate for Middle/Junior High School Students

Academic/Educational	Career	Personal/Social
• English Language Learner/ Acculturation Issues • New-Student Group • Special Needs (Learning Disability/Behavioral Disorder/Special Education) • Stress Management • Study Skills/Organization • Test Anxiety/Test-Taking Skills • Transition to Middle School/ Junior High • Transition to High School	• Career Exploration • Defining Values and Interests • Exploring Personal Assets	• Anger Management • Bullying Prevention • Dealing With Peer Pressure • Diversity/Appreciating Differences • Familial Issues and Transitions (e.g., Step Siblings, Parent Divorce) • Cultural Adjustment Issues for ESL or ELL Students • Friendship/Relationships • Learner/Acculturation Issues • Grief/Loss • Self-Esteem and Assertiveness • Social Anxiety/Social Skills

are regularly connected to the school population and have their finger on the pulse of the school. School counselors may find themselves with a unique need given an international, national, community, or school tragedy or event such as September 11 or a suicide. On those occasions, school counselors can be a strong support in attending to student issues by facilitating small groups focusing on the specific needs of the school community. Grief groups can be conducted in response to a teacher's or student's death, a parent's military deployment, or a community tragedy (e.g., the death of coal miners trapped in a mine in West Virginia). Also helpful are groups to process student fears and concerns related to an act of school violence (Pérusse et al., 2009).

Table 7.1 provides a list of common group topics identified under the subheadings of academic, career, and personal/social developmental domains (see ASCA's [2005a] National Model). Note that there may be topics that individuals in middle and junior high school may face that are not included in this table. Not all student counseling needs are appropriate for group counseling or school counseling services. As indicated in chapter 4, group members must be screened to ensure that their needs are best addressed in group counseling rather than by a community mental health professional. Additionally, group leaders must be careful to address only group topics that are well within their scope of practice. Adequate supervision and training in group work is a necessity. Students who require group experiences that are more therapeutic in nature or where students may be at risk to themselves or others are best served outside of the school by a trained community counselor or therapist.

Skills Needed

Almost anyone who has assisted a middle or junior high school student will tell you that a sense of humor and patience are a must. Not only does humor help school counselors cope with the many challenges of working in the schools, research points to the benefit for students as well. The Humor Styles Questionnaire (HSQ) was used to study a nonclinical population, ages 12–15, to measure adolescent humor. The study found that scores on the HSQ were predictive of both depressive symptoms and adjustment (Erickson & Feldstein, 2007). Although not all of us have the wit of stand-up comedians, humor can be integrated into group work through the use of fun activities, icebreakers, role plays, and a willingness to allow yourself and students to be silly at times.

In addition to being able to look at the comedic aspects of life and education, the group leader at this level must be savvy about the obstacles that middle and junior high school students face and understand their impact on group work. Although chapter 5 expounds upon the specific skills pertinent to being an effective group leader, special considerations at this level relate to the needs of this age group. The tasks and skills previously discussed have different implications when working with students at the middle/junior high school level. This is an awkward age for many teens. For example, some students at this level go unnoticed, yet are in need of attention and support. What manifests as the class clown or a behavioral issue may be a student in need of support. The same behaviors that may frustrate educators in the classroom may be a student in need. It is important to be thoughtful about the behaviors exhibited and consider what might be going on in that student's life as well as how that behavior impacts the group as a whole. Students at this level are significantly influenced by peers, which can be a powerful force for group work if encouraged. Group leaders can be instrumental in encouraging students to move into a working stage (Corey et al., 2010), where they are a strong influence on the group process and each other. They can, for instance, facilitate the use of peer pressure to be a support, rather than a stressor for students. Aronson (2004) summarized important traits of a leader of an adolescent group in this way: "In addition to a very healthy sense of humor, the ability to provide consistency, stability, and constancy in the face of provocation and aggression is critical" (p. 176). In practice then, professional school counselors facilitating groups need to consider the leadership tasks in light of the developmental needs and challenges that this age group is experiencing.

Flexibility and Adaptability   Adams's (2008) appropriately titled article, "The Scary World of Middle School," captures the essence of how many students view this level of their education. It is an intimidating time for many, and group counseling has the potential to be a support if facilitated in a way that is flexible and adapts to the changing needs and concerns of middle school/junior high school students. Flexibility and adaptability are important not only in group planning and preparation but throughout the group process as well. During pregroup planning, effective group leaders are mindful of the needs of multicultural and diverse learners. For example, students with special needs may require accommodations, including an accessible group meeting location, interpreters, or a reduced group size. Group members whose culture values collectivism over individualism may respond more favorably to dyad/triad sharing or activities rather than individual sharing within the group. Group leaders should adapt to meet the needs of the group members in an effort to effectively meet the group goals and objectives. This may require a revisiting of group topics and activities if it becomes apparent that a change is needed.

Group Management   This age group is testing the limits as they move from childhood to adulthood, so group leaders need to be especially clear regarding the structure of the group and participation expectations. Group leaders will want to include group members in the formation of group rules as students have a strong desire for autonomy and exerting influence. On a more basic level, group leaders need to encourage participation while remaining generally on task. More challenging for the leader is to demonstrate flexibility and the use of advanced group skills in order to draw out those students who may be shy or feel embarrassed to share. Further, the skill of blocking is especially relevant with this age group for multiple reasons. For example, leaders need to manage and "cut off" students who tend to overshare personal or family information or dominate group discussion, leaving little room for the more reticent members to voice their issues and contribute to the group. Students at this age may need assistance figuring out boundaries and appropriate limits of self-disclosure. The student who shares too much may become embarrassed and withdraw or terminate from the group.

Linking and modeling appropriate behavior are two other key leadership skills when working with this developmental level. Affirming normalcy is so important at this age when students often feel isolated or that they are all alone in dealing with a particular issue. The group leader can encourage group members to share how they relate to what each other is going through and facilitate group support for each other. Similarly, members are often unsure how they are supposed to act in group. Early adolescents are especially sensitive to being the "odd duck" and doing something wrong. By modeling appropriate sharing, listening to others, or carefully choosing how an activity is presented to the group, leaders can demonstrate what is expected or acceptable for group participation.

By middle school/junior high, most students have experienced the devastation of betrayed confidence. Feeling emotionally safe is an important need for this age group; as such, effective group leadership always emphasizes the importance of maintaining confidentiality. Leaders can help encourage confidentiality by allocating time during pregroup interviews and group meetings to make it clear that confidentiality is a member expectation and identifying possible consequences (perhaps decided by group members) for breaking this rule. Leaders should model the "what's said in group, stays in group" mantra and explicitly share the limits of confidentiality and how such situations would be handled. For example, the group leader might explain that group topics may be shared with teachers or parents but group content would not. The group leader could share how an inquiry by a parent, principal, or teacher would be handled. When limits of confidentiality are discussed, leaders need to inform the members that if something is shared in the group that would warrant a report, they are required to divulge that concern to a relevant person outside of group (e.g., administrator, parent). Specifically, members should be informed that the group's confidentiality policy will not apply if an issue related to student safety arises (i.e., harm to self or others). Should a subpoena be served involving a group member, this issue is discussed with the student, his or her caregiver/guardian, and the school administrator. In the event that confidentiality must be sacrificed, group leaders should talk to the affected student individually prior to sharing the concern outside of the group.

Another aspect of emotional safety to be considered is conversation and actions within the group. Group leaders have an ethical responsibility to attempt to maintain a secure environment for group participation (see chapter 4 for details). A leader may need to block or redirect group members who are not demonstrating respect or are being hurtful toward others. The leader may choose to address this individually with the offender after the meeting or during the group process by asking the other members what they thought of the offender's actions or comments. Also, if the leader feels the recipient/target of the offensive words or actions would be comfortable, the leader may ask the student how it felt to be the recipient of what was said or done. How this is handled is largely decided based on the group members and dynamics. How a situation might be addressed during the first meeting where group members are just beginning to get to know each other may be very different from how a situation might be addressed after members have progressed to a working stage and are able to share openly and challenge each other.

Equitable Treatment   Group leaders can be intentional about attending to the needs of historically underserved students in their school by running small groups for students of color; gay, lesbian, bisexual, and transgendered youth; or lower SES (socioeconomic status) students to address barriers to learning and provide support (Pérusse et al., 2009). School counselors must reach out to students with special needs—a population often overlooked regarding group membership (see chapter 9). Chapter 10 elaborates on the importance of group offerings specific to the needs of multicultural populations as well as groups focused on advocacy and diversity appreciation.

Logistical and Public Relations Issues

From their personal experience, some readers may consider the elementary years as the most "group-friendly" level for school counselors in terms of planning, as secondary schools have added layers to negotiate, such as the drive for academic rigor, achievement testing, after-school sports, and class scheduling. Nowadays, in the age of high-stakes testing, many teachers and parents are less than enthusiastic about consenting to their students missing class time in order to participate in small groups. Nevertheless, groups must be included as a responsive service for middle and junior high school students. Although all three of the authors have conducted and enjoyed groups at each level, we consistently find groups with young teens to be the most eventful. Whether it is attributed to the "raging" hormones or social pressures, there is no denying that there are many variables consider. As such, this is an ideal grade level in which to conduct a variety of groups that attend to personal/social, career, and academic issues.

This leads to the vital issue of public relations (PR) work for professional school counselors whether they are operating from a comprehensive school counseling program perspective or not. Middle/junior high school counselors must educate faculty, administration, staff, and parents/guardians regarding the role of the school counselor

Small groups starting this October!

1. **High school and beyond** (we'll be exploring life in high school and even college or technical school)

2. **Girls' GO Group** (Young women!! Do you want to discuss your concerns? Here's a place for you.)

3. **School survival skills** (Okay, be honest, school isn't so easy for some students; want to talk about it and do better??!!)

Want to find out more about these six week small groups?? Just come to the Counseling Center at lunch or after school. No prior experience necessary! Give a group a try!

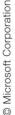
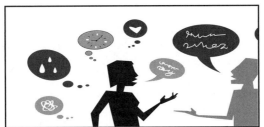

Middle Valley Junior High
COUNSELING CENTER

FIGURE 7.1 | Sample promotional flyer announcing upcoming small groups.

and the importance of group work. School counselors can lean on ASCA's (2005a) National Model to inform school and community members about the preventive focus of school counselors and how small-group counseling fits within this model. Collaboration with classroom educators and other school staff will help counselors find the most suitable way for small groups to meet students' academic, personal/social, and career developmental competencies (see Anderson, 2009; Beesley, 2004; Clark, Flower, Walton, & Oakley, 2008; Marlow, Bloss, & Bloss, 2000; Rowley, 2000; Shoffer, & Briggs, 2001; and Simcox, Nuijens, & Lee, 2006, for additional discussion regarding collaboration in middle/junior high schools). A sample PR flyer for group offerings is shown in Figure 7.1. Other logistical concerns counselors will need to think through include student composition, timing of groups, how long the groups will last, and so on.

Composition   School counselors should exercise caution when considering group composition. It may work well to include members from different grades if students are similar in maturity level. Extreme differences in intellectual ability, comfort in social situations,

TABLE 7.2 | Group Composition Considerations for Middle School/Junior High Groups

Group Composition

Mixed Gender
- Diverse perspectives are enjoyed.
- An opportunity is provided to model healthy interactions among girls and boys.
- There is an economy of resources (time, materials, space) when running one group together instead of separately.

Gender Specific
- Some students feel safer to share in single-gender groups.
- An opportunity is provided to model healthy interactions.
- Curriculum and activities may be more focused on gender.
- Gender-specific interests may be explored.

or maturity could lead to difficulties for more vulnerable students (Thompson & Henderson, 2007). Obviously, there are some specialized groups (such as transition to high school) that may be more appropriate for one specific grade. There are various perspectives on mixed-gender groups during the middle/junior high years. Anecdotal evidence seems to suggest that the focus is more easily maintained with same-gender groups, but this is not an absolute. Research indicates additional counseling benefits to females in all-female prevention-type groups (Chaplin et al., 2006). As with any issue of consideration relating to group logistics, it is always a good idea to assess the appropriateness of members during the pregroup interview process. After meeting with both males and females, you might decide that a mixed-gender group would work well or the interviews might lead you toward running two separate groups.

Table 7.2 lists a few considerations of mixed or gender-specific groups. Regardless of your decision, it is important to note that the potential for more than friendship interests in mixed-gender groups is not the only factor to consider. Romantic feelings or attraction may be evident in same-gender groups as well or may not be true for either, as many students are focused on friendships, academics, sports, or the arts at this point in their development. In any case, group cohesiveness is one of the most important tasks for groups with young adolescents to establish trust, create group norms, and generate a sense of mutual belonging (Akos et al., 2007).

Timing and Location   Other logistical considerations include when to meet, where, and for how long. School culture should be considered when choosing the time and location of your group. Although many middle school counselors are able to negotiate times during class periods to meet with their groups, others find it helpful to meet before or after school or during lunch. Transportation may be an issue if the group is scheduled to meet outside of the typical school day (before or after), as this age group most likely relies on school or parent/guardian-arranged transportation. Rotating the group meeting schedule is a good idea so that the same subject or class period is not missed weekly. In order to maintain confidentiality to the extent possible, it is important to meet in a location that is private. A classroom where a teacher remains to do some grading, a corner of the lunchroom or library, or other public location is not a good choice. Be aware of the windows and doors of the selected meeting location and make sure that they are closed to avoid distractions and ensure privacy. Many counselors also feel it is beneficial to use a "do not disturb" sign on the door, although be sure to avoid signs that say "group in session" or any wording to indicate the nature of your meeting.

Group Duration   The length of the group meeting time can be increased at this level. Unlike elementary groups, students at this age are able to maintain focus for a greater duration of time. Regrettably, many new counselors are apprehensive about meeting for an entire class period or block (e.g., 45 to 50 minutes). Often educators with limited or no previous group experience fear that they will not be able to fill this much time and that group members will spend a bulk of time staring at the walls or each other. To avoid this, new professionals often elect to meet for a shorter time period, such as 30 minutes. Although it is possible to conduct a relatively effective group session in a half hour, it can be problematic. Keep in mind that you will often need the first 5 or 10 minutes to get everyone together and situated—especially if you are meeting during lunch and students are eating at the beginning of group. You will also spend the last few minutes summarizing and closing the session and reminding group members of the number of sessions left and details of the next meeting. For school counselors who elect a shorter group time, this leaves very little opportunity for activities and discussion. We encourage each group leader, if able, to utilize a 45- to 50-minute time frame for your group. After years of running and teaching group counseling courses, we have yet to hear a preservice school counselor complain about having *too* much time during his or her group meetings. Regardless of the concerns or fears you may anticipate about your first few groups, the time does pass quickly.

Table 7.3 provides a typical time schedule for a middle/junior high school group session. Keep in mind that the first and last group meetings may look significantly different as you allow for more time for creating group rules or summarizing the group experience and facilitating closure. Also note that this is intended to be a guide, not a rigid schedule. Group needs may arise that encourage an extension of one or more group activities or discussions or a truncation or deletion of another.

Collaboration   This topic was mentioned earlier, but collaboration is so vital to successful group leadership that it should be addressed more in depth. When it comes to partnerships with coworkers in a school, it really is the small things that count. Classroom educators are eager to understand the benefits to students regarding small-group participation. Chapter 2 provides extensive evidence for why groups are conducted in school settings. We encourage readers to peruse this information before approaching your colleagues on running groups in the school. Having some research evidence to back up this responsive service is always a good practice.

Once educators understand the advantage to the student and the potential indirect impact on academic success, many will become a supportive ally in the establishment and continuance of small groups in schools. What may seem on the surface as unnecessary trivialities are actually important to consider when collaborating with school staff

TABLE 7.3 | Typical Time Schedule for Middle School/Junior High Group Meetings

Group Phase (Time Allotted) and Content

Opening (5–10 minutes)
Use this time to welcome students to the group session, briefly check in to see how students are doing, and introduce the group meeting topic for the day. You may utilize an icebreaker activity such as "fist to five," where each group member indicates how he or she is feeling that day through a hand signal of a fist (not a great day) to showing all five fingers (great day) or anything in between.

Activity (10–15 minutes):
This aspect of the group meeting focuses on a discussion, activity, or experience addressing a group objective. If the group topic is friendship skills, this may consist of breaking into dyads or triads to talk about what qualities are important to group members in a friend, completing a questionnaire related to friendship issues, or role-playing various friendship/conflict situations with the group members. Consider this part of the group meeting the "lesson."

Process (10–15 minutes)
Use this segment of the group meeting to discuss what group members learned during the activity or ask questions. When questions are directed to the group leader, the group leader can redirect the questions back to the group by asking what others think of the question or if anyone has an idea about how to respond to the question. The group leader can link responses by making comparisons to when students may have felt similarly about a situation or aspect of the activity.

Closing (5–10 minutes)
This aspect of the group process is often overlooked or rushed due to inadequate time management, yet it is a key part of the group experience. During this time, members are asked to reflect on what they have learned and set goals for the next meeting. The leader may choose to share an activity that members can practice outside of group prior to the next meeting. A go-around could also be facilitated during the closing wherein each group member can share one thing he or she learned during the meeting and/or one goal that he or she would like to accomplish by the next meeting. Remember that this is a transitional part of group where students are preparing to return to class and academic expectations. If the group was a particularly emotional meeting, the leader will want to attend to any unresolved needs during this time to ensure that students are ready to transition back into the classroom. This may require that the leader follow up individually with a particular student if there is a need or concern that cannot be attended to briefly within the group process. This is also a good time to remind students when the next group meeting is and how many meetings are left.

and parents/guardians to make small groups a success at your school. The following are several key recommendations:

- Be sure to connect with classroom teachers and other school staff regarding a needs assessment of students at your school.
- Include classroom educators in the referral process for small groups.
- Because limits of confidentiality preclude the school counselors from sharing group progress unless there is risk of harm to self or others or a subpoena involved, ask

students what is appropriate (or if it is okay) to share with their teachers about their group. The counselors might preface this conversation with the group members by saying, "Each of your teachers gave me permission to run this group. They are excited about this opportunity in our school and are eager to hear how things are going. What can I tell them about our group, given our group rule of what is said here, stays here? Would you consider this an exception to that rule, given their important support?" It is important that the school counselor follow this conversation by explaining that details will not be shared, only what group members give permission to tell. Members need to know that group is a safe place to share.

- Remind classroom educators when and where group is being conducted. As with all school staff, teachers are very busy. A simple reminder (or two) is appreciated. Many school counselors find that placing reminder notes in teachers' mailboxes on the day of the group is helpful. Of course, an email reminder or having an office assistant come to the classroom with a note at the beginning of the period when the group is meeting is helpful to ensure that the teachers know where their students will be (or where they should be) during the particular class period.

- Let teachers know when the group is over. To illustrate the importance of this rec-ommendation, a middle school counselor recently explained what happened when she failed to notify the relevant instructors. A teacher approached the school coun-selor and asked how a group was going about 3 weeks after the group had ended. One of her students was participating in the group and the teacher was particularly concerned about this student's progress. In the initial discussions with the teachers, the length of the group was covered but somehow the teachers were not informed when the group was to end. The "creative" (and devious?) female group member had continued leaving the classroom during the group meeting time period, using the time instead for "social" time with peers (i.e., cutting class). Regrettably, her teacher thought she was still attending the group. Needless to say, when the teacher discovered the reality of the situation, she was clearly frustrated and a bit upset. The group counselor was visibly very embarrassed. Since then, notes to each teacher prior to the last group meeting reminding her or him of when the group was ending are distributed. A personal "thank you" note sent to each educator thanking him or her for supporting the group experience is always welcomed.

- Consider school culture and schedule when planning the logistics of your group. Do after-school groups tend to work best? How about lunch groups? If you plan on conducting the group experience during class time, is it possible to shift the times around from week to week to avoid having the students miss the same class each week? Sometimes this is more hassle than it is worth, but again positive PR is vital to successful group leadership

- Attempt to link your group with state and school learning goals. Although each state is relatively unique regarding what it calls or names its learning goals, it has them. In other words, emphasize that the state learning goals will be addressed in the group and share this fact with academic stakeholders when soliciting educators to refer students for group participation. School staff, parents, and guardians will be interested in how the group will support students' academic success.

- The aforementioned are time-tested recommendations that will hopefully encourage a positive experience running groups in middle and junior high schools.

A comprehensive "to do" list is not what we are intending here, but rather we provide suggestions as you initiate groups with early teens. We also encourage to you to consider in your planning and implementation the norms of that school (school culture) regarding group work. It may be that you must pave the way for this important intervention, or reshape the vision of small groups, given your predecessors at that school. Either way, all school counselors want and need the support of school staff and parents/guardians to help make small groups as effective as possible. How do school counselors use group exercises to foster middle/junior high student growth? This question is answered next.

Using Activities to Mobilize the Group Experience

In addition to using student pairs and threesomes (referred to as dyads and triads), sample practical vignettes, and role plays, there are a number of practical activities for groups at this level. Whatever exercise you choose, it is important to create "buy-in" from group members regarding the activity and how it relates to the larger group goals that they have committed to. You do not need to convince them; just briefly explain the link between what you are doing and group goals. You might choose to let the group share their perspective on the connection as well. The group leader might say, "We are here to learn about friendship—each of you has shared that it is important to you. Now, I would like you to pair up with the person next to you and take the slip of paper I am passing out to each pair. Read the vignette, talk to each other about friendship qualities that you are able to identify, and be prepared to share two of them with the group." After the group has had a chance to share, the leader might encourage members to think about the activity and what it has to do with the group goals. A go-around is then facilitated for members, allowing them to individually share about how they are feeling. Always be authentic, caring, and clear with expectations. Another good idea is to keep directions simple and share one directive at a time. You might notice in the example above that the group leader facilitates the activity and later comes back to discuss how it relates to the group goals instead of asking the pairs to do the activity and think of how it relates at the same time. These two directives are presented separately to avoid confusion or having students feel overwhelmed.

Popular culture provides fodder for rich discussions related to adolescent life experiences and has been utilized effectively for therapeutic purposes (Enfield & Grosser, 2008; Finamore, 2008; Iwamoto, Creswell, & Caldwell, 2007; McNulty, 2008; Oliver, 2007; Saldaña, 2008; Schlozman, 2000; Schmidt, 2009). Using books, music, television shows, movies, or related resources can be a powerful way to relate to this age group and may encourage group member participation. To illustrate a concept for group discussion, the group leader might choose to talk about a current movie or television series and how friendship, study skills, bullying, or other issues are evident in the example used. Be considerate of members that may not or choose not to have access to media by encouraging group members to share with the rest of the group lyrics of a song or the plot of a television show or movie prior to using it as part of a discussion or activity.

Art and music activities can be integrated into group work. You might ask students to draw or paint during group, make a collage, or write a poem or lyrics to a song (or rap) that is related to the group topic. For example, encourage students to choose a "theme song" to share with the group and explain how it relates to their life. One activity that has been used in the past with self-awareness groups is to have students make a "soundtrack" of their lives in which they choose songs that represent different stages in their lives as well as where they hope to be in the future. This could be either a "play list" written down or an actual music compilation.

Students, particularly female, seem to appreciate nonacademic "quizzes" as evidenced by the number of them published in various teen magazines. Group leaders can utilize such quizzes to encourage members to consider whether or not they, for instance, have engaged in bullying behavior, been involved in a controlling relationship, or have solid study skills—any topic relevant to group goals. This type of activity is particularly useful if the group leader makes it clear that the "quiz" will not be graded or turned in but rather used as background information for discussion. Group members should feel safe to answer honestly and free to share with the group what they are comfortable sharing.

It bears repeating here that group leaders should be aware of the types of challenges that middle and junior high school students are experiencing when considering the type of group (e.g., support or growth, skills based, psychoeducational groups) being offered. Knowing this information provides guidance for the leader as he or she plans group activities that work well at this age group. Although briefly discussed above and in chapter 5, recall that some activities are especially constructive for this age group, such as working in dyads and triads and using role plays or vignettes to discuss issues related to the group topic. Breaking students into smaller units allows them to first "test the social waters." Sharing for an audience of one or two makes opening up to the entire group a little bit easier. Group members can also present ideas as a dyad or triad creation rather than an individual thought or opinion, which often feels safer for group members. Using role plays or vignettes with fictitious characters regarding issues related to the group allows group members to discuss and share ideas about the topic without feeling as if it is personal or they are self-disclosing too much. Sharing about "Juan" being bullied or preparing for a future career feels less risky for some than telling about their own concerns and fears. Group members are often more likely to give genuine and much-needed feedback to a fictitious role-play or vignette character than a classmate or school friend. After all, "Juan" will not get mad at you for suggesting that he could make better relationship decisions. Keep in mind that although activities serve as an important catalyst to help move the group through the various stages of the group process, ultimately it is the helping relationship between the members and the leader that has the potential to impact the group in a most significant way. In short, catalysts are only one tool in the small-group counselor's toolkit. Use them carefully, ethically, and after much practice.

What does a middle school group really look like? Next, we overview an actual group conducted with early teens.

SAMPLE REAL-WORLD GROUP[1]

You may have noticed from Table 7.1 that the personal/social focus included quite a few potential topics. It is not uncommon for students at this age to struggle with how to make friends and how to be a good friend. Given this issue's prevalence, it seemed to be the logical choice for an example of small-group counseling with early adolescents. Our intention is to help guide you through the group-planning process.

---

[1]The authors appreciate the contribution of Richard Cleveland, elementary school counselor, Everett School District, Washington.

When facilitating groups for the first few times, many find it helpful to have a large three-ring binder or other organizational structure with which to keep track of each week's activities and materials. It should be said that it is highly unlikely that you will be able to cover all the material that you plan for several reasons: (a) Activities usually take longer than you expect, and (b) groups have a way of going in directions other than planned. For those of you who have a background as a classroom educator or are a planner by nature, you will need to take a deep breath, relax, and become comfortable with the notion that your group plan will serve as a framework only and that your group in the end may look very different from what you had intended. Most beginning professional school counselors include significantly more activities and discussion topics than needed, often finding that they used only half of what they had planned. Although a formal group proposal would be much more extensive, below is an example of a brief outline that would serve as a foundation for a more substantive group plan/curriculum.

Sixth-Grade Boys Friendship Group

Group Rationale   The counselor at Riverview Middle School has identified six Grade 6 boys who are "new" to the school. All of these students moved into the area either this year or toward the end of last year. Students were identified through the following means: teacher referral, parental referral, or counselor identification through interaction with the student.

Learning how to make and keep friends is especially relevant for sixth-graders, as they are new to Riverview. Making friends and having sustaining friendships will support their transition to middle school.

Group Objectives   Objectives for this group will be:

- to establish rapport and trust with students
- to create an environment where students feel comfortable sharing
- to teach basic friendship skills (i.e., making friends, keeping friends, etc.)
- to facilitate relationship between group members

Group Logistics   Six group sessions will take place on Wednesday afternoons from approximately 1:10 p.m. to 1:55 p.m. Initial meeting/interview sessions with individual students will begin the week of January 21st, and the first group session will take place January 28th.

Group sessions will take place in the school counselor's office. If for some reason this room becomes unavailable, group will take place in the testing room located next door.

Group sessions will utilize *Teaching Friendship Skills, Intermediate Version* (Huggins, Moen, & Manion, 1998), a part of the ASSIST curriculum.

Group Procedures   Group sessions will proceed in the following format:

- greeting, welcoming, visiting
- reviewing topics covered last session
- introduction of session topic
- activity/discussion

- review of topic learned
- closing, dismissal to class

Although flexibility within session meetings is to be expected, the only real departures from this format will be the first and last sessions. The first session will concentrate more on getting to know one another and implementation of an icebreaker activity. The last session will review all that has been learned and celebrate the growth accomplished by the group. The group's 6-week outline will be as follows:

Weekly Schedule

Week 1, January 28th
   Thinking, Feeling, Doing (Behavior)
   Lesson based on work of Smead (1995) identifying and exploring differences between thoughts, feelings, and actions.

Week 2, February 4th
   The Way to Show You Are a Friend
   ASSIST Lesson 3: teaching keys to good listening skills

Week 3, February 11th
   Giving and Receiving Compliments
   ASSIST Lesson 5: teaching how to give and receive compliments in a sincere manner

Week 4, February 18th
   Making a New Friend
   ASSIST Lesson 6: teaching six steps for initiating conversation with an unknown peer

Week 5, February 25th
   Being a Good Friend Isn't Always Easy
   ASSIST Lesson 7: learning and understanding how to deal with some of the common difficulties encountered in friendships

Week 6, March 3rd
   Wrap-Up, Review, and Celebration
   Review of skills and information learned and consideration of applicable domains (i.e., class, recess, middle school, extracurricular, etc.); celebration with fun food and games

Group Evaluation   Anonymous evaluation forms will be given to student participants to rate the group experience and the student counselor's performance. Separate evaluation forms will be distributed to the school counselor and individual teachers for group participants to assess any noticeable differences in student postgroup behavior. Table 7.4 is an example of a postgroup evaluation tool.

Postgroup evaluations should be developmentally appropriate. Language and response options will vary depending on the population being served. For example, an evaluation for early readers may contain a series of cartoon faces ranging from unhappy to happy in response to evaluation questions. For students who are more verbal, open-ended questions may be useful. The take-home point is that group leaders should

TABLE 7.4 | Sample Group Evaluation Form

Sixth-Grade Boys Friendship Group Evaluation

Circle the number that best represents your feelings right now.
I liked being a part of this group.

1	2	3	4
Strongly Agree	Agree	Disagree	Strongly Disagree

I felt comfortable sharing in group.

1	2	3	4
Strongly Agree	Agree	Disagree	Strongly Disagree

I learned how to be a better friend during this group.

1	2	3	4
Strongly Agree	Agree	Disagree	Strongly Disagree

I learned ways to deal with friendship problems during this group.

1	2	3	4
Strongly Agree	Agree	Disagree	Strongly Disagree

I would like to be a part of another group in the future.

1	2	3	4
Strongly Agree	Agree	Disagree	Strongly Disagree

What are two things you liked most about the group experience?

What are two ways to improve the group experience?

consider their audience when creating or using group evaluations to ensure that they are user-friendly and will elicit useful data to inform future group offerings.

SUMMARY AND CLOSING REMARKS

Facilitating groups at this developmental level can be rewarding both for the school counselor and for the student members, but the challenges of maintaining group focus and being productive are daunting. This chapter summarized the leadership steps needed to conduct effective middle and junior high school groups. Group logistical considerations, intervention strategies, and hands-on examples were overviewed.

Middle school and junior high students need assistance with a variety of issues relevant to promoting educational, social, and career success. For educators who have difficulty seeing the connection between students' personal/social challenges and their ability to focus on classroom lessons, this level can prove to be a wonderful example. Show us a student in despair over a recent relationship breakup or a family crisis, and we will show you one who is struggling to maintain attention in class. This is also an age group that may be beginning to think more seriously regarding the career or educational opportunities that await them after graduation. The reality of high school is beginning to set in, and many students realize that this is a key time to begin thinking of what interests them professionally and vocationally. On a similar note, this is also a time when some students begin to struggle academically. As with all levels, the stakes are high and students begin to feel the pressure. For some teens, academics came easy during the elementary years when classroom educators may have had a more directive pedagogy. As teachers encourage increasing autonomy in the classroom, some students struggle with balancing self-discipline and academic rigor. Thus educationally focused groups are timely.

Overall, groups facilitated in middle/junior high schools are useful ways to support academic success while also attending to the personal/social, career, and academic needs of students (Akos et al., 2007). School counselors have a rich and diverse spectrum of topics to choose from when considering what types of groups may be useful to this population, and students are often eager to participate. Transition is the theme for this age group—both academically and personally. Middle/junior high students experience transition to and from this academic level as well as personally as they transition from childhood to young adulthood. As indicated throughout this chapter, this time of transition can be scary for students, and group counseling provides a venue for peer and school counselor support.

CHAPTER 7 SUPPLEMENT

The following are useful references concerning small-group counseling for early teenagers:

Akos, P., Hamm, J. V., Mack, S. G., & Dunaway, M. (2007). Utilizing the developmental influence of peers in middle school groups. *Journal for Specialists in Group Work, 32*, 51–60.

Aydlett, A. E. (2006). *Dealing with deployment: A small-group curriculum for elementary and middle school students.* Alexandria, VA: American School Counselor Association. (Provides group curriculum for students who are experiencing loss of parent/ caregiver due to military deployment.)

Blum, D. J., & Davis, T. E. (2010). *The school counselor's book of lists* (2nd ed.). New York: Wiley. (See section on small-group counseling.)

Guindon, M. (Ed.). (2010). *Self-esteem across the lifespan: Issues and interventions.* New York: Taylor and Francis. (Addresses key issues relevant to group work)

Hughes, F. P. (2009). *Children, play, and development* (4th ed.). Thousand Oaks, CA: Sage. (Covers developmental issues from birth through adolescence.)

Lowenstein, L. (2006). *Creative interventions for children of divorce.* Toronto, Canada: Champion Press. (Small-group activities when working with students who are experiencing divorce.)

Portman, G. L., & Portman, T. A. A. (2002). Empowering students for social justice (ES^{2}J): A structured group approach. *Journal for Specialists in Group Work, 27*, 16–31. (Journal article with group counseling recommendations to promote awareness of social justice issues.)

Smead, R. (1990). *Skills for living: Group counseling activities for young adolescents.* Champaign, IL: Research Press. (Various group counseling activities are provided.)

Taylor, J. V., & Trice-Black, S. (2010). *Girls in real life situations, grades 6–12: Group counseling activities for enhancing social and emotional development.* Champaign, IL: Research Press. (Group topics and activities specific to female students.)

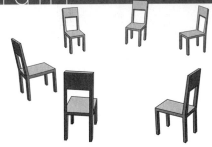

Groups for High School Students[1]

VIGNETTE

Case Vignette: High School Group for New Students

Ms. Brown had spent several years in her district as an elementary-level school counselor. She enjoyed leading groups, and had several predeveloped groups regarding
social skills, test-taking skills, and so forth. After being hired at South High School,
the principal notified Ms. Brown about several students whose parents had recently
emigrated from Latin America. The principal encouraged the counselor to put together
a group that would help connect these students to each other and to the school.
Ms. Brown conducted a literature search and found some applicable resources; she
wanted the group to be a safe place where students could share their own experiences.
Ms. Brown prepared her group proposal (action plan), leaving time for conversations
that the students could extend as long as they were productive. The main activity for
each group session was for students to draw from a basket a 3 × 5 card that had a
word (e.g., *family*, *marriage*, *school*, *college*, *friends*) written on it. The students would
take turns talking about the cultural differences between their home life and what they
experienced at school. Students could also explore what they wanted their futures to
look like in regard to these topics. Each group session would focus on one word or
theme. At first, Ms. Brown was uneasy at the thought of the group being less structured
than her other experiences. She even created some backup exercises just in case. But
after three sessions, the leader noticed that the conversation flowed freely and that
there were many rich discussions where the students were active and engaged. The
group wrapped up after seven sessions, and Ms. Brown found that there was enough
interest from other immigrated students that she ran several similar groups.

ADOLESCENTS AND SCHOOL-BASED GROUPS

The media often portray high school students as lost, disconnected, and full of teen
angst. Although it is true that adolescence is a time of physical and emotional growth
that can contribute to strife at school, at home, and with peers, the transition into young

---

[1]Practical content was provided in part by Jenna Bates, high school counselor, Bremerton High School,
Washington.

adulthood is also a time when teenagers begin to explore who they really are, who they want to be, and how they fit into their world (Rose, 1998). There is a trend in the adolescent development literature that suggests the importance of focusing on strengths and building assets in young persons' lives (Akos & Galassi, 2008; Benson, 2003; Lerner et al., 2005; Lerner, von Eye, Lerner, & Lewin-Bizan, 2009). The positive youth development literature fits well with the American School Counselor Association's (ASCA, 2005a) National Model and its call to see strengths, be preventive, and serve all students. Running small groups at the high school level is a productive way to meet these goals as the groups can be positive, preventive, empowering, and a healthy way for adolescents to build social skills (Bemak et al., 2005; Rose, 1998; Ripley & Goodnough, 2001; Wilson, 2003; Zinck & Littrell, 2000). Additionally, groups for higher-risk students may be implemented at the high school level (see Bruce, Getch, & Ziomek-Daigle, 2009, and Kayler & Sherman, 2009). This chapter explores the dynamics of high school small groups, suggests skills that professional school counselors need to lead small groups with adolescents, and presents a case study of implementing a study and social skills group in a high school.

USE OF THEORY AND RESEARCH TO GROUND HIGH SCHOOL GROUPS

Implementing theory and best practice research is important at all grade levels. Specifically, researchers have explored the efficacy and practice of groups at the high school level (Bauer et al., 2000; Bemak et al., 2005; Berg et al., 2006; Jacobs et al., 2009). High school group counselors need to be familiar with their students developmentally, culturally, and academically. For example, adolescents tend to privilege peer relationships, which can be used as a strength when recruiting high school students into a group. Most, if not all, high school students wonder about career, college, and life after graduation. Thus there are several best practice curricula that help high school students explore the world of career and work (see Ciborowski, 1994; Gibbons et al., 2006). Moreover, Bemak et al. advocated for counselors to champion causes and students that are often overlooked in traditional education. Group leaders can run groups for diverse students, including gay–straight alliances, underachieving performers, and students with learning and emotional differences. Deck, Scarborough, Sferrazza, and Estill (1999) noted that small groups benefit special needs students by bringing them together in a less academic environment and providing a space in which to teach and learn from peers. Arman (2002) added that small-group work that "employs cooperative learning, behaviorally based interventions, social skill training, and the use of play therapy are [sic] effective to assist developmentally different students to connect with peers, feel a sense of belonging at school, express feelings, and to form a self-identity" (p. 2).

Of course, high school groups are not just about academic and social skills; groups support the members in their emotional and interpersonal domains. Unlike with younger students, group leaders are afforded the opportunity to go a bit deeper with their group members by integrating counseling theory and techniques more fully into the group experience. High school students have the cognitive ability to process some of the more advanced skills that theories such as Gestalt, rational emotive behavioral therapy (REBT), and solution-focused brief counseling (SFBC) explore. For detailed descriptions of various counseling theories and techniques, see chapter 3 (also see Henderson & Thompson, 2010; Vernon & Davis-Gage, 2010). Situated within their theoretical context, we review next some of the key group counseling techniques used in high school groups.

What Groups Look Like in High Schools

High school students often ask reflective questions such as, "What am I going to do with my life?" These students are often thrown into a world where they are starting to consider many important questions such as being in romantic relationships, launching from their family of origin, and deciding what to do after graduation. All these questions come up during a time when they may have a heightened sensitivity to how others see them and how they view themselves. Taking a systems view (e.g., Bronfenbrenner, 1977), small groups may become a small world, a microcosm, of what is happening in the larger context of school, home, and community. High school students appreciate a safe place where they can find their voice, feel supported as they are making decisions about themselves and their relationships, and feel empowered to enter the "adult" world.

High school groups are both much the same as and very different from groups at the elementary and middle/junior high levels. Just as with the younger students, having an action plan and developmentally appropriate activities is fundamental to the success of the group. However, adolescents are capable of higher level thinking and have the ability to think critically about themselves (Rose, 1998). Thus group leaders assist members to explore issues at a deeper level, to encourage open and honest discussions around difficult subjects, and to feel empowered. Whereas activities such as worksheets, role plays, and assignments are of the utmost importance to keeping a group productive with all age levels, asking specific and thought-provoking questions to create a group conversation is the key when working with high school students.

Integrating counseling theory and technique is important when asking questions and leading conversations that create change. For example, when leading a career group about career options a counselor could have the students make a hypothetical budget based on a desired career. This reality testing is important in choice theory (Glasser, 2000). It is not just activities that can be steeped in theory. Counselors must have one ear bent toward theory while engaging the students in conversation. Students working on their budgets may exclaim, "I will *never* be able to afford a great car and a condo with a view if I pick this job." The leader informed by REBT (Bistaman & Nasir, 2009) would be able to hear the possible faulty thinking within that statement and respond, "You say 'never,' but I'm wondering, is it possible to set up a savings plan or revise other areas of your budget so you can afford a car and a home?"

Counseling experts recommend that small-group leaders avoid several pitfalls, including having too much "fluff" in their sessions, asking vague questions, and using activities that are too long or not meaningful (e.g., Jacobs & Schimmel, 2005). Any of these issues tend to derail the group experience and may even lead to high school students losing their enthusiasm and interest in carrying on. Counselors must support members with the openness and flexibility needed to create strong and positive relationships (G. Corey, 2008; M. S. Corey et al., 2010). Establishing a balance between group structure and leadership elasticity helps facilitate change. In short, secondary-level group counselors foster an environment where students can feel like they are giving their own direction to the group, but there are also clear organization and planned activities.

In order to give direction while letting the group form its own dynamic, leaders can ask thoughtful questions to empower students to set their own direction. SFBC (Brasher, 2009; Cooley, 2009; Nelson, 2010) has several techniques that could be used as icebreakers and activities. A leader may want to begin the group by asking a version of the miracle question, "If we were to have a great group today, what is something that you would be doing to make that happen?" This could help students focus on their goals and their behaviors, which should coalesce these unique individuals into a team. During group sessions, leaders may extend important conversations by asking about exceptions or inquiring how members can do more of a behavior that works: "Each of you has stated that you don't think it is possible to study for 10 minutes without listening to your iPod, but I've heard several of you say that you do better when you have some peace when you study. What did you do to make peace happen?" These strengths-based and solution-focused questions help members learn from one another while keeping the conversation active and fluid.

Strengths-based developmental research indicates that teens need person-to-person connections (Bosworth & Walz, 2005; DeLucia-Waack & Donigan, 2006; Galassi & Akos, 2007). A common way to build strong intergroup relationships (e.g., between members) is for the leader to ask about what is happening in the adolescents' world. Even if a school counselor thinks she or he is current on adolescent ways and inter-ests, the students may see anyone who is old enough to have graduated from college as ancient. It may be a good idea to embrace being an outsider to the teens' world and take a "you educate me" approach to what is trendy and cool. This may involve establishing rapport by asking about current music (e.g., have the students make you a mix CD), what movies they have seen, or what they like to do outside of school.

Striking a delicate balance between creating meaningful and authentic relation-ships among group members while, at the same time, not allowing the group to swerve too far off task is a challenging role for group leaders. As you can imagine, adolescents have a propensity to socialize, so keeping things moving in a constructive fashion is a managing skill requiring significant practice. In short, attempt to establish rapport among group members while also indicating that you have various enjoyable learning activities planned for sessions.

Sample Group Topics

Adolescents today face many complex issues and challenges, and school counselors strive to meet the needs of the students they serve. Although counselors often have a good idea what personal/social, educational, and career development issues their students are encountering, it is best practice to conduct a needs assessment early on in the school year. What's more, gathering relevant ideas from the professional counseling and psychological research literature is essential to effective group leadership. As an example, McEachern and Kenny (2007) outlined a transition to postsecondary school and/or work for high school students with disabilities. In brief, look at current research on adolescence and conduct a needs assessment. The findings from both activities will provide you a relatively clear picture of what small groups to offer in the fall and winter semesters (Jacob & Schimmel, 2005).

There are many possibilities for high school small groups, including:

- test and other anxieties (http://www.amazon.com/Anxiety-Workbook-Teens-Activities-Worry/dp/1572246030/ref=pd_sim_b_4)
- social skills building (http://www.amazon.com/Social-Success-Workbook-Teens-Skill-building/dp/1572246146/ref=pd_sim_b_6)
- anger management (see anger management for teens: http://www.amazon.com/Anger-Workbook-Teens-Activities-Frustration/dp/1572246995/ref=pd_sim_b_2)
- body image (see Go Grrrls: http://www.amazon.com/exec/obidos/ASIN/0393703487/qid=990127346/103-9966528-5963014)
- career/college concerns (http://www.amazon.com/Pursuit-My-Success-Teens-Developing/dp/0982345208/ref=sr_1_4?s=books&ie=UTF8&qid=1286917440&sr=1-4)
- living in changing families (http://www.amazon.com/Divorce-Workbook-Teens-Activities-Breakup/dp/157224657X/ref=sr_1_1?ie=UTF8&s=books&qid=1286917485&sr=1-1)
- asset development (http://www.search-institute.org)
- at-risk issues (see Bemak et al., 2005; Zinck & Littrell, 2000)

As noted in chapter 3, you will want to avoid topics that are beyond the scope of a professional school counselor. For instance, you would want to refer students with diagnosable mental health issues such as chronic depression or eating disorders to community mental health (or other) resources.

Skills Needed

As we have explored earlier with small-group leadership with lower grade–level small groups, high school groups also require a well-honed skill set. As we have touched upon in this chapter, high school groups are a suitable place to implement advanced counseling techniques. A group focused on changing families may have members who need to process some unfinished business as a result of someone abruptly leaving or joining the family. Group leaders who have been trained to use the Gestalt technique of the open chair (Barlow, 1981) may invite students to place an empty chair in the group circle. Students could take turns talking to the chair, a representation of the changing family, about what it felt like for them when the family was altered. Hearing other group members process this family change can help normalize the feelings that others in a similar circumstance share. Moreover, as discussed in chapter 6, using stories is a good way to connect counseling and the school's academic goals (Eppler et al., 2009). Although picture books may not be appropriate for high school students, group leaders could invite members to bring in journals, stories written for other classes, or excerpts from texts they have read. The process of using these stories is similar across the age span: Students are able to talk about their thoughts, feelings, and behaviors as related to what is going on in the narrative.

Although it is not within the scope of the professional school counselor to provide family therapy, high school group leaders may incorporate some creative and qualitative family assessments (e.g., family maps, community maps, timelines) into the group process. Eppler and Weir (2009) examined families, using these non-numeric family assessments in K–12 settings. High school students have the ability to reflect on family patterns and connections to community, and to think about how problems and solutions have changed over time. Adolescents tend to enjoy these types of activities. For example, group members could draw a family map or genogram to explore how other family members have solved a problem or learned a new skill. These solutions can be shared with other group members to build the members' toolbox of coping responses. Community maps or timelines can explore the collaborations that students have with nonfamilial supports, community resources, places of worship, and so on. Groups can examine where the members' time and energy are going and if there need to be any changes to promote healthy outcomes. By creating an ecomap in group, a student who spends a lot of time involved in sports and community recreation may find she draws a community map where her energy is extended away from her. She may find more balance if she is able to brainstorm with other group members ways to keep physically fit and civically active while still allowing time for herself and her schoolwork.

Not only do counselors possess the effective theory-based technique skills and facilitation skills summarized in chapter 5, they also possess these characteristics:

Flexibility and Adaptability   Group leaders at any level, and especially in high schools, must be able to go with the flow without imposing their agenda (Bemak et al., 2005; Berg et al., 2006). High school students from all walks of life want ownership and independence. For instance, it would be a mistake to assume that students with special needs or who are at risk may not be as independent as their peers and that they do not want to take control over some aspects of their lives (Bauer et al., 2000). All students connect well when they feel empowered to direct the conversation and give input on activities. This does not imply that group leaders are passive, but they do need the skills to guide the group while still giving the adolescents the sense of autonomy. For example, a leader could have two or three discussion questions written on a large sheet of paper, and the group could vote about which question to discuss first.

Flexibility is a necessary skill when leading high school groups because there tend to be various disruptions: school assemblies, sporting events, special classes for standardized testing, and so forth (Greenberg, 2003). Group leaders must have the skill to be able to schedule group meetings, knowing that there will be unavoidable absences. Also, it is necessary to show adaptability when collaborating with the teachers. It would be detrimental to a student's grade to miss 7 weeks of one class period. Professional school counselors need to find times to meet that accommodate the students' academic work and the teachers' need for students to be in class.

Cultural and Developmental Awareness Skills   Akin to cultural and developmental awareness in other grade levels, it is imperative that group leaders are aware of and knowledgeable about the many developmental, cultural, gender, and other differences among high school students (Bemak et al., 2005; DeLucia-Waack & Donigan, 2006). Many adolescents are sensitive to issues of social justice, and group leaders from all backgrounds can cultivate and build on this natural curiosity. Leaders of high school groups can be more overt about how students think and feel they are being perceived. For example, a group leader may feel some tension in the group and want to explore how culture plays a role in this dynamic. This leader could state, "I notice that we all communicate a little differently. I'm from an African American family and I tend to be up front with what I think. I'm wondering how your family or culture reacts when something is on your mind." This candidness and curiosity helps build transcultural relationships among group members and between the participants and the leader.

Group Management   In our experiences, one of the main challenges of working with a high school group is the ebb and flow of students' motivation levels. Students may not express an interest in joining a group unless they think it is relevant to them (Rollnick & Miller, 1995). Group leaders can encourage teens to connect with the group by explaining its benefits. We all are motivated to do things that make sense to us; we are less likely to continue even an appropriate behavior if we believe that it is purposeless. Motivational skills can be used in group management by asking students what they have learned, what they like about the group, and what they would change. Group leaders will want to address these questions not only at the first and last sessions but also at regular checkpoints along the way. Like in other grade levels, rewards (e.g., those used in token economies) may be used for students who show active engagement and are motivated to work on the group's goals. Also, teachers and counselor may collaborate on a behavioral plan to encourage students to sign up for and attend a group (see Dobson, 2010, for a description of behavioral techniques).

One enjoyable management technique for adolescents is the sticker challenge. The leader can bring in two stickers for each student. The stickers should be at least the size of a half-dollar. The leader will have a discussion question prepared that relates to the group topic. For instance, a career group question could be "My family thinks going to college is ..." Before the discussion, each student is given two stickers with the instruction that the conversation will be about 10 minutes and they can speak only twice. Each time students speak, they must put their sticker someplace visible (e.g., on their shirt or on a folder in front of them). The leader encourages the students to not just answer the question but to also respond to what others are saying. After the discussion, the leader can debrief the activity with questions such as these: What was it like to want to have input but not use up all your stickers before you gave the answer to the discussion question? How did you interact with others even after you had used both stickers? What was it like for quieter members to talk more and more vocal members to talk less? In general, this sticker activity helps the facilitator manage the group dynamics by keeping all students involved and motivated while also providing content (i.e., the information shared in the discussion) relevant to meeting the group's goals.

There are multiple ways to direct the interchange among group members. For instance, setting limits and boundaries is a central task in keeping a high school group constructive and moving forward to constructive ends. At times, the counselor may need to "sit back" and let the group facilitate itself, especially when members are fully engaged and talking in a productive manner. If students are maintaining the group's focus, then the group leader should empower them to continue. However, if the group veers off track, the leader's responsibility is to refocus the members back onto an activity or different conversation.

Relationship Building   Adolescents may be more likely to engage in the small group if they trust and respect the group leader. As such, small-group leaders must have personal relationship-building characteristics such as effective communication (e.g., listening, reflecting, summarizing), authenticity, honesty, and empathy (see chapter 5 for discussion of these and other skills). They should also model appropriate self-disclosure in order to be relational without blurring professional boundaries. Teens already receive much unsolicited advice from teachers, caregivers, and friends; therefore, school counselors need to avoid jumping in too quickly when offering their perspectives or feedback.

Although many adolescents are not as angst-ridden and disconnected as popular media may suggest, at times there may be a student who shows signs of being resistant to the group process. Leaders need to consider the meaning behind the student's reservations (M. S. Corey et al., 2010). You may ask that student to join the group for a few sessions to see if he or she notices any benefit. Remind all members that participation is voluntary. If a student is quiet in session, you may encourage the member to participate by giving him or her an opportunity to speak up. Asking gently, "What is it like for you to be here?" may open the door for the student to share any concerns. The group leader's goal is to understand the students' perspectives while offering them support for joining the group (M. S. Corey et al., 2010). Moreover, group leaders need to remember that not every student will connect with the group. Although counselors strive to offer services to all students (ASCA, 2005), a group setting may not fit with the needs of every individual.

Facilitation Skills   Even when you have a caring relationship with the students, there are times when the group conversation may seem stuck. During these periods, leaders may need to do a quick check-in, asking themselves: Do I have reasonable expectations for how quickly this group will bond? Am I asking meaningful questions? Am I providing activities that engage the group? On the other hand you, as a leader, may be doing great work, but the group could still seem to lack energy. During these times it is helpful to have ideas to use to work with challenging groups and problematic student behavior. For example, you may want to concentrate on your facilitation skills (G. Corey, 2008; M. S. Corey et al., 2010; see also chapter 5) and revisit pertinent theories and associated techniques (Henderson & Thompson, 2010; Vernon & Davis-Gage, 2010, and chapter 2) for suggested interventions.

When groups are not flowing, another good place to check in with is the larger school context. What is the climate of the school? Are there state tests adding anxiety to the students' lives? How are these affecting individual members and the group as a whole? Is there an assembly or an altered bell schedule that is negatively impacting the timing of the school day?

After assessing context, leaders can move to checking in with the group members. You want to determine if any changes have occurred since the last group session. Did someone fail an important exam? Did a student's family get an eviction notice? Even something that may seem "trivial" to us may affect the students' outlook.

In short, by building relationships by assessing personal and contextual variables, group leaders are better able to appreciate the students' worlds. However, even with a heightened level of understanding, blocks or challenges when running a group may still exist. Should a leader notice that there seems to be a break with one or more of the students, listen to the language that the student uses. Adolescents are known for interpersonal drama affecting the group dynamic. Table 8.1 overviews various problem behaviors that one or more group members may present and some suggestions for how the group leader may intervene.

Equitable Treatment　Educators often hear adolescents say "Life's not fair." Although human justice is elusive, high school students thrive when they perceive that they are being treated impartially and with cultural sensitivity (Bemak & Chung, 2004). Group leaders should be transparent in their attempts to treat students equitably. At times, one group member may have more to share than others. It is fine for one student to have the floor as long as it is not a pattern in the group. Additionally, the group leader needs to be vocal after the student has spoken. Leaders can remind members that each student will be afforded an opportunity to speak and that the goal is to balance the time allotted among members over the entirety of all the sessions. Moreover, leaders need to be aware of how much they interact with group members. Strengths of all students should be pointed out. It may be easy to identify the helpers' strengths or those of the student who keeps the action flowing. Adolescents take note of these subtle cues, and that may have a significant effect on the group process.

Logistical Issues

Groups at the high school level require significant planning for the following reasons: (a) so students do not miss the same class period every week, (b) so teachers can be notified of the students' excused absences, and (c) so the group leader's expectations are obvious to the student members. Group leaders need to think about whether the group will be open (students can come and go from session to session) or closed (group membership remains the same for all group sessions). Because school-based groups are time limited (six or seven sessions), it is generally a good idea for the sessions to be closed (Jacobs & Schimmel, 2005). While setting goals and creating the group's activities, the group leader should plan for what will happen if group members do not want to talk, what will happen if a member breaches confidentiality, and how to facilitate the activities.

Pregroup Reflection

- What will you do if the group members are silent?
- What is your plan to explain confidentiality?
- How will you decide what happens if confidentiality is broken?
- What types of activities may work well with the students you serve?

Students at the high school level either may be referred to the counseling office or may self-refer. Some students may be hesitant to inquire about counseling services. Professional school counselors ought to be visible and make the services offered known.

TABLE 8.1 | Problem Behavior and Possible Group Leader Interventions

Problem Behavior in Group	Group Leader Intervention
One student speaks for everyone ("Everyone knows that!")	Solicit feedback from the group: "I'm glad we are a team, and I want to hear what others have to say."
One student speaks for another in the group ("She already knows that.")	• Solicit feedback from the individual and/or group. • Ask the member to make an "I statement": "I hear that you think Sal agrees, but before we get to Sal, I'm wondering what you think."
Seeking approval from leader or other members (e.g., member says something like, "I agree with Ms. Brown.")	Point out behavior in a gentle way: "I notice that you tend to agree with almost everything I say. What would happen if you didn't agree with something?"
Focuses on issues occurring outside the group context (e.g., student says, "My brother …")	Refocus on the here and now: "Remember, we can't change others. What is it like for you when … ?"
Withdraws or uses silence	Find meaning in behavior: "I notice that when we start taking about [topic], you are pretty quiet. [Silence]. What is the silence telling us?"
Blames others for problems (e.g., member reminds the group, "You know I have a foster mom.")	Provide feedback and encourage ownership: "Yes, I understand that having a foster mom has been a big transition for you; I'm wondering what the group has done to help make transitions a bit easier."
Person believes he or she can't change (e.g., member indicates, "I was born like this.")	Clarify with questions and/or help members change language: "How has being 'like that' helped?" or "I'm hearing you say you 'can't' change. What does the group think about someone being one way forever?"
Acts passively or in a nonparticipatory way (e.g., overuses comments like: "Pass." "No idea!" "This sucks!")	Process disconnection in the group: "I'm noticing that it is becoming easy to pass. What do the group members think when one or a few of us doesn't share?" or "How can we motivate everyone to get involved?"
Shows incongruent behavior (e.g., member says, "It's cool …" even though he or she shows tension on face)	Provide feedback: "I hear you saying that you are okay with your mom's new boyfriend, but I see you giving a fake smile. Tell us about that; what is the grimace saying that you may have a hard time saying?"
Dominates group	Give feedback and/or block: "Hey, I'm glad you are into this group, but I want to make sure others have a chance to speak up. Let's hear what you have to say after a few other members tell us what they are thinking."

Hey! New Small Group is forming...

- Want to do better in school?
- Want to learn how to set goals....AND meet them???
- Want to meet some cool, new people?

If you answered YES to these questions, sign up in the counseling office to be part of a new small group. See yah there!!!

© Microsoft Corporation

FIGURE 8.1 | Promotional poster announcing small-group formation.

Group leaders should consult with teachers in order to connect with students who may benefit from the group. Another way to encourage students to join a group is to post signs around the building letting them know about upcoming sessions. Figure 8.1 is one example of a "promotional" sign that a school counselor posted before she led a study and social skills group.

These signs need to be easy to read, inventive, and fun so they attract diverse students. After the student has expressed interest, the next step is for the leader to connect with the teachers. Figure 8.2 is an example of a school counselor–teacher communication.

Obtaining buy-in from the teachers is key, as they are an essential resource for supporting students and providing background information. Ripley and Goodnough (2001) suggested that schools allow students to miss class without penalty. However, districts have regulations governing student absences. Professional school counselors must advocate and educate the administration and teachers about the importance of small groups in order to gather support for students to miss class assuming they make up the work (Ripley & Goodnough, 2001).

Pregroup Interview

Before group sessions can begin, the group leader should conduct a brief (10–15 minute) pregroup interview with each potential group member (Hines & Fields, 2002). These screening/interviews allow the group leader to decide whether or not a student would be a good fit for the group. Through potential group members' answers to specific questions, the group leader assesses whether the student might benefit from the group experience and whether he or she will contribute positively to the group. The interviews also serve another purpose: They ensure that participants give their informed consent to participate in the group process.

First, the group leader should begin with an introduction. The counselor may want to give a brief background by saying, "Hi! I'm Ms. Shallenberger and I'm one of the counselors here at the [name] High School. You may not have talked to me before because I tend to work with students who have last names beginning with E and F, but I am starting a group to help students gain study and social skills. You signed up in the office, and I'm curious about what made you want to join the group."

SCHOOL LETTERHEAD

Date [mm/dd/yy]

Hello Colleague,
    You are receiving this letter because a student of yours, [student name], has agreed to participate in a counseling group titled [name]. This is an educational opportunity for your student to gain [goals].
    The group will begin on [date], running for 6 consecutive weeks. The group will last for approximately 40 minutes on [day and time]. A rotating schedule will be put into effect so that on some days, students will miss a few minutes of second period, and on other days, they'll miss a few minutes of fourth period. Students will be signing contracts during the first session, where they will commit to making up any class assignments they miss as a result of their participation in the group.

Objectives for the group are listed below:
[List objectives]

I am looking forward to having your student as a member of my counseling group. If you have any questions related to this group, feel free to contact me. My phone extension is: [___] and my email is [schoolcounselor@xyzschooldistrict.edu].

Thanks so much for your cooperation!

Sincerely,

FIGURE 8.2 | Counselor–teacher communication regarding formation of new small group.

    After listening to the student, briefly inform her or him about the structure of the group, stating: "We will be doing some talking as a group and we will work on various projects together. One project may be to make a mural." Then the leader could ask, "Does this sound like a group that might be helpful for you?" Solicit feedback from the student by asking what their initial thoughts are about the group. Then, depending on the age of the student, state requirements, and district policy, the counselor would give the student the caregiver permission letter. We advocate that all students receive and return a signed letter (see Figure 8.3 for an example of a permission letter).

Group Evaluation

Evaluation of the group process serves two integral purposes. First, if the group leader is able to acquire feedback from group members, the information will be helpful in modifying the group for future use. Second, group appraisals can promote the school counseling program in general when these student evaluations are shared with administrators and school staff (Jacobs, & Schimmel, 2005). If the member evaluations are viewed by anyone other than the group leader or school counselor, the group leader is ethically responsible for removing the names to protect students' confidentiality (Greenberg, 2003). At the close of the final group session, formal evaluation surveys will be distributed to and then collected from all members of the group. These can then be

Sample Parent/Guardian Permission Letter

To the parent or guardian of _____,

　　Your student has asked/been asked to participate in a school-based counseling group exploring study and social skills.

　　This is an exciting and valuable experience for your student to gain additional academic and social support. The group will take place on [day] from approximately [time]. This time will rotate slightly each week so that students are not missing out on the same few minutes of classroom time. The first group meeting will be held on [date], and will meet weekly until the closing group session on [date]. Student participation is completely voluntary, and students understand that they are free to end their membership in the group at any time. To gain the most benefit from the group experience, it is hoped that each student will attend all six sessions.

　　The leader of the group will also respect and maintain the confidentiality of each student. This will be the case unless the leader is ethically or legally obligated to limit confidentiality. An example of this would be if a student threatened to cause harm to him- or herself or another student.

　　If you agree that your student may participate in the group, please sign below and return to the school counseling office by [date].

I have read, understand, and agree to the above information.

Parent/Caregiver Signature: _____ Date: _____

FIGURE 8.3 | Parent/guardian information and permission letter.

compared to group members' responses during the pregroup interviews. For example, group members are asked whether they have any goals in mind during the initial interview. In the formal assessment, members are asked about goals once again. For evaluative aims, these responses can be compared at the end of the group process. A sample member evaluation survey is provided in Figure 8.4.

High School Group Example: Academic and Social Skills Small Group

Small groups focusing on students' learning specific academic success strategies contribute positively to student school behavior (Brigman & Campbell, 2003; Webb, Brigman, & Campbell, 2005). Research indicates that not only are groups more effective than individual counseling when related to underachieving students' success but the most productive counseling groups are those that include study skills instruction (Cook & Kaffenberger, 2003). The key purpose of the Academic and Social Skills for Success Group is to assist underachieving high school students to increase their overall school performance. Groups such as these assist students who are falling behind their peers to receive additional social and academic support. Below is a description of an actual psychoeducational group recently led by a practicing high school counselor. Each of the crucial areas of group design and implementation are outlined, beginning with the core group objectives.

Name: _____   Date: _____

Academic & Social Skills for Success

Student *Pregroup* Self-Evaluation

Directions: Rate yourself on a scale of 1 to 5 on each statement below. Follow the rating system listed here:

5 = Strongly Agree 4 = Agree 3 = Unsure 2 = Disagree 1 = Strongly Disagree

1) I listen carefully and follow directions.	5	4	3	2	1
2) I actively participate in class discussions.	5	4	3	2	1
3) I know when and how to ask questions when I'm uncertain or don't know.	5	4	3	2	1
4) I work well in small groups.	5	4	3	2	1
5) I get along well with others in class.	5	4	3	2	1
6) I read all assignments and understand what I read.	5	4	3	2	1
7) I complete work assigned on time, avoiding getting no credit.	5	4	3	2	1
8) I have at least one dependable study friend in each class whom I can call for help.	5	4	3	2	1
9) I have a good system to help me recall important facts and concepts (e.g., outlining).	5	4	3	2	1
10) I have a study plan to prepare for tests that I use a few days ahead of the test.	5	4	3	2	1
11) I keep track of my test grades and other course grades.	5	4	3	2	1
12) I know how my teacher calculates my final grade.	5	4	3	2	1

FIGURE 8.4 | Sample group evaluation survey ("pretest").

Group Member Objectives   The major objectives of this academic success group are relatively straightforward. Participants will:

- develop positive social relationships with other members of the group,
- develop a clear academic goal,
- learn to ask good questions and feel comfortable doing so in class,
- learn at least one strategy for successfully accomplishing a reading assignment, and
- learn at least one strategy for successfully accomplishing a mathematics assignment.

Basic Format and Procedures   Within each week's session, the format will generally include the following:

1. Welcome to the group and greet each other.
2. Update grade monitoring forms, and complete sentence fragments related to goals.
3. Review prior week's session and report on current goal fulfillment stage.
4. Present new material and skills to be learned.
5. Review ratings on self-evaluation forms.
6. Close the session and preview next week's topic.

Content of Group Meetings   Each group meeting has relatively clear goals and is focused on a topic(s) with accompanying content. Here we detail how a real-world high school group was structured and conducted. You will notice that the group leader attempted to follow best practices outlined in previous chapters. As you read over the weekly sessions, make note of group leadership skills illustrated by the high school counselor.

- **Session 1.** The goals of the first session were to establish rules, review confidentiality, introduce group members, and begin to share initial thoughts regarding study and social skills. Jenna, the high school counselor and group leader, wanted to attend to the group cohesion so she assigned students to dyads, directing each pair to introduce themselves and ask each other about their favorite subject in school. Before the dyads broke off from the larger group, members were also instructed to notice their commonalities. After the pairs talked for about 5 minutes, the leader modeled for the group how to appropriately share, providing some limited self-disclosure. She introduced her interest in running a group to combine study and social skills by saying:

   > When I was in high school there were limited opportunities for me to think about what I was already doing well and things I needed to improve on in both my friendships and my work at school. Sometimes we focus on one thing or the other, but both are so important at this time in your life. Also, looking back now I see that having good social and study skills really helped me after I graduated.

   At the same time, the facilitator asked all members introduce their partner to the larger group. (Recall that members do have the right to "pass" if they so choose.)

   After introductions, a discussion ensued about naming the group and creating group rules and norms. First, members brainstormed a group name, with the leader writing down each suggestion and the group eventually voting on their favorite. Subsequently group rules were explored, with Jenna suggesting:

   > Let's make this group a place where everyone feels comfortable sharing about studying and friendship. In order to do that, it is a good idea for everyone to be on the same page about what happens in a group. What do you think would help to make this a good place for all to share their thoughts?

   The group came up with several appropriate suggestions. Jenna made sure that the list included these "universal" guidelines: Avoid negative comments about others; members have the right to pass when asked a question; and confidentiality must be maintained. (A common expression used is, "What is said in the group stays in the group.") Of course exceptions to the confidentiality guideline were explained (e.g., self- or other harm would have to be reported). As the purpose of this high school group was to empower students to have a voice and share their thoughts, Jenna had students lead most of the discussion, while at the same time carefully facilitating the conversation to include best practice group norms and rules.

   Because this group was conducted with high school students, the leader opted to run a discussion-based group that included some structured activities promoting knowledge and awareness of study and friendship skills. Moreover, to obtain a "reading" of the members' initial understanding of the subject matter, during the first group meeting a "pretest" evaluation questionnaire was distributed and individually completed. Afterward, the members were requested to share one or two questions that they felt were most important to them. Effectively using this discussion time, Jenna attempted to link group members' responses (i.e., to find common themes) and to talk about common themes found in the students' responses. Members were told to expect various group activities throughout the coming weeks, indicating that these exercises should enhance intergroup communication and personal sharing about what they were thinking and learning. Although not as overt as talking about the activities, the leader also planned to implement SFBC techniques when she probed the students for more information.

To close the initial session, the group leader changed the focus to personal goal setting. The counselor suggested that students think about what they would like to learn and change about themselves over the course of the next few weeks. Anticipating perhaps some member anxiety about sharing of goals, Jenna let the students know that the next week's discussion would start with the students sharing about their goals and what changes they were already making to reach a goal. This "delaying" strategy allows the students some processing time in between group meetings and sets the stage for Session 2. After positively reinforcing group members with sincere comments about the students' attendance and involvement, the leader further encouraged them by telling them that she was looking forward to next week's group and seeing them again.

- **Early Stages: Sessions 2 and 3.** During the beginning group stages, the high school counselor wanted to build a strong connection among students and to encourage them to learn new social and academic skills. Again, Jenna balanced having structured activities and techniques stemmed from theory with allowing members to facilitate the conversations around these important topics. Discussed previously, a useful strategy with high school students is to adopt a "one-down" position in group. To illustrate this, Jenna encouraged the members to explore those situations that were meaningful and relevant to their lives. Lulls in the conversation were appropriate times for the insertion of an activity, thus keeping the group productive.

  Two of the activities Jenna had on hand for use in the early sessions included (adapted from Brigman & Goodman, 2001):

  1. A relaxation and visualization exercise: Students were instructed to get in a comfortable position, think about a calm place, and then visualize themselves working on a goal that they had set for themselves. After several minutes of guided relaxation, the leader brought the group members together to share their images. Students were asked to point out positives of each other's images in order to build up a set of options that could work when the student encountered stressful situations (e.g., taking a test).

  2. Assertiveness training: Members role-played asking questions in class and clarifying information the teacher had given, and brainstormed when it was a good idea to speak up and when it was better to wait to ask a question. The group leader facilitated linking this assertiveness in the classroom to being a strong

friend. Jenna talked with the students about when to be a listener, when to ask questions, and when to speak up for yourself.

During the early stages, the school counselor noticed that several group members were quiet. This reluctance to speak up was due in part to other students tending to dominate the conversation. Deploying group counseling skills, the leaders was able to block and redirect the conversation to the more silent group members. For example, when one student answered several questions in a row, Jenna thanked the student for being involved and asked if a member who had not yet shared would be brave and go first on the next question. The leader effectively used the go-around technique, where members took turns sharing in the order that they were sitting in the group circle. Limits were set regarding how long answers should last, pointing out that the views of all group members should be voiced.

- **Middle Stages: Sessions 4 and 5.** The middle stages of the group were used to query deeper into strengths necessary for effective study and social skills. Compared to the earlier group stage, the leader spent less time at the beginning of each session building rapport. In the first few sessions, Jenna would open the group by asking a more general question about what they had learned or something they had noticed that was different from the week before. In the middle stage of the group, Jenna voiced more direct questions related to the day's focus. Activities related to the topics included (from Brigman & Goodman, 2001):

  1. Social Strengths: The leader gave the students five fill-in-the-blank statements about social connections. For instance, "When people talk to me, I like to _____"; "I trust people who _____"; and "I am willing to listen to others if _____." The statements were written on a note card or a sheet of paper. Students then came back to the group and shared what they had written. The school counselor reminded the group members of their rules (e.g., this is a safe place to share). Students were allowed to agree, disagree, and/ or comment on responses as long as they followed the group rules of no negative sharing ("put-downs") or interruptions. During this activity, Jenna worked to build on the group dynamic, finding similarities and affirming differences in group members' opinions. To model how to find one's strengths, the leader asked the members to comment on what they liked about some of the responses shared.

  2. Reading Strategies: Students were instructed to bring in a reading assignment from one of their classes. As a way of linking classroom academics with the group experience, students reviewed what they had learned in the group that had helped them with this assignment. Group members were asked to think about the skills they had learned in group and how those techniques might be applied to reading both at school and in their "real world." Again, the primary intent here was to have the members establish a clear link between what they had learned in group to an academic requirement. To make the learning even more relevant, the leader brought in a clipping from the high school newspaper and related some of the reading strategies to understanding how effective reading skills can help both in and out of the classroom.

3. Math Skills: Group members were also asked to bring their math book to group. The students were given a math checklist to help tackle difficult problems. Examples from the checklist included: drawing out a picture of the problem, finding out the specific question that needed to be answered, and writing out steps that could help the student answer the problem. In order to link these problem-solving skills to friendship skills, Jenna asked if the students could think of any way that these math skills could help them become better friends. Students answered that they could help tutor their friends. Students were further encouraged to think about ways these skills could assist their friendships that did not include math homework. The group arrived at these valuable ideas: Ask friends good questions and get to know their friends well in a similar way to understanding what was being asked in the math problem.

- **Late Stage and Termination: Sessions 6 and 7.** In order to prepare for ending the group, the leader spent the last two sessions reflecting on and validating the group members' growth both individually and as a whole. Starting in Session 5, Jenna reminded the group that there were only two sessions left; during the sixth session, she talked about the last session, indicating that the last meeting would be a time of celebration to affirm their group accomplishments. The wrap-up included a balance between continuing to provide new skills for the members to learn and reflecting on what had been learned. Activities useful for these later sessions included:

1. Spotlight: Group members were each given a large piece of paper, at the top of which they wrote their names, and then they passed the paper to the left. The other members took turns writing a strength about that member. The leader requested that members not comment on physical appearance but instead focus on personality traits such as "hardworking" or "shares openly."

2. Signs of Learning: Group members were each given two note cards and instructed to write something they had learned from another group member. Students were not to identify whom they were addressing so no one felt left out if their idea was not included. Members all placed their cards in the middle of the circle. Each took a turn reading one card out of the pile and discussing that particular strength.

The last session had a celebratory theme where group members could bring in a healthy snack to share and a CD of "school-sanctioned" music to play during the last session. During this time, group members filled out the "posttest" evaluation survey (see example in Figure 8.5). It essentially mirrors the pregroup version, but with additional questions. Before saying goodbye, members were given the opportunity to review the changes they observed in themselves. The leader also provided positive reinforcement for each member's contributions and thanked everyone for their participation.

Part of the struggle of ending the group is for the school counselor to maintain the boundaries that were initially established. Often group members who have enjoyed the experience ask to continue with the group for additional sessions. Leaders may struggle with wanting to meet the students' needs while also understanding that a good ending transition is part of an effective group process. Setting limits to connect with the students while also encouraging them to find their own support is an

Name:_____   Date:_____

Academic & Social Skills for Success
Student *Postgroup* Self-Evaluation

Directions: Rate yourself on a scale of 1 to 5 on each statement below. Follow the rating system listed here:

1. Overall, my experience in this group was: Very Helpful Helpful OK Unhelpful (circle one)

Directions: Rate yourself on a scale of 1 to 5 on each statement below. Follow the rating system listed here:

5 = Strongly Agree   4 = Agree   3 = Unsure   2 = Disagree   1 = Strongly Disagree

	5	4	3	2	1
1) I listen carefully and follow directions.	5	4	3	2	1
2) I actively participate in class discussions.	5	4	3	2	1
3) I know when and how to ask questions when I'm uncertain or don't know.	5	4	3	2	1
4) I work well in small groups.	5	4	3	2	1
5) I get along well with others in class.	5	4	3	2	1
6) I read all assignments and understand what I read.	5	4	3	2	1
7) I complete work assigned on time, avoiding getting no credit.	5	4	3	2	1
8) I have at least one dependable study friend in each class whom I can call for help.	5	4	3	2	1
9) I have a good system to help me recall important facts and concepts (e.g., outlining).	5	4	3	2	1
10) I have a study plan to prepare for tests that I use a few days ahead of the test.	5	4	3	2	1
11) I keep track of my test grades and other course grades	5	4	3	2	1
12) I how my teacher calculates my final grade.	5	4	3	2	1
13) I enjoyed meeting new people while participating in the group.	5	4	3	2	1
14) I clearly understand the concept of goal setting and am able to set my own goals.	5	4	3	2	1
15) I am now capable of asking good questions in class.	5	4	3	2	1
16) I gained new skills that will help me tackle any reading assignment.	5	4	3	2	1
17) I gained new skills that will help me tackle any math assignment.	5	4	3	2	1

18) Things I appreciated about being a member of the group:

_____

_____

_____

19) Things about the group that I feel might need some improvement:

_____

_____

_____

20) Anything other comments you want to make?

_____

_____

_____

FIGURE 8.5 | Sample group evaluation survey ("posttest").

important issue for professional school counselors to be aware of and work on in the final stages of the group.

Following the end of the group, students were encouraged to individually meet with the leader to briefly discuss their experience. Any need for additional counseling, support, or a potential mental health referral was assessed. Again, the counselor encouraged each group member to apply his or her learning to school and home life.

GROUPS IN PRACTICE

Reflection Questions for High School Groups

- Think about running a group at a high school. What strengths do you have that will help you facilitate the group at this level? What limitations are you worried about or feel you may need to work on?
- One of the challenges of leading high school groups is finding the balance between having appropriate activities and creating a strong discussion dynamic. How do you see the balance between these two pieces of a group? How would you know if it is okay to leave out or stop an activity if the conversation seems productive?
- It can be challenging to prepare the group curriculum for each week's session. What resources are available to help you guide the group sessions?
- Collaboration within high schools is important, and it is hard to balance how much to share and how much to keep private. Imagine having a conversation with a teacher of one of your high school group students. How can you balance sharing information about the group without breaking confidentiality?

SUMMARY AND CONCLUSION

This chapter explored the world of high schools students as holistic individuals who are developmentally ready to look at themselves in new ways. They are ready to explore intimacy issues, choose a job or college, and possibly distance themselves from family members whose job it has been to care for them. Best practice and theory-based high school groups are supportive in helping adolescents transition into adulthood and graduate from high school. A primary task of adolescents is to know themselves and others at a deeper level. The group example shared one counselor's journey of encouraging her students to build on their social and academic skills, promoting healthy behaviors in both school and life. Obviously, tailoring and conducting small groups for this population are challenging tasks, but the obstacles are well worth working through. To observe, firsthand, adolescents changing and growing is a joy and honor.

CHAPTER 8 SUPPLEMENT

USEFUL RESOURCES TO CONSULT

Bruce et al. (2009) outlines a small group with African American students designed to increase achievement test results.

Kayler and Sherman (2009) detailed a small-group intervention with at-risk ninth-grade students to increase study skills and grade point average.

The Missouri Center for Career Education has numerous resources and curricula that are readily adaptable for high school groups: http://missouricareereducation.org/curr/cmd/guidanceplacementG/elearning/

Lessons to assist students to acquire skills for school success are available at: http://www.schoolcounselor.org/rc_files/275/Academic.pdf

Activities, exercises, and icebreakers for groups are available at: http://counselorsroom.com/SC_Group.php

Small Groups for Students With Special Needs

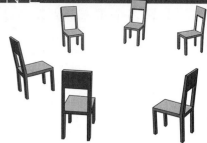

INTRODUCTION

Groups with diversity provide all students, as Bandura (1986, 2001) suggested, with opportunities for modeling, feedback, and experiences with individuals who are in some ways unlike themselves. Blending students of varied histories, skills, and abilities into a single group provides opportunities for peers to learn from each other, while, at the same time, increasing their awareness and appreciation of individual and subgroup differences. Not only does the concept of diversity include students of color, language, ethnicity, and other differentiating background variables, it also speaks to students with special learning needs. Depending on the topic and membership, students with special needs may benefit from group experiences that include general education students and vice versa. Groups focusing explicitly on the special needs of particular students may be appropriate when it is less productive to include other learners. The point made here is not intended to suggest that such students with learning challenges should be separated or isolated into "special needs only" groups. Rather, research and anecdotal evidence indicate that students with atypical learning needs often benefit from *both* heterogeneous member groups as well as more targeted group counseling support (e.g., Chen & Han, 2001; DeRosier, 2004; Tarver-Behring & Spagna, 2004). In fact, DeRosier suggests that the "availability of a multipurpose group intervention to meet the needs of diverse groups of children may enhance the likelihood that children will receive such services in schools" (p. 200).

Given the number of factors that influence the health of a small group, professional school counselors must think through carefully how the group is composed, whether it is blended or not. The screening of potential members is therefore crucial to making this decision. If you are planning on running a blended group, the school counselor should consider these important questions during the pregroup screening: Will the potential group member from the general student population demonstrate sensitivity to the needs and characteristics of students with special needs, and will he or she contribute to the group's overall vibrancy and productivity? Such issues and others are explored in this chapter. Specifically, topics discussed here include the skill set needed to facilitate effective groups with students with special needs, the importance of collaboration among educators, legal and ethical considerations, and various logistical issues. Several practical examples and recommendations are also provided as well.

Before moving on, however, let's define what is meant by the notion of "students with special needs." In this chapter, the label refers to students receiving special education services (SPED) as well as to student groups that may be particularly at risk or who are often underserved through small-group interventions. These latter groups of students with special needs may include, but are not limited to, English language learners (ELL) or English as a second language (ESL) learners, gifted and talented students, individuals with minority sexual orientations, students with substance abuse issues, and so on.

SMALL GROUP WORK FOR STUDENTS WITH SPECIAL NEEDS

The sad reality of small groups for some special needs populations is that they are infrequently conducted (e.g., Tarver-Behring & Spagna, 2004). Although it is wise for novice group counselors to begin their experiences with less challenging student populations and group topics (e.g., making friends), as school counselors become more experienced they begin to conduct small groups that address the needs of *all* students. Although some SPED and ELL classrooms are in part self-contained, these students should not be excluded from professional school counseling services. Regrettably, experience suggests that in self-contained learning environments, often the ELL or SPED classroom educators fulfill the various roles of, among others, teacher, counselor, and community liaison. Before discussion goes any further, here's a school example to consider.

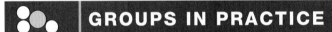

GROUPS IN PRACTICE

Small-Group Scenario: High School Group with ELL Students

One of this text's authors, Cher Edwards, recently conducted a small group with ELL students at a local high school in collaboration with one of the professional school counselors (PSCs) in the building. Because of Cher's interest in working with diverse students, the PSC asked her to come in to lead the group. The group's focus was on anger management and friendship skills. Evidently, there were two predominant immigrant groups at the school that were at odds with each other, and the situation had escalated into violence. Cher wondered to herself, "How did it get to this?" When she talked with the students, it became clear that they were unaware of the school counseling resources available. Cher asked who they went to when they had a personal/ social, academic, or even career question or concern, and their response was "our teacher." It was evident based on these interactions with the ELL students that most of the students knew that the school counselor existed and even knew the role of the school counselor. Sadly, what was also apparent is that these students felt that the counselor's' guidance services were "not for them."

SKILLS NEEDED

With this troubling scenario in mind, school counselors need to be clear regarding their role as group leaders: that they are there for *all* students. Back in the late 1990s, 1 in 10 students was diagnosed with a disability (Glenn, 1998); however over the past 10 years, the number of U.S. students enrolled in special education programs has increased to 30% (National Education Association, 2010). Despite this large rise in the prevalence rate over 10 or so years, the amount of time school counselors allocate toward specifically serving this population is relatively low (Studer & Quigney, 2003). PSCs must be therefore be intentional about creating groups to meet the needs of students who are often overlooked or even marginalized. When appropriate, collaborate with school staff to learn how to best meet the needs of a special population.

School counselors must be familiar with the key players likely to serve students with special needs (see Trolley, Hass, & Patti, 2009, for details). These individuals and their functions are overviewed here. First, SPED teachers, sometimes referred to as resource room instructors, are certified/licensed educators specifically trained in special education. These teachers work closely with other support staff, including "therapeutic" support staff (e.g., occupational, speech/language, physical, psychological), classroom aides, the school psychologist, the 504 coordinator, students receiving special education services, and their parents/caregivers. Therapists are professionals who provide specific supportive services to students. These services may be provided within the school building or by a community agency, and the therapists may or may not be employed by the school district. The 504 coordinator or committee is an individual or group charged with responding to inquiries about accommodation plans for students with disabilities and creating those plans. Section 504 of the Vocational Rehabilitation Act of 1973 addresses the rights of individuals with disabilities. In schools, this law requires that students who have a documented physical or mental impairment that substantially limits a major life activity have equal access to programs or activities receiving federal support, which includes most public schools (Baumberger & Harper, 2007).

The school psychologist is an individual who is hired by a school district and often serves more than one school. This professional may have a variety of duties, some of which are similar to those provided by a school counselor. Although the duties of school psychologists may look different at various schools and districts, their role related to special education is more standardized. School psychologists are typically responsible for, among other related activities, the testing and assessment of students identified as potentially in need of special education services or other accommodations.

Furthermore, school psychologists often work closely with special education/resource room teachers and provide recommendations to guide the formation of a student's individualized education program (IEP). An IEP is a legally binding document that commits to specially designed instruction (SDI) to accommodate an identified student with a disability in receiving free and appropriate public school education (FAPE) in the least restrictive environment (LRE). Essentially, this means that students with disabilities have a legal right to education without additional cost to the family and in a way that supports their academic needs in the least restrictive or alternative way possible. For example, if a student's needs are specific to math, and the need warrants support beyond an accommodation to the general education curriculum (in that case the student may have a 504 plan), an IEP will be created to document the plan for SDI in the least restrictive way possible. In practice, this may mean that the student is a part of the general education (what some refer to as "normal," although we discourage the use of the labels *normal* or *abnormal*) curriculum and is released for SDI for math instruction only.

In short, identifying the key players who support students with special needs is the first step in creating the solid partnership needed to ensure that this population is included in small-group offerings. For a more comprehensive resource on the role of school counselors specific to working with students with disabilities, refer to the chapter supplement.

COLLABORATION

As mentioned above, school counselors know that collaboration is an important part of being a supportive presence in the schools (McWhirter et al., 2007). With students with special needs, teamwork is imperative. As well trained as school counselors are, the breadth of student needs is too great to be an expert in every area. Collaborating with special education teachers, school psychologists, special education support staff, and parents/caregivers allows for the consultation and support necessary to be an effective group leader when offering groups that include students with special needs. In addition to providing expertise specific to various populations, collaborating provides the opportunity for school counselors to promote both school counseling as a profession and school counseling interventions.

Collaboration is also a key component of Response to Intervention (RTI) and Positive Behavioral Interventions and Support (PBIS)—two schoolwide systems that can be utilized independently or in concert to support academic success and reduce behavioral challenges for all students, including those with special needs (U.S. Department of Education, 2010b). RTI utilizes a three-tiered model integrating interventions to focus on prevention, screening, data-based decision making, and progress monitoring (U.S. Department of Education, 2010b). Similarly, PBIS, also referred to as SWPBIS (Schoolwide Positive Behavioral Interventions and Support), is a "decision making framework that guides selection, integration, and implementation of the best evidenced-based academic and behavioral practices for improving important academic and behavior outcomes for all students" (Sugai, n.d., p. 1). ASCA (2008b) identified the role of the professional school counselor as a stakeholder in the development and implementation of such interventions, specifically citing small-group counseling as an appropriate preventative and responsive service. School counselors can collaborate with all educational stakeholders to support RTI and PBIS through the utilization of specific strategies appropriate during group meetings. In practice, this means that school counselors leading groups should be aware of what specific strategies are employed to support positive behavior of the students *outside* of group and follow through *during* the group (e.g., redirection, use of manipulatives, etc.).

SPED Teachers

These educators may be more likely to refer a student to a small group if they are assured of the school counselor's commitment to and willingness to serve students with disabilities. Similarly, as SPED teachers and school staff are creating IEPs and 504 plans, they may be more likely to include school counseling interventions if they are aware of what school counseling services can and will be offered that address the educational goals for students with special needs. Additionally, school counselors might partner with a special education teacher to provide an in-service to all school staff regarding the identification and referral of students with special needs and services available (e.g., small groups). Other opportunities for collaboration include speaking at the parent–teacher association (PTA) meetings or offering a parent information night to inform students and their families of community and school resources that may be of support. School counselors can work to gain the trust of students with disabilities by being intentional about being present in SPED classrooms for needs assessment and classroom guidance. Needs assessment will ensure that needs specific to this population are identified when considering school counseling services to meet the needs of all students. For groups that focus on self-referral, students with special needs may be more likely to consider group participation if they have had a previous connection with the school counselor.

Families of Students with Special Needs

Collaborating with parents/caregivers and students receiving special education is a less formal process, but equally as important. In practice, this means that school counselors connect with these groups by providing services to reach out to this often underserved group. In fact, partnering with families is a vital way to promote academic success (Lam, 2005). School counselors may add a link on the school counseling website specifically for students and families with special needs, provide information on community support resources, or facilitate parent/caregiver meetings to share with families of students with special needs materials on relevant topics (e.g., transition, peer relationships, study skills). The important aspect of this collaborative relationship is creating awareness for families that school counselors are committed to supporting the academic success of all students, and making a connection with the families so that when a parent or caregiver of a student with special needs receives a permission form for group participation, it is not their first interaction with the school counselor. Keep in mind that parents, like students, are a diverse group of individuals with varying levels of comfort with counseling-related services and school systems. Parents and caregivers may have quite a few questions regarding their student's involvement in small groups and the potential benefit of such an experience. Encourage family participation through the sharing of group topics and auxiliary materials (e.g., take-home activities that include the family) to encourage parent/caregiver involvement in group work. Be sensitive to family preferences regarding descriptors used for their students and disabilities. Congruent with professional expectations, person-first language should always be used—that is, referring to individuals prior to their disability or exceptionality (e.g., students with a disability versus disabled students). For additional discussion of person-first language and other disability etiquette considerations, Parette and Hourcade (1995) provide a useful resource for school counselors.

School Psychologist

Collaboration between school counselors and school psychologists is pertinent to providing more comprehensive and prevention services to students (Pérusse et al., 2009; Staton & Gilligan, 2003). Similar to the interventions suggested in partnership with special education teachers, school counselors and school psychologists can partner to facilitate staff in-service trainings and parent/caregiver meetings to provide resources for families of students with special needs. School psychologists are also a great resource to co-lead small-group counseling groups for students with special needs given their common skill base in group counseling (Murphy, DeEsch, & Strein, 1998) and knowledge of disabilities. Popular choices for such a partnership are groups focused on social skills acquisition for students diagnosed with Asperger's or an autism spectrum disorder (see McGuire, 2009, for research regarding the efficacy of group interventions for this population as well as a strengths-based model for group work, and Okada, Ohtake, & Yanagihara, 2010, for potential group activities when working with this population).

Others

For students with special needs focused on medical issues (e.g., HIV positive, obesity, etc.) collaborating with medical professionals may also be helpful when considering small-group offerings that may be of support (McCabe & Shaw, 2010). When considering facilitating groups for special populations aside from students receiving special education services, consider school staff primed for collaboration such as the gay–straight alliance (GSA) advisor, multicultural club advisor, the school drug and alcohol specialist, school nurse, or related professionals. These individuals may provide formal support such as referrals for group participation or informal support such as recommendations related to specific needs of a particular population.

LEGAL AND ETHICAL CONSIDERATIONS

Collaboration is a professional expectation for best serving the needs of students with special needs, but it may also be an ethical or legal mandate. The Individuals with Disabilities Education Improvement Act of 2004 (IDEiA—formerly IDEA; U.S. Department of Education, 2004) specifies that school districts provide students with disabilities an FAPE in an LRE. In response, states review federal guidelines and interpret them in the form of state law (seen as revised or administrative codes). Additionally, school districts draft their own policies and procedures reflecting federal and state laws to ensure compliance and best practice. Federal and state laws dictate the legal right of students with disabilities to an FAPE that includes a range of support services including school counseling interventions (Bowen, 1998). Professional and ethical guidelines also address the importance of school counseling interventions for students with special needs (ASCA, 2010). The *Ethical Standards for School Counselors* (ASCA, 2010) is clear that school counselors have a responsibility to address the personal/social, career, and academic needs of all students, including those with special needs. The ASCA (2010) position statement regarding students with special needs acknowledges the rights of students with special needs and the history of this population as an underserved group related to educational services and support. The position statement also identifies the disproportionality related to representation of students of color, ELLs, and individuals of low socioeconomic status receiving special education services, and encourages professional school counselors to advocate for and serve students with special needs, including the provision of small-group counseling.

In addition to intentionality, advocacy, and collaboration, school counselors facilitating groups for students with special needs should possess group skills that can effectively meet the needs of diverse students. As such, counselors must be able to conduct groups with not only students in special needs classrooms but also students of color and diverse sexual orientation. Clearly, sensitivity and awareness of these issues are critical. Cultural competency, which includes cultural awareness, knowledge, and skills (Pedersen, 2003), necessitates that professional school counselors consider their own value system, biases, prejudice, and worldview and the impact these might have on group leadership.

To be proficient at running groups for particular special needs issues requires that group leaders be well prepared. For example, if you want to lead a psychoeducational group for students with substance abuse concerns, a visit to an Alcoholics Anonymous (AA) open meeting could be useful. In this way, you would obtain a sense of the AA community and culture and key issues to address in the group experience. If you plan on facilitating a group that includes students with Asperger's syndrome, for example, beforehand you might attend a workshop and research the topic further. There may be groups for which you are unprepared to lead, such as those of a more therapeutic nature and outside the scope of practice of a professional school counselor. In such cases, it is important to be aware of community resources appropriate for students with special needs to ensure a supportive referral.

To reiterate the importance of pregroup preparation, remember that each student's experience and background are relatively unique. You may feel inclined to conduct a group for students who are ELL, receiving special education services, identify as gay, lesbian, bisexual, or transgendered (GLBT), or have drug and alcohol issues. Perhaps part of your decision to do so relates to personal identification with one of the aforementioned groups. Although close experience can sometimes provide instant empathy and a rich experiential pool to draw from, it can also lend itself to additional challenges. For example, keep in mind boundary and countertransference (i.e., the counselor overidentifies with the client and "sees" him- or herself in the client) issues in these situations. Counselors who have personal experience similar to group members may have a hard time setting limits as to how much to help and self-disclose, and, as they recall their own journey related to the topic at hand (e.g., substance use, coming out, being bullied, etc.), may find themselves relating personally to the struggles of the student. These situations refer to those beyond where there is basic empathy to those that impact the counselor's ability to maintain a professional relationship. In cases where there is this potential, some counselors find it helpful to have a cofacilitator and/or consultant for additional support. In brief, make sure you have specific professional training in addition to real-life experience.

Although there may be benefits and challenges to having firsthand experience with the group topic, it is certainly not a requirement. As discussed in greater detail in chapter 10, there are many variables that contribute to group member satisfaction, including establishing rapport and a therapeutic alliance with the group leader as well as the cultural competency and general counseling competency of the group leader.

LOGISTICAL ISSUES

Aside from additional skills, there are logistical considerations as well. Most of these are well documented in earlier chapters; however, groups for students with special needs may require supplementary resources. School counselors will use their collaboration and advocacy skills, communicating with the administration regarding the importance of group work and what needs may be evident. An example of an additional resource that might be needed is funding for interpreters for families who are non-English speaking. All group consent forms and other paperwork need to be translated into the family's language so genuine informed consent can be obtained. Special co-facilitators and accessible meeting locations are just a few other considerations to keep in mind. Additionally, accommodations may need to be made for individuals with visual and or hearing differences. For instance, the group curriculum may need to be translated into Braille, and an interpreter may need to be present as well.

Sample Groups Targeted for Students with Special Needs

As mentioned earlier, research shows that students with special needs can benefit from small-group counseling (Leichtentritt & Shechtman, 2010; Shechtman & Pastor, 2005; Stephens, Jain, & Kim, 2010). The following sections will address the unique needs of various special populations within K–12 school settings and recommendations for best practice. Although there are many special needs within our schools, below are a few examples, presented in alphabetical order, of student groups that may benefit from a small-group counseling experience.

It should be noted that these populations are identified by their status as *at risk* (also referred to as *at promise*) and/or as a potentially underserved group. Although these individuals may have counseling needs beyond the scope of the school counselor, they may often benefit from small-group counseling. As indicated in chapter 4, pregroup screening is extremely important to ensure that students are receiving appropriate services and that school counselors are not overstepping their role. Remember, even though these students may have specific needs (e.g., recovery, coming out, etc.) associated with personal/social issues, the role of the school counselor related to each of the domains of school counseling (career, personal/social, academic) is through the lens of supporting academic success. With this in mind, group leaders may benefit from being well informed about the unique needs of students with special needs when leading groups. For example, school counselors may choose to facilitate groups focused on academic success, which includes students experiencing academic challenge due to substance use; however, the group does not target recovery issues but rather prevention and how substance use impacts academic achievement. Being aware of the specific challenges and needs of students with substance abuse issues can help the school counselor make good decisions about the students' appropriateness for small-group participation as well as what groups may be of support. For those issues outside the scope of the school counselor, the student can and should be referred to community agencies and resources. In the event that a student is receiving therapeutic support from a community agency while participating in a school counseling group, it is suggested that a release of information be signed so that the school counselor may inform the community counselor of the student's involvement in the school-based group and encourage collaboration to further support the student.

Drug and Alcohol Issues

Kelly and Juhnke's (2005) chapter titled "Addictions Prevention and Intervention Within Schools" points to the significance of substance abuse issues for today's students.

Almost 29% of high school students surveyed reported binge drinking within the past 30 days. These students were also more likely to report poor school performance, health risk behaviors, sexual activity, cigarette smoking, dating violence, suicide attempts, and drug use (J. W. Miller, Naimi, Brewer, & Jones, 2007). Reducing substance use has been associated with increased school attendance (Engberg & Morral, 2006). Considering the long-term impact of school attendance (i.e., graduation, career opportunities), school counseling interventions focused on prevention and current use are imperative. Brief interventions have been shown to be effective when working with adolescents with substance abuse issues (Winters, Leitten, Wagner, & Tevyah, 2007). Small-group work can provide support as that brief intervention in school settings.

Given the potential frequency of contact and accessibility to the student, an important responsibility of school counselors is to support students so they do not relapse into drug and alcohol use (Burrow-Sanchez & Lopez, 2009; Fisher & Harrison, 1993). In fact, three high-risk situations—negative emotional states, interpersonal conflict, and social pressure—account for 75% of reported relapse events (Cummings, Gordon, & Marlatt, 1980). Recent research also notes the school environment itself as a potential trigger for substance abuse: "Much like neglectful or dysfunctional school climate, the physical aspect of schools in disrepair may have a detrimental impact on student behavior, including substance using behavior" (Grana et al., 2010, p. 388). As such, counselors can focus on these topics within small-group work to support student abstinence and prevent use. Small groups focusing on conflict resolution, self-esteem, and peer pressure may have indirect benefits for substance use prevention as well. If you conduct small groups with African American students with substance abuse issues, a good resource is Brinson (1995).

Gifted and Talented

Despite ASCA's (2004c) recommendation that school counseling interventions should be prevention focused, let's face it, some school counselors spend a majority of time putting out fires; they are reactive rather than proactive. In schools where this is the case, gifted/talented and other "nonproblem" students often are un- or underserved by school counselors. To meet the academic press in many schools, groups are conducted for students in need of, for example, organizational or study skills. Because the highly capable population is largely not in this category, school counselors tend to focus their groups on the struggling learners. Of course, the gifted and talented have significant needs that merit group interventions. At the forefront of these needs are social and emotional issues (Sunde Peterson & Raye, 2006). In fact, Tessier (1982) many years ago declared that "problems of gifted students include a lag between intellectual and physical/social development, manipulative tendencies, intellectual laziness, work avoidance, low self-worth, alienation, and pressure for success" (p. 43). In response to such concerns, PSCs can provide small groups focused on social skills, self-esteem, career exploration, school success, and stress management.

Bullying is identified in the literature as one of the social issues of concern for gifted populations. In a pertinent study of 432 gifted eighth-graders from 16 different school districts in 11 states, 73% of males and 63% of females indicated they had experienced either physical or verbal bullying or both (Sunde Peterson & Raye, 2006). Interestingly, some of these same participants (33% of males, 22% of females) also reported engaging in acts of bullying during kindergarten through eighth grade. The researchers recommended small-group work focusing on both prevention and intervention, noting the benefits of group counseling (e.g., the opportunity for learning communication skills and finding commonalities). Other benefits of small groups mentioned by the authors included improving interpersonal skills, learning to appreciate others' perspectives, learning to problem solve, and learning to express feeling appropriately (Sunde Peterson & Raye, 2006).

In Randall's (1997) summary of research related to gifted females, major difficulties experienced by this population were identified, including cultural, social, psychological, educational, and parental challenges. One particular study, spanning eight decades, indicated these concerns to be consistent throughout the time period (Walker, Reis, & Leonard, 1992). Specific issues identified in Randall's literature review included a lack of awareness of career options, social challenges associated with being gifted, and a tendency for females who had multiple strengths to spread themselves too thin. Apparently they do this because of the "Superwoman Syndrome," wherein the highly capable girls seem to think "I am good at and enjoy so many things, I should do them all" (Callahan, Cunningham, & Plucker, 1994, p. 100). Randall goes on to report that "gifted girls may be the most ignored population in our schools" (p. 48) and recommends that group counseling include peer support, time to share frustrations and challenges, and opportunities to celebrate successes. Group counseling is also recommended for gifted culturally diverse students (e.g., see Robbins, Tonemah, & Robbins, 2002, for a sample group for gifted Native American students). Group leaders working with this latter population are encouraged to consider both academic and nonacademic needs, embracing issues such as self-concept, relationships, culture, life satisfaction, and future goals (Ford-Harris, Schuerger, & Harris, 1991; Humes & Clark, 1989; Tessier, 1982).

Sexual Minority Youth

Sexual minority is a term often used to describe students who identify as GLBT (gay, lesbian, bisexual, or transgendered) (Davies, 2006; Goodenow, Szalacha, & Westheimer, 2006). As with any marginalized minority group, the potential for lack of services to address their unique needs is a real issue (P. Griffin, Lee, Waugh, & Beyer, 2004). A 2006 published qualitative study of gay, lesbian, and bisexual (GLB) youth indicated that participants felt judged by school counselors and teachers, felt unsafe at school, and had concerns regarding the lack of preventative services for suicide and risk assessment for GLB students (Rutter & Leech, 2006). Additional research looking at the experiences of 202 sexual minority youth in 52 schools indicated that those students in schools with GLB support groups experienced lower rates of victimization and suicide attempts than those without such support (Goodenow et al., 2006). Similarly, Davies (2006) cited schools as unsafe for GLB students, indicating that discrimination and bullying are prevalent and often result in self-harm or suicide. In addition to isolation, harassment, bullying, depression, and suicide, additional concerns for GLBT students include family rejection, homelessness, truancy, school withdrawal or dropping out, and substance use and abuse (Satterly & Dyson, 2005).

Research further points to the need for school reform and supportive factors for GLBT students in our schools (Mayberry, 2006). Small groups, not necessarily specific to GLBT students but rather intentional regarding inclusion, can provide such support. For example, bullying prevention programs for all students can include curriculum specific to this population; friendship groups can attend to healthy relationships, which are also important for GLBT students; and self-efficacy groups can challenge negative self-perception or identity. When including GLBT students in groups open to non-sexual-minority youth, it is imperative that pregroup interviews are utilized to screen for group members who may perpetuate bullying and harm to GLBT students within the group.

Support groups are essential for this population. Satterly and Dyson (2005) encouraged advocacy to come from a strengths-based perspective, focusing on the assets of GLBT students, resiliency issues, and existing supportive factors in the school. For example, Muller and Hartman (1998) provided a 15-session group plan for sexual minority youth. The article highlights the importance of small-group work for GLB students and provides topics, activities, discussion catalysts, and recommended speakers to attend to the challenges of this population.

Students Receiving Special Education Services

To reiterate, students with disabilities benefit from group counseling, and school counselors must be more intentional to include them in their group work (Tarver-Behring & Spagna, 2004). In a 2006 published study (Monteiro-Leitner, Asner-Self, Milde, Leitner, & Skelton), 102 rural school counselors were asked to share their perception of their roles as professional school counselors, the time they actually allocated to various activities, and the time they felt they should allocate to various activities. The 26 activities presented in the survey were based on the ASCA (2005a) National Model guidelines for professional school counselors. Interestingly, the issue of special education elicited the most responses. Respondents indicated they were very involved (up to 50% of their time) in the administrative aspect of students receiving special education services. Although the issue of small-group counseling was mentioned for the general school population, it was not indicated as being related specifically to those students receiving special education services (Monteiro-Leitner et al., 2006). Given the substantial amount of time that some counselors spend related to special education testing and paperwork, it makes sense that counselors focus on the preventive aspects of these students' needs as well.

As with any population in our schools, those receiving special education services are a diverse group. In the midst of this uniqueness is a frequent need for personal/social support in addition to academic assistance. Frye (2005) underscored this point, stating that "current research suggests a number of personal/social difficulties that come with a diagnosis of a physical disability, emotional disorder, or learning disability" (p. 442). Small-group counseling is indicated as an important intervention for this population, specifically focusing on behavior, social skills, and self-esteem (Frye, 2005).

Transition challenges, particularly the transition from high school to postsecondary education and careers, are identified as another significant need for students receiving special education services (Milsom & Hartley, 2005; Scarborough & Gilbride, 2006; Trolley et al., 2009). Despite this concern, research indicates that school counselors often fail to provide such support and report feeling unprepared to do so (Milsom, 2002).

Studies also point to higher dropout rates and lower likelihood of college attendance for this population than their peers without disabilities (Fabian & MacDonald-Wilson, 2005). Small-group counseling can provide much-needed support for the transition needs for students with disabilities (Scarborough & Gilbride, 2006). Below, an example of a school-based group designed for students with special needs is provided. School counselors considering starting a group for students with special needs should research additional group curriculum and activities. For example, Mannix (1993, 1998) provides great resources related to social skills group work for both primary and secondary students with special needs that include an abundance of lessons, activity sheets, and worksheets for group use.

GROUPS IN PRACTICE

Small-Group Scenario: High School Group for Students Receiving Special Education[1]

Most groups deployed for specific student subpopulations can be used with most high school students. Nevertheless, students receiving special education often need the group to be further individualized to their specific needs. For example, in a recent group conducted in a Washington State high school, members were selected from the SPED population. Based on previous research indicating that a significant percentage of students with special needs regularly exhibit a negative sense of self-worth and low self-esteem (Brennan & Brennan,1999; Butler & Marinov-Glassman,1994; Pijl, Skaalvik, & Skaalvik, 2010; Ryba & And, 1995) and transitional challenges (C. Griffin, 2010; McEachern & Kenny, 2007; Sun, 2007), the school counselor designed the group with this overarching aim in mind: Members were to gain new skills and behaviors that might help their identity development and personal adjustment, as well as contribute to higher self-esteem. It was assumed that if students developed these skills, their transitional issues would decline.

Specifically, the small group was developed for six students classified as having specific learning challenges (e.g., learning disability, attention deficit disorder, or attention deficit hyperactivity disorder) and who were currently receiving SPED services. Group topics included learning how to identify and discuss strengths and weaknesses and how to better communicate their feelings, thoughts, and ideas about this topic more effectively. Group members were provided with the opportunity to practice how to give and receive positive feedback, and acquired various techniques to deal effectively with the transition from high school to the real world, including personal goal setting, motivation, and self-determination. For detailed information on the group rationale, weekly objectives, logistical considerations, materials needed, procedures, evaluation tools, and so on, refer to the chapter supplement.

---

[1]This real-world example was graciously provided by Lorraine Bettelyoun, school counselor, Washington State.

OTHER PRACTICAL CONSIDERATIONS

When it comes to meeting the needs of special populations in your school, you may not know where to begin. As discussed in earlier chapters, a formal (i.e., survey) or informal (observation, teacher or other staff recommendations) needs assessment can serve you well to identify populations in your school that would benefit from small-group counseling. As with any population being served, it is imperative that you also thoughtfully consider your own personal values and biases prior to working with an individual or group. As mentioned above, even though having personal experience with a group topic may be particularly useful, it can also be a hindrance if appropriate boundaries are not clearly defined. Similarly, not having experience with a specific special need, such as being gifted, having a substance abuse issue, or dealing with other unique challenges, does not prohibit you from being an effective helper and advocate for that population. Prior to running a group for a population with a specific special need, it would behoove you as a school counselor to familiarize yourself with the culture of such a group, keeping in mind that some information provided may include stereotypes and that not all cultural norms apply to everyone within a group. It is important to be aware of resources frequently used within a group, such as Alcoholics Anonymous (AA), Narcotics Anonymous (NA), or Alateen (Alanon for teenage populations). It is necessary to be open and honest; students are savvy and can spot an imposter or a fake. In our experience, students are more concerned with your commitment to being a support, being genuine, and being willing to ask respectful questions rather than your being an expert on a topic or being a member of a particular group.

SUMMARY AND CONCLUSION

Students with special needs are ideal candidates for small-group counseling. Through this school counseling intervention, students may learn skills to support their academic, personal/social, and career goals and achieve academic success. In addition to important skill-building opportunities, group counseling provides this population with much-needed peer support, a sense of normalcy, and opportunities to practice new skills. This chapter provided an overview of the relevance of group work for students with special needs as well as the professional, legal, and ethical mandates relevant to working with these populations. Key players in the lives of students with special needs were identified including recommendations for collaboration. A small-group scenario was provided to share an example of a small group appropriate for students receiving special education services (additional detail is provided in the following chapter supplement), and the chapter concluded with a few practical considerations to guide your work as a school counselor to support the needs of all students. We hope this chapter encourages consideration of how your work as a group counselor might include students with special needs and elicit intentionality when assessing and planning for the needs of your school population.

CHAPTER 9 SUPPLEMENTS

Supplement 9.1: Additional Published Resources   When conducting group with students in SPED, it is a good idea to read up on the topic before proceeding. Consider perusing the first two texts, for they provide both an excellent overview of the various laws that impact students with disabilities and important considerations for school counselors working with this population, and then reading through more specific articles.

- *Assisting students with disabilities: A handbook for school counselors* (Baumberger & Harper, 2007)
- *The school counselor's guide to special education* (Trolley et al., 2009): This article provides user-friendly descriptions of various special education categories (specific learning disabilities, speech and language impairments, emotional disturbance, mild mental retardation, and development delay) and how to counsel students according to their classification:
- "Counseling with Exceptional Children" (Tarver-Behring & Spagna, 2004): This is an example of an article addressing a group for high-functioning students in SPED.
- "A Brief Group Counseling Model to Increase Resiliency of Students with Mild Disabilities" (Arman, 2002)

Supplement 9.2: Sample Group with High School Students in SPED   What follows is a summary of an actual 7-week group conducted with high school students in SPED. The title of the group reflects its primary foci: Self-Esteem and Transition for High School Students. The major components of a group action plan discussed in chapter 3 are included here. Much of this plan can be adapted to students with other special needs.

Rationale. Adolescence is a time of identity development, when many teens have difficulty developing a strong sense of self (Carrell, 2000). Having a positive, realistic self-esteem (i.e., how one feels and thinks about his or her self-worth and competence) contributes to one's ability to deal with life's challenges, learn from experiences, and live cooperatively with others (Currie & Wadlington, 2000). Regrettably, due to a lack of success throughout their schooling, many students with disabilities have a low self-image and pessimistic ideas about their aptitudes (Currie & Wadlington, 2000). This small group will attempt to increase the self-esteem of students with disabilities, contributing to a higher likelihood of success in members' high school and post–high school endeavors.

Overall objectives. The group objectives were as follows:

- to establish trust and rapport
- to contribute to an environment where group members can feel safe and comfortable sharing their thoughts, feelings, and behaviors
- to increase understanding of self-esteem and its connection to their future
- to increase understanding of their strengths as well as areas in need of improvement
- to increase ability to give and receive positive feedback
- to increase ability to develop and meet realistic goals
- to increase understanding of motivation and self-determination and how these relate to their future transition from high school to the "real world"

Weekly objectives. Here the objectives for each session are outlined.

Week 1: Getting to Know the Group
Students will get to know each other, learn how the group functions (including norms and rules), review confidentiality, clarify expectations, identify how they fit in the group, and develop trust of other group members and the group leader.

Week 2: I Am Someone Who
Students will clarify aspects of their self-identity.

Week 3: A Personal Symbol/Objects Like Me
Students will increase self-awareness by describing themselves in relation to chosen objects, clarify who they are and what they value in relation to the chosen objects, and increase self-awareness by listening to feedback from others.

Week 4: Strengths and Limitations
Students will affirm their capabilities and enhance their self-esteem, learn that others share areas in need of improvement and that having differences is not "shameful," increase their self-awareness and ability to assess themselves realistically, and learn to value their unique strengths and to see that there are many kinds of valuable personal characteristics.

Week 5: Me and My Future/Success and Failure
Students will clarify how they see themselves in the future regarding "success" and "failure."

Week 6: Gain with Goals
Students will differentiate between short-term and long-term goals, distinguish between realistic and unrealistic goals, and learn how to establish short-term and long-term goals.

Week 7: Final Goal Setting and Celebration
Students will develop a long-term goal and the short-term goals to reach it, discuss their group experience, and celebrate their growth and progress.

Logistics. Students were recruited through their school's study skills classes. The SPED teachers were approached and asked for a list of students who might benefit from a group on self-esteem. The level of these students' learning difficulties was relatively mild. From this list, the group leader conducted screening/pregroup interviews and selected six group members (see interview questions in Procedures section). The leader also arranged a tentative meeting place, the school's conference room. The group met during Period 6 on block days for approximately 45 minutes.

Procedures. To ensure that the teacher-recommended group members were appropriate for the group, the group leader led screening/pregroup interviews. These individual interviews including the following questions regarding group member expectations, confidentiality, informed consent, and potential harm to students (adapted from Smead, 1995):

- The topic of the group is self-esteem and post–high school transition. Does this sound like something that you could benefit from?
- The group leader is a graduate student, enrolled in a group counseling class and under the supervision of both a university supervisor and the school counselor in this building. Is that clear?

- The group will meet on block schedule days, during sixth period, from 1:10 to 1:55. Will that work for you?
- You will be expected to come on time to group and stay the entire session. Can you do that?
- As a group member, you will have the responsibility to attend all sessions unless you talk with me ahead of time and arrange to not come to a session or to leave the group. Can you make this commitment to the group?
- If you have academic work to make up, you will be responsible to do so. Are you prepared to take that responsibility?
- The other group members will be male and female _____ High School students, Grades 10 through 12. Are you comfortable with that?
- To participate in the group, you must give your written permission, and obtain the written permission of your parent or guardian. Would that be feasible?
- As a member of the group, you will be required to share some of your personal thoughts, feelings, and behaviors, but only those you choose to share. Nobody will force you to share things that are private to you and that you do not want to share. Are you comfortable with that?
- As a member of the group, you have a responsibility to explore yourself and develop goals to make positive changes in your life. Can you commit to this?
- As a member of the group, you must give other members the freedom to share their personal thoughts, feelings, and behaviors, without interrupting or ridiculing them. Can you do this?
- The group leader has the responsibility to make every effort to protect the safety and well-being of all group members, including safety from physical and verbal harm. Can you abstain from physically or verbally harming another group member?
- By being in the group, you open yourself up to be pressured by other group members to take risks. It is part of the group leader's job to make every effort to keep other members from pressuring you against your choice. Are you comfortable with that?
- In group, all members must agree to keep what is said in group confidential. This means that no member tells what anyone else says or does in the group. The other group members will agree not to tell what you say or do in group, and you must agree not to tell what they say or do in group. Because we do not always have control over what other people say or do, we cannot be sure everybody will keep this promise. At the beginning of each session, to help everyone remember I will remind everyone of the confidentiality rule. Does this sound reasonable to you?
- There are some times when the group leader would need to share what you say with other adults, such as your parents or guardian. These times are as follows:
  - If you say you are going to harm yourself or someone else.
  - If you say anything about child abuse happening to yourself or someone else.
  - If a court (judge) tells the group leader she or he needs to share some information with them.
- Does that make sense?
- You have the right to leave the group at any time, provided you discuss this with the group leader. You are expected to be at every group meeting, but the leader understands that sometimes unforeseen circumstances occur. Is that clear?

- Between group sessions, the group leader can discuss only issues of confidentiality or a serious problem, but not issues that are related to the group. Those issues must be dealt with during group sessions. Does that seem reasonable?
- Sometimes, you might have practice to do outside of group between sessions. Will you do that?
- Are you seeing any other counselors for counseling in a group or individually?
- Would you give your permission for the group leader to videotape one or more sessions?

After the interviews, the group leader answered the following questions about each member (adapted from Smead, 1995):

- Does the student seem to understand what the purpose and goals of the group are?
- Does the student appear to want to participate in and be a productive member of the group?
- Does the student have some positive behaviors/attitudes that might serve as a model for some of the other tentative group members?
- Does the student seem to be making the decision to join the group independently or under the influence of others?

Based on the interview and follow-up questions, the group leader provided each prospective member with a parent/guardian permission form to return as soon as possible. They were reminded that they could not be part of the group until the form was returned.

Evaluation procedures. To formally assess students' progress toward understanding and developing self-esteem, group members and their teachers will be given evaluation forms following the last group session (see the following samples adapted from Greenberg, 2003). Also, group members will complete a pre- and posttest regarding their knowledge of self-esteem (see the following sample adapted from Huggins, Manion, & Moen, 1994). The pregroup survey was administered before the first meeting in the students' study skills class. Posttesting occurred during the last session.

Group Member Evaluation Form

Name: (Optional)

Directions: Please circle "Y" for "YES," "N" for "NO," and "MAYBE" for "NOT SURE."

1. Did the group talk about things that were interesting to you?
   Y   N   MAYBE

2. Did you participate frequently in the group discussions?
   Y   N   MAYBE

3. Was the group helpful to you?
   Y   N   MAYBE

4. As a result of being in this group, do you have a better understanding of what self-esteem means?
   Y   N   MAYBE

(continued)

Group Member Evaluation Form (*continued*)

5. As a result of being in this group, do you have a better understanding of yourself?

   Y   N   MAYBE

6. As a result of being in this group, are you more aware of things you can do well and things you need to improve on?

   Y   N   MAYBE

7. As a result of being in this group, are you able to define your personal goals more clearly?

   Y   N   MAYBE

8. As a result of being in this group, do you have a better understanding of your motivation to pursue goals?

   Y   N   MAYBE

9. As a result of being in this group, do you have a better understanding of what other teens are dealing with?

   Y   N   MAYBE

10. Do you feel you have accomplished something as a result of being in this group?

    Y   N   MAYBE

    If **YES**, what have you accomplished specifically? (Write your comments here.)

    If **NO**, what do you think prevented you from accomplishing anything? (Write your comments here.)

    If **MAYBE**, what do you think might have contributed to you accomplishing more? (Write your comments here.)

11. Would you want to be included in another group someday?

    Y   N   MAYBE

12. Please list any things about the group or activities you especially liked. (Write your comments here.)

13. Please list any things about the group or activities you especially disliked. (Write your comments here.)

Thank you for your time!
Ms. B ☺

Group Member Self-Esteem Knowledge Pre- and Posttest Survey

Directions: On the line before each statement, please write "T" for TRUE, "F" for FALSE, and "?" for "DON'T KNOW."

1. _____ Every person is good at some things and not good at other things.

2. _____ Everyone has some things to be proud of.

3. _____ It is okay to praise yourself.

4. _____ You are different from most people in the world.

5. _____ Everyone makes mistakes.

6. _____ It is important to like yourself.

7. _____ The only way to like yourself is to be perfect.

8. _____ Thinking and saying good things about yourself is bragging.

9. _____ We cannot learn from our mistakes, so it is best to just ignore them.

10. _____ How you feel about yourself affects everything you do in life.

11. _____ Someone can get low grades in math and still be very intelligent.

12. _____ People like you better if you are self-confident.

13. _____ Most people think you are great.

14. _____ You will do better at things if you encourage yourself instead of criticizing yourself.

15. _____ A person who gets low grades in reading is probably not very smart.

16. _____ The only way to like yourself is to be perfect at the things that are important to you.

17. _____ It helps you to be continually thinking about your mistakes.

18. _____ Being different from everyone else in the world makes you special.

19. _____ There is no such thing as a worthless human being.

20. _____ Before you start something difficult, it is helpful to think about all the possible ways you might fail.

21. _____ Every single person has some strengths and some weaknesses.

22. _____ Telling yourself you are going to fail at something increases your chances of failing.

Teacher Group Evaluation Form

Teacher Name:

Name of Student:

A seven-session group dealing with self-esteem has just concluded. Your student listed above participated in the group. I would appreciate your input regarding his or her personal growth and any change you may have noticed in this student as a result of the group experience. Your answers to this evaluation will be kept confidential. They will be used only to help me assess the effectiveness of this group and to make any needed changes for future groups. Any comments will be especially appreciated.

Using the following *scale from 1 to 5*, please rate each student on his or her progress toward each of the following objectives:

5 = *a lot* of change/improvement
4 = *much* change/improvement
3 = *some* change/improvement
2 = *little* change/improvement
1 = *no* change/improvement
0 = *cannot say/no opportunity to observe*

1. To increase their understanding of self-esteem and its connection to their future

   Progress toward objective: _____

   Comments:

   _____

   _____

2. To increase their understanding of their strengths as well as their weaknesses

   Progress toward objective: _____

   Comments:

   _____

   _____

3. To increase their ability to give and receive positive feedback

   Progress toward objective: _____

   Comments:

   _____

   _____

4. To increase their ability to develop realistic goals for themselves and make plans to meet these goals

   Progress toward objective: _____

   Comments:

   _____

   _____

5. To increase their understanding of motivation and self-determination and how these relate to their future transition from high school to the "real world"
Progress toward objective: _____
Comments:

_____
_____

6. General growth and progress in matters pertaining to self-esteem (i.e., confidence, self-awareness, self-expression, motivation).
Progress (*using the same scale*): _____
Comments:

_____
_____

Thanks for your time!

Session topics and procedures outline. All sessions were adapted from the following resources: Carrell (2000), Khalsa (1996), Peterson (1993), and Vernon (1998).

Week 1: Getting to Know the Group[2]
Objectives:

- The students will get to know each other.
- The students will establish how the group functions (including norms and rules).
- The students will review confidentiality.
- The students will clarify their expectations and apprehensions for the group.
- The students will identify how they fit in the group.
- The students will develop trust of other group members and the group leader.
- The students will begin a discussion of self-esteem.

Materials:

- Large piece of butcher paper and markers

Procedure:
Getting to Know Each Other

- Group members sit in a circle.
- The group leader explains that one way to help remember someone's name is by associating it with something about them.
- An example is given as the group leader introduces herself: "My name is Ms. B and I like to go to concerts for fun."
- The members are asked to take turns doing the same and then repeat the name and special interest of the group member who preceded them (and any others that they can remember).

---

[2]Specific handouts and information referenced in this supplement can be obtained from the authors.

- If a group member cannot remember the name of the preceding member, he or she should be encouraged to ask that member his or her name and special interest.
- Continue until all members have introduced themselves and stated a special interest.
- Ask if any of the members can state all of the names and special interests of the other students.

Establishing Group Norms and Rules (Including Confidentiality)

- The group leader explains the importance of establishing norms and rules for groups.
- The group brainstorms rules for the group as the leader writes them on a big piece of butcher paper.
  - The leader makes sure to suggest any of the rules that were discussed in the pregroup interview.
  - The leader makes sure to include rules and limits of *confidentiality*.
- The leader asks each group member to agree to the rules.
- If there is any disagreement, the group discusses it.

Clarifying Expectations and Apprehensions of the Group

- The leader asks each member to discuss his or her expectations for the group and one apprehension.
- The leader reinforces appropriate self-disclosures and attempts at sharing feelings.

Discussing Self-Esteem

- The leader asks the members what self-esteem means to them.
  - The leader provides definition or adds to the members' definitions:
    - Self-esteem is how we feel about ourselves.
    - Self-esteem is how we think others feel about us.
- The leader asks the members, "What are some ways we can feel about ourselves?"
- The leader asks the members, "Why do you think we feel the way we do about ourselves?"
- The leader asks the members, "Do you think our self-esteem can change?"
- The leader asks the members, "What could make our self-esteem change?"
- The leader asks the members, "How high is your self-esteem on a scale from 1 to 10?"
  - The leader should take note of the ratings and re-ask this question at the last session.
- The leader asks the members, "How do you feel others feel about you?"

Summary of the Session

- The leader reviews the session.
- The leader asks if any members have any questions.
- The leader answers questions if necessary.
- The leader thanks the group members for their participation.

Week 2: I Am Someone Who
Objectives:

- The students will clarify aspects of their self-identity.

Materials:

- Copy of "I Am Someone Who" Sorting Board (Handout 1) for each student
- Copy of "I Am Someone Who" Sentence Strips (Handout 2) for each student
  - Cut apart and in envelopes
- Glue stick for every student

Procedures:

- The leader checks in with the students, asking each how their week is going.
- The leader introduces the lesson by eliciting responses in gestures.
  - If they really know "who they are," they are to raise both hands in the air.
  - It they have some idea of "who they are," they are to raise one hand in the air.
  - If they are unclear of "who they are," they are to keep their hands in their laps.
- The leader distributes the "I Am Someone Who" Sorting Board (Handout 1) and Sentence Strips (Handout 2) to each student.
- The students independently read the Sentence Strips and glue them to the appropriate categories on the Sorting Board.
- When the students are finished sorting, the leader invites them to share their results with a partner.
- The leader facilitates discussion regarding the process.
  - How easy was it for you to do the sorting?
  - Did you and your partner have similar Sentence Strips in the various categories?
  - Were any items particularly difficult to categorize? If so, which ones?
  - On the basis of this activity, do you know yourself as well as you thought you did?
  - What, if anything, would you like to have in the "Very Much Like Me" category that is not there now?
  - How about the "Not at All Like Me" category?
  - On the basis of your responses to the last two questions, what things would you like to change about yourself? Is that possible? How can you do it?
    - Invite the students to share specific examples.
  - Suppose you cannot change anything. Can you accept yourself how you are currently? What can facilitate acceptance?
  - What did you learn about yourself from this activity?
  - The leader and group members summarize the session.
    - *In preparation for the next session, the leader prompts the students to bring an object from home that "symbolizes" them.*
    - *The object might be something that represents who they are or what they value, or it might be something that "sums them up."*
    - *It must be something that they can touch, hold, and show to the group.*
    - *If the object cannot actually be carried to the group, a photograph or drawing will suffice.*

Week 3: A Personal Symbol/Objects Like Me
Objectives:

- The students will choose an object from home or one from those provided that is most like them and tell why they chose it.
- The students will listen to others' self-perceptions and give feedback thoughtfully and sensitively.
- The students will increase self-awareness by describing themselves in relation to the chosen objects.
- The students will clarify who they are and what they value in relation to the chosen objects.
- The students will increase self-awareness by listening to feedback from others.

Materials:

- Students' objects brought from home
- Carefully chosen objects such as a box of matches, a sponge, a red ball, a clown doll, an old tennis shoe, a mask, a rock, a pine cone, a puzzle, a heart-shaped box, a whistle

Procedures:

- The leader reviews briefly what was learned last week and checks in with students on how their week is going.
- The leader begins by asking students to show the group their personal symbol brought from home and explain why it represents something about them.
  - For students who did not bring a symbol, they can choose one from those provided by the leader.
  - The students respond to the self-perception described by group members by giving feedback to that member.
- The leader asks, "Is there anyone who would have had a much different symbol a few years ago?"
  - Allow time for discussion.
- The leader asks, "Is there anyone who would have brought the same symbol to group a few years ago?"
  - Allow time for discussion.
- The leader and students summarize the session.
- The leader closes the group by thanking members for sharing their symbols and giving honest and appropriate feedback.

Week 4: Strengths and Limitations
Objectives:

- Through articulating personal strengths, the students affirm their capabilities and enhance their self-esteem.
- By sharing their personal limitations with peers and getting feedback, the students learn that others have similar differences or challenges and that having limitations is not "shameful."
- The students increase their self-awareness and ability to assess themselves realistically.

- The students learn to value their unique strengths and to see that there are many kinds of valuable personal characteristics.
- The students learn that they do not have to apologize for their strengths or their limitations.

Materials:

- List of possible strengths on butcher paper
- List of possible limitations on butcher paper
- Piece of paper and pen for each student

Procedures:

- The leader reviews briefly what was learned last week and checks in with the students on how their week is going.
- The leader prompts the students to fold the paper in half lengthwise, and brainstorm a list of their personal strengths on the left side of the paper, labeled *strengths*.
  - The leader tells them to think of the things they can "count on" or "have confidence in" or "trust" about themselves, both as they interact with others and when they are alone. The leader might also ask, "What do you think other people value in you?" or "What do you think other people would say your strengths are?"
- Before the students start to write, the leader shares her or his own list of strengths and/or offers suggestions from this list:

organized	a good listener
responsible	kind
compassionate	energetic
personable	even-tempered
patient	an eager learner
athletic	a good dancer
helpful	not moody (even-tempered)
intelligent	good sense of humor
dependable	organized
tolerant	nonjudgmental
self-confident	creative
witty	verbal skills
mechanical gifts	mathematical skills
musical talent	good with elderly people
artistically talented	good with young children

- The leader tells the students that affirming their capabilities is good practice for the future, when they will need to speak or write about themselves with confidence during job interviews and on college and scholarship applications.
- The leader prompts the students to share their lists.
- The leader prompts the students to list their limitations on the other side of the paper.
  - The leader tells the students to think of the characteristics, habits, or "flaws" that get in the way of things they want to do; that cause problems in their relationships; that keep them from being their best.

- Before the students start to write, the leader shares her or his own list of challenges/limitations and/or offers suggestions from this list.

a procrastinator	hot-tempered
a gossip	disorganized
impatient	irresponsible
messy	mean
a poor listener	critical
naïve	easily depressed

- The leader tells the students that being able to describe their limitations is an important step in learning to deal with them and/or compensate for them.
- The leader prompts the students to share their lists.
- Time permitting, the leader prompts the students to discuss why they might have more limitations than strengths listed.
- For closure, the leader asks the students which strengths and limitations seem to be common in the group. The leader asks, "How did it feel to talk about your strengths and limitations with other group members?"

Week 5: Me and My Future/Success and Failure
Objectives:

- To clarify how the students see themselves in the future regarding "success" and "failure"

Materials:

- A copy of "Me and My Future—Rank-Order" Worksheet (Handout 3)
- A pen or pencil for each student

Procedures:

- The leader reviews briefly what was learned last week and checks in with the students on how their week is going.
- The leader introduces the lesson by discussing the fact that the students are reaching a point in their development where they are naturally beginning to think about who they are and how they see themselves in the future.
- The leader distributes the "Me and My Future—Rank-Order" Worksheet (Handout 3) to each student.
- The leader asks the students to think seriously about how they see themselves in the future and to complete the worksheet.
- The leader prompts the students to discuss their rankings with the group.
- The leader asks the following discussion questions:
  - Was it difficult to rank the items on the worksheet? If so, what about the process was difficult?
  - Which issues did you have to think of the most?
  - Are there other issues that you think should have been included on this list? If so, what and why?
  - What did you learn about yourself by doing this activity?
  - If you had completed this worksheet a year ago, what might have been ranked differently? Why?

- If you were to do this worksheet in the future, how do you think your rankings might change? How come would they change?
- When you think about the future, what is your image of yourself?
- How do you define success?
  - Having positive relationships?
  - Contributing to someone else's happiness?
  - Having someone's respect?
  - Knowing that you have done the best in your life?
  - Being able to appreciate life?
  - Being able to put your natural talents and abilities to use?
  - Being content with what you have?
- What will make you feel successful when you are 20? 30? 50? Retired?
- What might make you feel like a "failure" when you are an adult?
- How do you feel when you think about your future?
- For closure, the leader asks the students for a summary of anything new the students have learned or thought about that day.

Week 6: Gain with Goals
Objectives:

- The students will differentiate between short-term and long-term goals.
- The students will distinguish between realistic and unrealistic goals.
- The students will learn how to establish short-term and long-term goals.

Materials:

- A copy of "Gain with Goals" Worksheet (Handout 15) for each student
- Pencil and paper for each student
- A sheet of butcher paper and a marker for each dyad
- Masking tape

Procedures:

- The leader reviews briefly what was learned last week and checks in with the students on how their week is going.
- The leader introduces the lesson by asking the students to define the word *goal*.

  Goal = a plan, purpose, or object of effort or ambition

- The leader asks the students to explain the difference between short- and long-term goals.
  - Short-term goals = more immediate and usually lead up to a long-term goal
    - example: studying for tests to do well in classes and keep a good GPA
  - Long-term goals = more in the future
    - example: getting into a 4-year college after high school
- The leader asks the students who routinely sets short-term goals.
  - Have students describe one of their short-term goals.
- The leader asks the students who routinely sets long-term goals.
  - Have the students describe one of their long-term goals.
- The leader asks the students who routinely follows through on the goals they set.
  - What contributes to follow-through?

- The leader asks the students how they benefit from setting goals.
- The leader distributes the "Gain with Goals" Worksheet (Handout 15) to each student.
- The students work as partners to identify their responses.
- When the students have responded to the worksheet, the leader prompts them to discuss their answers with the group.
  - The leader clarifies and emphasizes the difference between realistic and unrealistic goals in terms of attainability.
- The leader asks the students to form dyads.
  - Each dyad gets a sheet of butcher paper and a marker.
  - Each student in the dyad needs to choose a long-term goal and brainstorm with his or her partner how to set short-term goals to reach it.
  - Dyads should discuss whether these goals seem realistic or unrealistic.
- Dyads who are comfortable share their long- and short-term goals with the group.
- The leader asks the following discussion questions.
  - How can you tell whether a goal is realistic or unrealistic?
  - What do you see as the major difference between short-term and long-term goals?
  - Why is it or is it not important to set goals?
  - What do you think prevents people from setting goals?
  - What do you think prevents people from achieving goals?
  - Who usually sets short-term goals?
    - Do you usually achieve them?
    - If not, what gets in the way?
  - Who usually sets long-term goals?
    - Do you usually achieve them?
    - If not, what gets in the way?
  - Describe a time in your life when you set a goal and it paid off.
  - Describe a time when you did not set a goal but wish you had. How might the outcome have been different if you had set a goal?
  - How can you apply what you have learned from this lesson to your life?

Week 7: Final Goal Setting and Celebration
Objectives:

- The students will develop a long-term goal and short-term goals to reach it.
- The students will discuss their group experience.
- The students will celebrate their growth and progress.

Materials:

- Pencil and paper for each student
- Treats for celebration

Procedures:

- The leader reviews briefly what was learned last week and checks in with the students on how their week is going.
- The leader reminds the students about long-term and short-term goals, as well as realistic and unrealistic goals.

- The leader prompts the students to think of a long-term goal for the remainder of the school year and the short-term goals to reach it.
- The students work independently and write their goals on their papers.
  - When students are finished, the leader prompts them to share their goals with the group.
  - The students discuss whether the goals are realistic or unrealistic.
- The students discuss one thing they have learned from the group experience.
- The students discuss one thing they have enjoyed about the group experience.
- The leader asks the members, "Now that we are done with the group, how high is your self-esteem on a scale from 1 to 10?"
  - The leader asks the students if their number has changed.
  - The leader asks why or why not?
- The leader thanks the students for their participation in the group and praises each of them for their growth.
- The group celebrates with a chance to eat and relax!

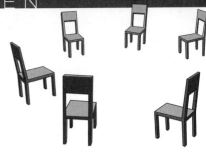

Small Groups for Students of Color: Multicultural Considerations

INTRODUCTION

When preservice school counseling interns are beginning their school-based practice, counseling a student from a different culture sometimes can be intimidating. Perhaps even more so, counseling a diverse group of students with major cultural differences that interns are unfamiliar with can be downright scary. Naturally, the student's counselees may have some fears as well, asking themselves, "Does this counselor really understand my world and where I come from? Can I trust her?" Perhaps some of this initial disquiet may arise out of a fundamental human misunderstanding: People frequently assume that those who look and talk like us share similar experiences, and that those who look and sound dissimilar from us experience life in different ways. To alleviate some of this mutual anxiety, school counselors can rely on rapport building, a basic skill they learned early on in their graduate education. If sensitively used, counselors and students should find shared experiences, providing a basis for establishing a common understanding and respect. Hopefully, in time, students will even feel a sense of acceptance, care, and support.

Although school counselors recognize that there are many definitions of the term *multicultural*, for the purpose of this chapter ethnicity is described as a primary variable contributing to culture. We would be remiss if we failed to acknowledge factors such as socioeconomic status, gender, sexual orientation, spirituality, and physical and mental differences as contributing forces in what creates the "lens" that each of us looks through. It should also be noted that the terms *multicultural* and *cultural* are used interchangeably as they relate to competency and counseling skills. Statistics taken from school districts around the United States indicate that today's schools are culturally diverse (U.S. Department of Education, 2010a). Despite the challenges of segregation that continue to exist in some schools, school counselors are more likely than ever to have the opportunity to learn from and be challenged by a diverse student population.

Counseling students of color, as suggested by the previous chapter, is somewhat unlike counseling students from privileged groups (e.g., dominant culture, male, high socioeconomic status, etc.). There are issues specific to individuals who have survived a history of racism, marginalization, segregation, and oppression that require awareness beyond basic group counseling skills. The idea that multicultural counseling and general counseling are unique constructs continues to be raised but is rarely addressed

(Cates, Schaefle, Smaby, Maddux, & LeBeauf, 2007; Coleman, 1998). Although great strides have been made in understanding these dynamics, there continue to be unresolved issues, specifically regarding the discontinuity espoused by some research-ers between general counseling competency and multicultural counseling competency (Cates et al., 2007; Coleman, 1998; Constantine, 2002). Numerous studies have pointed to the benefits of cultural competency when working with culturally diverse individ-uals (Carter, 1995; Collins & Arthur, 2010; Constantine, 2002; Fuertes et al., 2006; Ochs, 1994; Tomlinson-Clarke & Clarke, 2010; Ziomek-Daigle & Manalo, 2010). This chapter does not provide a handbook of what to do when working with culturally diverse students, but rather is a framework from which to guide your growth and development as a group leader.

Even as some nascent school counselors are fearful about working with students from diverse groups, other beginning counselors believe that if they know the history and culture of each student's background, they will be effective group leaders. Knowing the underlying themes found in cultural groups is clearly a first step toward multicul-tural counseling competency, but it is impossible to assimilate all the details about each student's cultural and familial story. Amazingly, some educators have reported working with students from over 60 ethnic groups in one school. Thus, in this chapter, we attend to important issues for students of color as identified in the following section, titled Special Considerations. Next, cultural competency and what it entails as well as con-siderations for working with culturally diverse students and group leader awareness are addressed. In the final section, actual field-based case examples and applications from the field are provided. The chapter supplement includes a multicultural counseling skills checklist as well as additional readings and resources that may be helpful when working with culturally diverse groups.

SPECIAL CONSIDERATIONS

Cultural competency for a group leader in schools requires that the school counselor be aware of and attend to issues specific to students of color (Astramovich, Forkner, & Bodenhorn, 2004; Delgado-Romero, Barfield, Fairley, & Martinez, 2005). Also at the forefront of important issues are those such as racial identity development, developmen-tal perspectives, group member/leader cultural differences, English-language learners, and first-generation students.

As we focus on the journey toward cultural competency, we may consider *why* culture is such an important variable for school counselors to consider in their group work. Culture is an overt and covert system of shared meaning; it helps us make sense of our world and our actions. Understanding cultural backgrounds furthers our self-understanding and how our perceptions, assumptions, treatments, and actions are influenced by the world in which we live. When we more fully understand our personal and cultural backgrounds and have knowledge of those in our interpersonal circles, we are better equipped to serve students of diverse histories and communities. Additionally, seeing the world through a lens that considers the dynamics of culture allows us to view the strengths and positives necessary to provide assistance, guidance, and support. For example, knowing that a child's family promotes interreliance among kin and extended family members may benefit school counselors as they attempt to recognize the student's need to be connected instead of labeling the child as "clingy" or "enmeshed."

When school counselors begin to observe differences between and among cultural groups, they may overlook the strengths and similarities of students. Developing a cultural lens is a both/and construct; counselors must see the unity within diversity without over- or underestimating the uniqueness of each child. All students have valuable skills and visions. Every child is influenced by political, economic, racial, and social contexts. We must foster the empowerment of families and schools by respecting the child's own experiences without placing our value system on those we seek to serve (Manning & Baruth, 2009). Thus, as mentioned above, one of the first steps is to establish rapport with each group member. When working with students of diverse backgrounds (typically these students belong to visible racial ethnic groups or VREGs), counselors seek to gather general data related to their:

- families' story and level of support for particular student,
- degree of language proficiency,
- educational history, and
- proximity to own and other cultural groups.

Gathering this data from multiple sources (e.g., teachers' input, student's cumulative file, student self-report) will help counselors know their students more fully, particularly their cultural frame of reference. Even with the best of intentions, school counselors would not be offering culturally relevant support if they asked a group member whose caregivers do not speak English to fill out a take-home worksheet that has not been translated into the caregiver's native language.

As counselors begin to discern the intricacies of their students, they are able to appreciate that a particular student's culture influences a myriad of dynamics in his or her life. Group members' personal backgrounds, family norms, and community standards influence their experience of pain, what they label as a symptom, how they communicate about pain/symptoms, their beliefs about the causes of suffering, and their attitudes toward helpers (school counselors), among other aspects related to group dynamics.

RACIAL IDENTITY DEVELOPMENT WITHIN A DEVELOPMENTAL PERSPECTIVE

As children grow, they develop personality and other traits that make each child relatively unique (Mistry & Sarawathi, 2003). Cultural, racial, and ethic development is a learned aspect of a child's comprehensive development. The sense of connection with a racial/ethnic group forms when one begins to negotiate boundaries in a pluralistic society (Hirschfeld, 1995; Jackson, 2009; Quintana, 1998). This development occurs throughout the life span. As children mature, they learn more about

- their own culture and history,
- others' cultures,
- self-identification,
- attitudes and values,

- use of language,
- feelings about the culture, and
- social preferences.

So, how do these processes develop? Like personality, cultural identity development begins at birth, is influenced by socialization, and is affected by experiences. This development continues throughout the life span. The process is nonlinear, and students can often get stuck in a place where they are not forming an identity or where they seek to deny their cultural identity (Hargrow, 2001; Salazar & Abrams, 2005).

There are several models for how adults apprehend their racial and ethnic development (Aldarondo, 2001; Atkinson, Morten, & Sue, 1998; Gay, 1999; Hargrow, 2001; Helms, 1995; Smith, 1991). Children's racial and ethnic development, however, cannot be understood using adult models (Quintana, 1998). Students' development is tied to their cognitive development; their understanding of culture is limited by their ability to understand ideas and understand how ideas relate to themselves. An adult may have the abstract-thinking capabilities to hypothesize why one person may like the adult for his or her humor, while understanding that another person, who is racist, will not like him or her no matter how much humor the adult uses. Young children do not have this level of abstract thought.

It is possible for children as young as 3 to recognize their own race. For VREGs it happens earlier, especially for children whose families prioritize ethnic and cultural socialization (Hirschfeld, 1995; Quintana, 1998). For children in a mixed ethnic setting, this development may occur under the age of 3. Quintana proposed that young children (ages 3 to 6) perceive physical properties of race such as skin color and believe that one can change (e.g., one can wash off his or her skin color). Children are likely to recognize their own ethnicity before that of others. For some, this may lead to feelings of rejection for those who are different.

Differing opinions exist in the literature related to children and their understanding of race (Mackinlay & Barney, 2008). One perspective indicates that throughout middle childhood, children are still largely concrete in their cognitive processing and tend to view racial identity as an external attribute (Hirschfeld, 1995; Quintana, 1998). Children understand race in literal terms: ancestry, customs, and language. For example, an early elementary school student may identify a "Chinese person" as someone who "eats rice" (Quintana, 1998). In late childhood and early adolescence, students are developing more complex thought and start to see ethnicity as an internal attribute. This new attitude leads to empathy and understanding of others. At this age, race and ethnicity are viewed as a social construct and schoolchildren are able to understand social justice involved in the treatment of others. Alternatively, more recent early childhood development literature has suggested that young children have a more complex view of race, similar to adults (Mackinlay & Barney, 2008; Van Ausdale & Feagin, 2000).

In adolescence, developing identity is linked to the emergence of a coherent sense of self. School counselors need to remember that it is possible for some students to get "stuck" in an early developmental stage and that stages are nonlinear in trajectory. Thus a child may have the cognitive and emotional potential to reach integration before adolescence. As teens begin to develop higher order cognitive abilities, thinking about self and others in terms of racial and ethnic identity becomes more complex. How students perceive themselves is often a result of how others perceive their group. This influences students' psychological well-being and their development of a positive cultural identity (Malott et al., 2010; Quintana, 1998).

CONDUCTING MULTIETHNIC SMALL GROUPS

Just as schools are becoming increasingly diverse (Roaten & Schmidt, 2009), so are the students participating in group counseling activities. If your school is representative of the changing demographics evidenced by the U.S. census data, it is more likely that the small groups conducted will be more ethnically and culturally heterogeneous than homogeneous. Although groups with a diverse membership can provide increased opportunities for students to learn from their peers and experience worldviews other than their own, ethnically heterogeneous groups present additional challenges for the leader.

Several themes have emerged in the literature regarding these potential leadership challenges. For instance, Cheng, Chae, and Gunn (1998) warned group leaders to be aware of the potential for racial and ethnic minorities to become scapegoats in the group counseling experience. Possible reasons for this scapegoating relate to the group members' "distinct racial characteristics; differing cultural beliefs; and lower political, economic, and social status in society" (Cheng et al., 1998, p. 384). Although school counselors facilitating groups should appreciate the value of cultural diversity in group composition, some student members may not share this welcoming attitude.

Although it is impossible to think through all the issues that may evolve in a multiethnic group, several considerations should be attended to prior to the formation of the group. When groups include a variety of ethnic and cultural backgrounds, the leader must be proactive in the screening process. Pregroup interviews allow counselors to determine a student's sensitivity to diverse groups. It should also not be assumed that all individuals within certain ethnic groups will automatically feel a positive connection. Various ethnic groups that may share the ethnic title of, say, "Native American" or "Asian" may have long-standing and historical dislike of one another.

Another variable to consider in multicultural groups is the individualistic and collective perspectives of various subpopulations (Friedman et al., 2010; Lee & Kelly, 1996; Trumbull & Rothstein-Fisch, 2008). Whereas many individuals from Asian and other collectivist-oriented cultures appreciate the holistic nature of group counseling, this perspective may be difficult or uncomfortable for students raised in a dominant culture that tends to be individualistic in nature (Pope, 1999). Additional recommendations for those facilitating multiethnic groups include consideration of concepts of time, commitment to schedules, level of emotional expressiveness, and the communication styles of potential group members (Acosta & Cristo, 1981; Portman, 2003). When it comes to cultural competence and meeting the needs of diverse students through group practice, the words of Johnson and Johnson (2005) are relevant: "The need for new ways to reach all students calls for acquiring new skills and reframing traditional professional competencies for school counselors" (p. 400).

To summarize, despite the potential challenges of facilitating a multiethnic group, the benefits far outweigh the difficulties. The opportunities for meaningful interaction that can occur within a group are necessary to create a genuine understanding of and appreciation for diversity within our schools. Groups provide a positive venue for thought-provoking discussions, relationship building, and a closer look at individuals who initially appear much different from ourselves—an opportunity to see our similarities and our shared experiences.

GROUP MEMBER/LEADER DIFFERENCES

Differences between the ethnicity of the counselor and that of the client, sometimes referred to as an "ethnic mismatch," are related to the group ending prematurely (Echemendía & Nuñez, 2004; Sexton & Whiston, 1998). One factor shown to outweigh this potential was the counselor's ability to establish a therapeutic alliance and adopt the worldview of the client. This proficiency, when working with multicultural populations, is attributed to the acquisition of cultural awareness, knowledge, and skills (Arrendondo et al., 1996). This perspective coincides with Davis and Osborn's (2000) citing the importance of the client's life outside of the counseling experience as relevant to the counseling relationship. Similarly, Lambert's (1992) findings identify the client's extratherapeutic factors as the most significant factor to client improvement.

Terrell and Terrell (1984) also addressed the issue of ethnic mismatch. Based on their study focusing on premature termination from counseling among Black clients, they determined that Black clients are more likely to terminate after the first session when working with a White counselor than when working with a Black counselor. The authors noted the chief concern related to this issue, noting that clients who do not return because they are unable to establish a working alliance and rapport with a counselor will not receive the benefits of therapeutic intervention.

Although cultural and ethnic differences between the school counselor and the group members have the potential to create challenges within the group process, research acknowledges that the cultural competency and sensitivity of the counselor is more important than ethnic group membership (Baruth & Manning, 2006; Esquivel, 1998; Esquivel & Keitel, 1990; Paniagua, 2005). It should be noted that although this chapter attempts to present an overview of key concepts important for working with diverse students in small groups, it is not intended as a stand-alone resource for cultural competency. We strongly encourage all school counselors to seek out additional personal, educational, and professional multicultural experiences.

ENGLISH-LANGUAGE LEARNERS

Linguistic diversity often proves to be a barrier to counseling services (McCall-Perez, 2000; Sue & Sue, 1999) and to interaction in the schools for students who are English-language learners (ELLs) (Esquivel, 1998; McCall-Perez, 2000). School counselors can assist in this process by attending to the special needs of this diverse group by being proactive with ELL students at the onset of group formation.

As briefly discussed in the previous chapter, the parents and caregivers of ELL students often do not speak English themselves. As the school counselor creates permission forms for the students to participate in groups, consider the best language(s) to use in the forms. Distributing the forms in English only could set the family up for role confusion and conflict. The students may be placed in a situation where they are required to be a translator or interpreter (Gibbs & Huang, 1989) of the form, which not only creates odd power dynamics for the family but also has the potential to impede the communication between the parents/caregivers and the school. Furthermore, if the student perceives the group as negative or it is something that he or she is not interested in, the likelihood of a direct translation of the permission form is minimal. That is, students may neglect to mention various aspects of the group or present it as something entirely different.

A suggestion that might seem rather obvious includes the language proficiency of the group leader. As one would expect, the school counselor leading a group would benefit from having a familiarity with the native language of the students participating in the group (Delgado, 1983). The degree of fluency necessary for the group leader is dependent upon the English proficiency of the group members. Throughout the years, school counseling students have approached the authors with questions regarding the use of interpreters in the group counseling process. Although there are different schools of thought regarding this practice, we would strongly encourage interpreters to be used only when there has been appropriate training for both the school counselor and the interpreter. Paone, Malott, and Maddux (2010) identified both risks and benefits of working with interpreters in the schools in their survey of 213 school counselors from across the country. Keep in mind that those individuals who practice as professional interpreters may not adhere to the same codes of ethics as school counselors and will be privy to the sharing of information within the group. Although a common language is important as part of the group process, the literature encourages creative approaches to sharing ideas and feelings within the group, including art, play, and other activities (Esquivel, 1998; Halperin, 2001).

IMMIGRANTS, REFUGEES, AND FIRST-GENERATION STUDENTS

Moving is stressful. Those who have experienced a move to a different state, or even across the country, know from experience that there are many changes associated with such a transition. Each area has new streets and highways to learn, new people to get to know, and often even a different dialect, slang, food, and culture that are indigenous to that particular state or part of the country. Imagine moving to an entirely different country where all of the aforementioned issues are experienced but amplified by a completely different language. Imagine that the apparent values and cultural norms you find yourself living in now vary drastically from your country of origin: There is no local market that sells the foods you know and love; there is no place to buy the skin and hair products you need; families look different; there is no place of worship that honors your faith tradition in the new community. What would this feel like for the student in your group? This is a tough question to answer, but it should be considered when including in your group a student who has recently immigrated to the United States.

Anatole France was quoted as saying, "All changes, even the most longed for, have their melancholy; for what we leave behind us is a part of ourselves; we must die to one life before we can enter into another!" (Ehrlick & Debruhl, 1996, p. 79). The most significant issue for learners whose families have immigrated to this country or are refugees is that of cultural transition. Individuals in transition are at an increased risk of serious illness and depression (Lee, Blando, Mizelle, & Orozco, 2007). Other issues often experienced include loneliness, frustrations with American culture, relationship difficulties (e.g., relating to peers), and those related to marginalization and discrimination (Smith, Chin, Inman, & Findling, 1999). Pedersen (1995) further discussed the rationale for the increased stress, also referred to as culture shock, associated with transitioning to a new culture. Several of the characteristics described by Pedersen focus on the uncertainty associated with behavioral cues, value conflicts, feelings of disorientation and dissatisfaction, and inadequate coping skills. Some of the stressors many immigrant and refugee families experience include changes in socioeconomic status due to job loss (many families leave stable employment for the chance of better opportunities in a new country), undocumented status, and cultural racism. Pedersen noted that refugees are particularly at risk of psychological difficulties as these individuals have not left their country voluntarily but rather were forced to leave. Many of these individuals have experienced significant trauma including abuse, torture, internment camps, and loss of family.

Students new to this country may be difficult to engage in school counseling–related services. The literature points to the stigma often attached to mental health–related services (Bernard, Naiyapatana, & Lloyd, 2006; Fu Keung Wong, 2007; Smith et al., 1999). School counselors can avoid the stigma by creating a group that focuses on opportunities to learn more about the school and community rather than one intended to attend to and provide support for the emotional challenges associated with the new changes—even though much of this can be achieved in the process of sharing information. Additional recommendations for minimizing stigma include being sensitive to where the group is located (neutral ground vs. counseling offices), limited use of psychological terminology, and avoiding use of scripted or in-depth emotional exercises. Utilizing cofacilitators, both male and female, can attend to the issue of differences in gender roles among various countries. Group members who may disrespect or feel uncomfortable sharing or being in a group led by one particular gender may be more likely to stay involved with one that has leadership inclusive of both gender perspectives (Smith et al., 1999). Group techniques employing storytelling and expressive art activities provide opportunities for students to share emotions in a safe and culturally relevant way (del Valle, McEachern, &Garcia, 1999; Esquivel, 1998; Mallott et al., 2010; Molina, Monteiro-Leitner, Garrett, & Gladding, 2005).

CULTURAL COMPETENCY

The counseling literature defines a culturally competent counselor as one who is culturally aware, has cultural knowledge, and demonstrates cultural skills (Arrendondo et al., 1996). Midgette and Meggert (1991) contended that attitude change is also a necessary component of becoming a culturally competent counselor.

Sue et al. (1992) noted the lack of multicultural training in the past, reporting that due to the monocultural training offered to counselors in the 1980s, most were ineffective when working with culturally diverse clients. Counselors void in cultural competence may risk "miscommunications and the undermining of a potential counseling relationship" (Arrendondo et al., 1996, p. 8). Miller and Garran (2008, p. 227) recommended a "relational, intersubjective, strengths-based approach to cross-cultural clinical practice," explaining that *relational* refers to the connection between the counselor and group members, and *intersubjective* is the "intersecting inner worlds" of the counselor and members. By "inner worlds" the authors are referring to all that we are as individuals—our worldviews. A *strengths-based* approach is one that considers all the supportive factors in an individual's life, or "assets" (Miller & Garran, p. 227), including a student's strengths, support systems, and potential (Galassi & Akos, 2007).

Research continues to provide evidence of the connection between multicultural counseling training and counseling competence (Carter, 1995; Constantine, 2002; Ochs, 1994). Pedersen (1991) suggested that most counseling could be regarded as multicultural considering that race, ethnicity, gender, sexual orientation, religion, class, and other factors influence our thoughts, assumptions, and behaviors. The literature supports the notion that cultural background will be incorporated into an individual's perception of self and her or his role in society. Davis and Osborn (2000) made reference to the importance of the client's current context, and advocate for counselors to focus on the client's life outside of the counseling experience. In a quest to identify factors that contribute to client improvement, the most significant were extratherapeutic factors, including characteristics that are integral to the client as a person (Fulton, 2005; Lambert, 1992). These extratherapuetic factors include all aspects of the person's identity, and although not specifically stated, include cultural identity. Lambert also made reference to the importance of awareness in counseling as it relates to the therapeutic relationship as a predictor of therapeutic outcome. Chung and Bemak (2002) saw the need to go beyond empathy to recognition and understanding, including incorporating, or at least being aware of, traditional or indigenous healing methods.

Therefore, school counselors will benefit by considering multicultural issues within the therapeutic relationships established in group counseling. Cultural awareness, cultural sensitivity, and cultural knowledge should not be assumed on the basis of the acquisition of basic clinical skills nor from identification as part of a particular cultural group. Cultural competence is not immediately attained from having the experience of being a part of a minority group. Although the experiences of oppression and discrimination experienced by people of color certainly provide a firsthand appreciation of sensitivity that White privilege does not afford, cultural competency embraces more than personal experience. Awareness of one's own cultural heritage, awareness of personal values and biases, being comfortable with cultural differences in relationships, and being able to provide culturally appropriate referrals are all components of cultural competency (Midgette & Meggert, 1991). Individuals of minority groups have most likely had to consider these dynamics of cultural competency on the very basis of being a part of a minority group; however, consideration does not equal comfort or competency. To assume that cultural knowledge, skills, and awareness are innate to within-group minority members may be premature based on the specific criteria set forth by such respected organizations as the Association for Multicultural Counseling and Development (Arrendondo et al., 1996).

GROUP WORK WITH STUDENTS FROM VARYING CULTURAL BACKGROUNDS

Are all White people the same? How about individuals from Asian heritage? Of course not. With this reality in mind, it is with significant caution that we write this section of the chapter. Although we believe that there are cultural norms that individuals within various cultures may or may not adhere to, we also contend that individuals within cultures are influenced by many factors outside of ethnicity (such as those mentioned in the beginning of this chapter). Karcher and Nakkula (1997) acknowledged this limitation, suggesting that "while these profiles can provide important information, they tend to reflect fairly simple generalizations that by their very nature fit no person exactly" (p. 219).

What we have found, and what other school counseling experts and practitioners have shared with us, is that it is useful to have a frame of reference from which to begin the counseling relationship when working with students of color. While acknowledging that students within cultures are very diverse, approach counseling relationships with sensitivity to cultural norms that often exist. In the following sections (in alphabetical order), we will share from the literature, from our personal and professional experiences, as well as from those who represent the various cultures identified. In an effort to create an awareness of various cultural groups, a few (and certainly not comprehensive) considerations for school counselors running groups are provided in Table 10.1 as summarized from a wonderful resource, *An Introduction to Multicultural Counseling for Helping Professionals* (Lee et al., 2007).

African American

Themes emerging in the literature regarding recommendations for African American students included encouragement for group leader awareness, community involvement, and attendance to issues relevant to the African American community (Bradley, 2001). In addition to the developmental challenges that most students face, many African American students continue to be strongly affected by societal racism and discrimination. Trust in counselors and the counseling relationship can be difficult to establish given this history of oppression (Lee et al., 2007). Although there are a number of challenges identified in the literature as relevant within the African American community (C. Bradley, 1999; Constantine, Miville, Warren, Gainor, & Lewis-Coles, 2006; Kenny & McEachern, 2009; Lee et al., 2007; Taylor, 1995; White & Parham, 1990), rather than listing these national trends, we strongly encourage school counselors who are considering running a small group focused on the needs of African American students to conduct a needs assessment to identify those needs that are perceived by the students themselves as most significant within their school.

Cultural values that influence many African Americans include the role of their family and spirituality in their lives. In a national survey, 84% of African Americans identified themselves as religious, and 77% said that the church was very important in their lives (Billingsley, 1992).

As mentioned previously, not all African American individuals identify with all, or necessarily any, of the values and traits mentioned in Table 10.1. Learning about culture requires much more than reading about a specific ethnic group. Although it

TABLE 10.1 │ Multicultural Considerations When Running Groups
with Ethnically Diverse Students

Tentative Generalizations about Major Ethnicities in the United States

African American
- Family includes relationships based on blood, marriage, and both formal and informal adoption and is often used as a solution to individual problems.
- Emphasis is on the present more than the future.
- Animated emotional expression is often used.
- Self-knowledge is revealed through symbolic image and rhythm.
- Interpersonal relationships that are cooperative are valued.
- Parables, folk verses, folk tales, biblical verses, songs, and proverbs contribute to their strong oral tradition.
- The counselor is cautioned not to interpret African American anger as simple transference.
- The student's feelings are a realistic response to the counselor as part of a social system that has historically proven inhospitable and deserving of mistrust.
- Low expectations, lack of role models, disregard for cultural diversity, and grouping or tracking practices all serve as potential barriers to academic success of African American students.

Asian and Pacific Islander
- Among the values that appear common to many Asian cultures are those of harmony, humility, and respect for family, authority, and tradition.
- To promote interpersonal harmony, emotional restraint, and indirect communication as opposed to confrontation are often preferred.
- Birth order and sex roles are strongly emphasized.
- Group needs often take precedence over the needs of the individual.
- Out of respect for authority, some Asian American clients may expect advice or specific direction from their counselor.
- Extended and nuclear families are valued.
- Comparisons between family members are often made as a means of encouragement and motivation.
- A more passive versus active approach to learning may be prevalent.
- One value associated with Japanese culture is termed *enryo*, which means to not dominate others in social situations. *Enryo* can easily be mistaken by a counselor who is unaware of Japanese culture as passivity or low self-esteem.
- Another Japanese value is that of *gaman*, meaning the endurance of hardships.
- Some Japanese have a somewhat fatalistic orientation to problems, called *shikata ga-nai*—literally, "it cannot be helped." This notion may originate in a Buddhist attitude toward living life without struggle.

European American/White
- Importance of work is a significant cultural value.
- There is a strong emphasis on individuality.
- Suppression of feelings is common.
- Distancing is used as a mode of coping with interpersonal conflict. European Americans may cope with interpersonal conflicts by distancing or cutting off the relationship (Lee et al., 2007).

Other important considerations include:
- Sense of hurriedness and need for time management have their roots in the German propensity for structuring time and relationships.
- The family is of great importance to many southern European Americans, and individual needs may come second.
- Families with Jewish cultural background value expression of feelings as part of family interaction.
- Polish and Greek American cultures may easily express emotions related to joy or sexuality, but other emotions such as anxiety or weakness may be censored.
- Assess the client's individual views of spirituality and do not assume that membership in a particular ethnic group implies religious convictions common to that group.
- Church activities and services may be utilized as a wrap-around service for the student and family in addition to school counseling services (Lee et al., 2007).

Latino(a)/Hispanic
- There is a long history of discrimination of Latinos and Latinas in the United States (e.g., linguistic discrimination).
- Loyalty to the family is highly valued among most Latinas(os). *Compadrazgo* describes a formalized system of kinship relationships that tends to be both hierarchical and patriarchal (Arrendondo, 1991).
- Children in the family are taught respect (*respecto*) and obedience to parents and adults in general. *Respecto* may surface in the counseling relationship as the student is unwilling to disagree, ask questions, or speak up in an effort to be respectful to counselor.
- Within Latino cultures, *machismo* has a meaning that is far different from the male chauvinistic stereotype typically associated with the word in the United States. In Spanish, the term originally referred to honor, loyalty, and the following of a gallant code of ethics, comparable to that often associated with knighthood and chivalry in European history.
- Religion and spirituality have a great influence on the lives of many Latinas(os).

Native American
- When referring to the ethnicity of a Native American student, it is generally best to use the name of the person's tribe, as many Native Americans most strongly identify themselves as members of a tribe versus Native American as an ethnicity.
- Counselors would benefit from taking time to understand family history when working with a Native American student.
- Storytelling may be a useful counseling resource when working with Native American students.
- Nonverbal communication is extremely important to Native Americans and should be attended to during counseling interventions. However, do not expect nonverbal signs of attention, such as head nodding or "uh huhs," as they are uncharacteristic for many Native Americans.
- Attention to how the counselor enters the room, the furnishings, and the presence of coffee or food can make the office seem more comfortable.
- Casual dress may be perceived negatively (e.g., as lack of respect).
- Silence is valued.
- Mirroring, or reflecting back a student's words, affect, or actions, is helpful when working with this student population.
- Native American children tend to speak more slowly and softly than White children.
- Prolonged eye contact may be considered disrespectful.

(continued)

TABLE 10.1 | Multicultural Considerations When Running Groups
with Ethnically Diverse Students (*continued*)

- Disclose who you are and where you come from before asking the student to self-disclose.
- Short stories are good ways to model self-disclosure.
- Ask questions, allowing the student to feel empowered.
- Family history is important to understand and give context to the student's experience.
- No one counseling theory is proven to be more effective when working with this population.
- The preferred characteristics of the counselor for this population are sincere, directive, problem solving, flexible, and informal with time frames.
- Nonverbal play and creative arts for children, spirituality, humor, storytelling, metaphors, imagery, modeling, and role play are recommended.
- Groups should be of the same gender.

is important to learn about the history of a people to understand their challenges and accomplishments, true cultural competency entails much more than knowledge. As with all of the groups discussed in this chapter, we are presenting just a few key concepts that have been shared with us and are presented in the literature. If an issue presents itself during the group process, we encourage group leaders to ask respectful questions, rather than make assumptions based on textbooks or other such resources.

Asian/Pacific Islander

The terms *Asian* and *Pacific Islander* often include a wide range of subpopulations: Chinese, Japanese, Koreans, Filipinos, Malays, Vietnamese, Cambodians, Laotians, Hmong, and Mien. And Hawaiians, Samoans, Tongans (Pacific Islanders), and Asian Indians also are sometimes grouped and counted with Asian Americans, although it should be noted that the history of Pacific Islanders is more similar to Native Americans than Asian Americans (Lee et al., 2007). When supporting Asian and Pacific Islander students in groups, the leader should consider the following the information.

Much of the literature focusing on the needs of Asian and Pacific Islander students attends to the group-oriented and collectivist perspective of many individuals who share this ethnic perspective (Heppner, 2006; I. Lee & Kelly, 1996; Lowe, 2005; Pope, 1999). With this in mind, group counseling may initially appear an ideal intervention for individuals of Asian descent. Although the group format may indeed be a supportive resource, the success of the group is largely determined by the expectations of the group leader and the interventions utilized within the group process. For example, many individuals of Asian heritage honor the group leader as an individual deserving respect and attention. Asian students in a group may feel that their responsibility to the group involves that of a listener, and that it would be rude or disrespectful to speak during the group session (Paniagua, 2005; Pope, 1999; Yu & Gregg, 1993). Due to the strong oral traditions of many Asian communities, the use of stories and images is often recommended when working with Asian individuals in group counseling (Sue & Sue, 1991). In practice, this means that although a group experience would honor the collectivist orientation of many Asian cultures, if the group leader is not sensitive to other traditions and values, the group may not be successful.

European American/White

The term *European American* is often used to describe individuals who have or whose families have immigrated to the United States from Europe. Many individuals who identify as White or European American have very little understanding of their cultural background or family history. The literature indicates the lack of emphasis on encouraging Whites to explore what it means to be White or to explore their own cultural identity development (Lee et al., 2007). There are many differences between individuals who have immigrated to the United States from European countries; however, there are also some important similarities that are worth noting, as they have shaped current American culture. These are presented in Table 10.1.

When involved in an ethnically diverse group and the topic of cultural diversity is discussed, many White students have expressed a sense of regret that they are not more familiar with their cultural history and European roots. Some White students believe that they do not have a culture (Kostelnik, 1999), and many are lacking in ethnic identity development (Ellis, 2004). White racial identity development theories have emerged (Ellis, 2004; Farough, 2006; Wong & Cho, 2005), providing European Americans the opportunity to associate a common experience for many White individuals to their own when exploring their ancestry. Primary themes that often evolve include guilt and confusion (Lee et al., 2007, Pedersen & Carey, 2003). Group counselors will want to familiarize themselves with identity development models as well as topics of ethnocentrism and privilege in an effort to understand this time of exploration in students' lives.

Latino(a)/Hispanic

As with other groups identified in this chapter, a broad term is used to represent people from a variety of cultural origins. Latinos and Latinas are people of Hispanic ancestry living in the United States. The term *Hispanic* is a designation of the federal government that includes people whose cultural origins are in Mexico, Puerto Rico, Cuba, and other countries including El Salvador, Guatemala, Honduras, the Dominican Republic, and Spain. Although diverse in representation and meaning, the terms *Chicano*, *Mexican*, and *Mexican American* are also used by individuals originating from Mexico (Lee et al., 2007). As with other aspects of multiculturalism, if in doubt, ask the student how she or he identifies.

In addition to the considerations presented in Table 10.1, the topic of *personalismo*, which refers to a preference for personal contact and individual interactions over more formal associations, seems especially relevant for group leaders. In a counseling group, this could mean a preference for more personal small talk and self-disclosure between group members and the group leader (Esquivel, 1998; Lee et al., 2007) as well as for an active group leader who is validating and supportive (Khantzian, 1986; Sue & Sue, 1999). To create an informal, personal atmosphere, the group leader may consider using her or his first name or a variation of such (Mr. Pat instead of Mr. Pat Jackson). In brief, creating an effective school counseling group with Latino(a) students may require some groundwork on behalf of establishing relationships *prior* to the formation of the group (Delgado, 1983). These relationships and personal connections affirm the concept of *personalismo* mentioned above.

Native American

There is significant diversity among Native Americans, a term that includes American Indians, Eskimos, and Aleuts (Lee et al., 2007). The literature acknowledges a long history of the utilization of group work for therapeutic purposes by Native American people (Garrett, Garrett, & Brotherton, 2001). Research focusing on the efficacy of group counseling with individuals of Native American backgrounds can provide recommendations for group leaders. Themes include the importance of a present-time orientation (Esquivel, 1998; Garrett et al., 2001; Portman, 2003), mutual respect, and harmony and balance (Lee et al., 2007; Portman, 2003).

Biracial/Multiracial

A group sometimes overlooked in the multicultural literature is those who identify as biracial or multiracial. Biracial and multiracial students are often faced with the difficulty of answering the question, "What *are* you?" regarding their ethnicity (Miville, Constantine, Baysden, & So-Lloyd, 2005). Furthermore, they are often placed in a position of having to "check a box" regarding which race or ethnic group they identify with, forcing them to disregard a parent's or grandparent's heritage by claiming only one aspect of who they are. Whereas information and training exists regarding the cultural norms and common concerns among various ethnic groups, fewer resources are available regarding the biracial or multiracial student. It is not sufficient to simply learn about the various ethnic groups comprising who the student is as a multiracial individual. The literature acknowledges issues and concerns specific to being biracial and multiracial (Sue & Sue, 2007).

Common themes and issues for biracial and multiracial individuals emerged in a 2005 qualitative study of individuals from a variety of mixed racial backgrounds (Miville et al., 2005). These themes included experiencing encounters with racism, the tendency to identify with a primary ethnicity or race in addition to being biracial or multiracial, adaptability to their surroundings, and open attitudes toward others. According to their research, parents are identified as the most influential factor in the development and expression of participants' racial identity. For those unfamiliar with multiracial identity development models, the article "Chameleon Changes: An Exploration of Racial Identity Themes of Multiracial People" (Miville et al., 2005) provides a concise overview of various biracial and multiracial identity development models. These models, as well as the aforementioned issues, are relevant when working with individuals of biracial or multiracial descent in small groups.

GROUP LEADER AWARENESS

The above descriptions are trends and characteristics that may apply to the students we serve. Consideration of each student's unique qualities is a necessity. How does the influence of culture, context, race, and gender converge in *this particular student's* life? Realistically, we will never know each student's full and rich description, yet we must openly acknowledge how culture affects students and our role as a group counselor.

Assessing Cultural Competence

There are many ways for us, as leaders, to assess our competence when working with diverse groups. For those who appreciate a more structured approach to assessing cultural competence, Holcomb-McCoy (2004) provided a thorough checklist that can serve as an assessment tool as well as an indicator of areas where additional training and supervision may be helpful (see chapter supplement). The key component of an effective group counselor who works with student groups is to be curious; we need to take an open stance regarding our students' culture. Although we may become familiar with trends within racial and ethnic groups, our students are the "experts" on their culture. It is up to group counselors to listen and remain open as to how their culture influences their behavior and functioning.

So, how does a group leader become intentional about cultural awareness? There are many germane aspects to culturally competent leadership. The first is to acknowledge that we do not know everything. On the surface, this may seem easy to comprehend. When asked about appreciating culture, it is simple to answer "I'm not biased" or "I honor diversity." However, when we are really honest with ourselves, we often realize that we make assumptions, have personal biases, and are affected by subconscious and internalized racism that influences our work with students (Miller & Garran, 2008; Watts-Jones, 2002). Becoming culturally competent is a journey, and the more we learn the more we realize that there is no end point in this voyage. Along the path, we add to our competency by asking questions, taking the one-down approach (Egan, 2009; Rogers, 1958), and becoming increasingly aware of the assumptions and biases that we hold.

Being genuinely interested and asking culturally informed questions are important tools not only for the group leader but also for the group experience. In the group process, it is critical to know the students as whole beings. Who are the members of the group through a psychological, biological, social, and spiritual lens? Group leaders can facilitate this knowledge by stating that they would like to know the cultural influence regarding the identified group issue (presenting problem). Being overt and asking to include culture as part of the discussion opens the door for rich discussion to occur. This should not happen only at the beginning of the group but throughout the group's life span.

One role of the group leader is to spark or mobilize conversations that enrich the cultural knowledge of others. Group leaders who assume a hierarchical approach (i.e., the stance that the leader will always know what is best for the group and the group members; see chapter 2 for a fuller discussion) limit the students' voices to inform themselves and others about what is important in their world. When group leaders ask questions, we admit that we do not know everything about culture and our students' lives. Does this make us seem unprofessional? No. In fact, we become skilled professionals by knowing when to take the one-down approach. Asking "How do you see and how does your culture see …" is more important than prescribing a solution that is invalid within a student's cultural norm.

Understanding Privilege

As group leaders, we must continually assess and reassess our assumptions and biases regarding the group counseling process. If we are from the same racial or ethnic background as our student members, does this help us to better connect with them? How may we limit our understanding of those we seek to serve by thinking that we already know their situation?

If we are of a different racial or ethnic background, are we open and curious about the similarities and differences between and among the group members and the group leader?

No matter what our cultural background, we all have levels of privilege when working with students. Specifically, European Americans must recognize the historical privilege they have held in terms of power and dominance over other groups. It may come naturally for a middle-class White female to say, "I worked hard to get into college so I'll encourage my college-bound discussion group to work hard so they can go to college," without realizing that, even with this best of intentions, this counselor could be perpetrating institutionalized racism. Because this White counselor had the *privilege* of living in a community with tax funding to support education, had familial expectations that education was a priority regardless of gender, and had the financial means to fund a college education, her hard work paid off. Students without such privilege often, even with hard work, do not have the opportunity to pursue their choice of education. Consider that context affects behavior, and we cannot apply interventions that are helpful in one situation to all situations. Instead of discussing the importance of hard work, it may be more important to lead discussions on finding economic and emotional support for college and how to choose a college that attunes to cultural diversity.

Privilege is a difficult concept for many to understand and, perhaps, accept. In a chapter titled "Why Is It So Difficult for People With Privilege to See Racism?" J. Miller and Garran (2008) discussed the role of privilege and its influence on racism as a social construct. To help us understand privilege, McIntosh (1989) provided counselors with examples of various aspects of privilege that many White individuals experience on a daily basis. Being able to find bandages (Band-Aids, e.g.) that match your skin tone, being able to buy toy dolls that look like you, or being expected to speak for your entire race are just a few of the examples provided in her article. You might ask yourself "What does privilege have to do with group counseling?" As a culturally competent professional school counselor, you'll want to be mindful of privilege within your group and its impact on group process.

Specific Recommendations

Again, most individuals who go into the school counseling profession do so because they want to help others. We would never intentionally run an ineffective group. Thus possessing a clear awareness of our historical privilege, biases, and assumptions is critical to successful group leadership with students of color. How do we do this? First, reading this chapter and others like it is a good start. Also, expand your knowledge by reading sources that interest you (e.g., ones found in our reference list or recommended in the chapter supplement).

Knowledge alone is not enough. Check in with your students to see if they feel there is an open environment regarding honoring cultural diversity. Students may be inhibited about talking to you directly, so you may want to provide confidential feedback forms. Debrief with group members during the meetings and after the final group session. Ask how you as the leader could add more cultural awareness to the group process.

You are not alone in your journey toward cultural competence. Seek collaboration and supervision as you add cultural awareness, knowledge, and skills to the groups you implement. Check in with other professionals and school counselors who are leading groups. Ask what is going well in others' experiences. Be curious about the strengths of others who lead culturally competent groups and share your own successes. Let's now take a look at some examples of school-based groups conducted with students of color.

CASE EXAMPLES

Case Examples and Applications from the Field

Miko's Silence

After attending a training regarding positive youth development, Ms. Cee, a White elementary school counselor, wanted to start a girls group for fifth-grade students. Her primary goal was to support the young women as they discover their developmental assets (e.g., positive values, hope for the future, strength in self). (For a complete list of developmental assets, readers may want to peruse the Search Institute's website [http://www.search-institute.org].) She asked the teachers to give her a list of candidates. After reviewing the candidates' academic files, Ms. Cee picked five girls with high academic honors to begin the group. The group consisted of four European American girls and one Japanese American girl. Ms. Cee began the first group session by asking the girls to draw a self-portrait that highlighted the feature the girls liked best about themselves. Ms. Cee noticed that Miko, the Japanese American student, drew a beautiful but abstract drawing that Ms. Cee could not interpret. When the students were asked to explain their drawings, the European American students explained that they had drawn big ears because they valued listening or muscular legs because they liked to run. Miko said nothing. During the next few sessions, Ms. Cee asked the girls to share something nice they did for someone else during the past week. When Miko's turn arrived, she said nothing. Near the end of the group, Ms. Cee was concerned that Miko was not making any progress toward the articulation of self-strengths and -assets. Ms. Cee decided that Miko would need extra help and support, and so she referred Miko to the school assessment team for further evaluation regarding social skills and personal assertiveness.

Although it is an admirable goal for Ms. Cee to want to promote her student's assets, Ms. Cee failed to recognize the cultural implications of asking Miko to share her strengths. If Ms. Cee had investigated more than the academic background of the students, she would have learned that this student is a first-generation student whose caregivers recently emigrated from Japan. Miko's caregivers adhere to traditional Japanese values and traditions. Thus Miko's cultural orientation does not encourage her to highlight her individual achievements. Miko talking about her achievements is seen in her culture as taking a "one up" position at the expense of the whole. For Miko to speak about her success, she would be contradicting community and family values such as modesty, interreliance, and interdependence. Additionally, if she highlighted her strengths, her family could interpret it as her shaming another family who did not share similar strengths.

Reflecting on this scenario, should have Ms. Cee excluded Miko from the group? Not in our professional opinion; it is important to have diverse groups. Some techniques that Ms. Cee could have employed would be to be thoughtful about what strengths the students' cultures value. Students could begin by talking about these strengths in generic terms and then talking about how they see the strengths within their systems (community, family, and self). Ms. Cee also could have used displaced communication to ask what strengths the students see in others. It may be easier for some students to talk about caregivers, teachers, and other significant persons instead of talking directly about themselves. This may have given Miko the chance to share strengths that she sees within her collectivist culture.

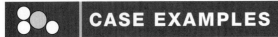

CASE EXAMPLES

Bruce's Career Choice

Bruce is a Native American high school senior. His school counselor suggested that Bruce join a small group regarding postgraduation choices. The group explored topics such as how to apply for college and interview skills for job applications. Each week the school counselor assigned activities for the students to complete in between sessions. The first assignment was for students to fill out a mock college application. The second assignment was for students to take an online career assessment. Weekly, the group would meet and discuss the assignments. Each time the group met, Bruce did not have his work completed. The school counselor assessed that Bruce was disinterested in the group and asked him to not attend future meetings.

Reflecting on this scenario, was Bruce disinterested? No, Bruce was not resistant; rather, the group meetings were not meeting his needs. Bruce lived with his extended kin on a reservation. If Bruce would unilaterally decide to pursue either a job or an education off the reservation, he would have been disowned by his family and community. For Bruce, it was important that his extended kin be a part of the decision-making process.

Had the group process been culturally sensitive, the group could have helped Bruce explore different possibilities. First, the group leader could have asked what factors were important in making a postgraduation decision. The group leader also could have asked who would help make the decision. The group could process the role of external others in life choices. Furthermore, the school counselor could have brought in take-home resources that were culturally appropriate, which Bruce and other students could have shared with significant others. Seeking culturally relevant resources such as those provided by the National Office of School Counselor Advocacy (NOSCA) and the National Center for Transforming School Counseling may be helpful for school counselors working with students like Bruce.

Low Attendance in Groups

A team of school counselors were discussing what groups to offer in the fall. The panel decided that a test-taking anxiety group, a friendship group, and a "say-no-to-drugs" group were all worthwhile for the students. The team of school counselors decided that it was vital for the groups to have six students each and to meet for 8 weeks. The groups would be "closed," and no members would be allowed to join after the group had started. Two weeks into the groups, the team met and discussed the fact that there were few students attending the groups. Each group had, at most, three students. The team was frustrated with their efforts and decided to postpone group meetings until the students showed more interest.

Reflecting on this scenario, although these school counselors were attuned to what groups the students needed, they did not know the school climate well enough to know that "closed" groups may not be effective when a substantial portion of the students are children of migratory workers. These students were hesitant to commit to long-running groups as they may relocate before the group ended. Additionally, many students were working during the first few weeks of classes and were not able to attend the first group meeting; this left them ineligible to attend future sessions. For school counselors work-ing with migrant populations, issues of flexibility and adaptability within the group counseling schedule should be considered.

SUMMARY AND CONCLUSION

In each of the above examples, the group leaders wanted to promote healthy outcomes in the students' lives. What prevented this from occurring was an inattention to the cultural dynamics at work. The counselors could have prevented and adjusted their mistakes by understanding cultural dynamics. Knowledge about cultural relevance and discussion about cultural norms could have helped the above groups become successful for all of the members.

We realize that cultural competency is a journey of cultural awareness, knowledge, and skills. In this chapter we have begun the discussion of looking at school counseling groups from a cultural viewpoint. Again, this is just a beginning. With continued infor-mation and an emerging awareness, you will develop what works in your school culture and with the students you serve. We acknowledge the limitation of our "lenses" through which we view the world and are grateful to those who have provided the literature and experiences on which we based our writing, enabling us to incorporate a variety of perspectives. For curriculum and activity examples that can be used for group work to promote awareness as well as identity development, see texts such as Pedersen's (2004) *110 Experiences for Multicultural Learning*. Malott et al. (2010) speak to the commit-ment required to meet the needs of today's multicultural student populations:

> One of the greatest challenges for school counselors today is identifying appropri-ate services for ethnically diverse youth who struggle to overcome the many bar-riers present to achieving academically. It is essential that school counselors are informed of empirically supported resources that will enable them to engage such students in effective, culturally congruent services. (p. 267)

This chapter addresses this concern and provides insights into how to best reach students of color through effective group counseling methods.

CHAPTER 10 SUPPLEMENTS

Supplement 10.1   Below is a useful tool developed by Cheryl Holcomb-McCoy (2004) to help school counselors assess their multicultural competence.

School Counselor Multicultural Competence Checklist
(adapted from Holcomb-McCoy, 2004)

Level of Competency 1 Low --- 4 Strong	Competence Dimension
	I. Multicultural Counseling
	1. I can recognize when my attitudes, beliefs, and values are interfering with providing the best services to my students.
	2. I can identify the cultural bases of my communication style.
	3. I can discuss how culture affects the help-seeking behaviors of students.
	4. I can describe the degree to which a counseling approach is culturally inappropriate for a specific student.
	5. I use culturally appropriate interventions and counseling approaches (e.g., indigenous practices with students).
	6. I can list at least three barriers that prevent ethnic minority students from using counseling services.
	7. I can anticipate when my helping style is inappropriate for a culturally different student.
	8. I can give examples of how stereotypical beliefs about culturally different persons impact the counseling relationship.
	II. Multicultural Consultation
	9. I am aware of how culture affects traditional models of consultation.
	10. I can discuss at least one model of multicultural consultation.
	11. I recognize when racial and cultural issues are impacting the consultation process.
	12. I can identify when the race and/or culture of the client is a problem for the consultee.
	13. I discuss issues related to race/ethnicity/culture during the consultation process, when applicable.
	III. Understanding Racism and Student Resistance
	14. I can define and discuss White privilege.
	15. I can discuss how I (if European American/White) am privileged based on my race.
	16. I can identify racist aspects of educational institutions.
	17. I can define and discuss prejudice.
	18. I recognize and challenge colleagues about discrimination and discriminatory practices in schools.
	19. I can define and discuss racism and its impact on the counseling process.
	20. I can help students determine whether a problem stems from racism or biases in others.

© Courtesy Cheryl Holcomb-McCoy, Ph.D.

21. I understand the relationship between student resistance and racism.
22. I include topics related to race and racism in my classroom guidance units.

IV. Understanding Racial and/or Ethnic Identity Development
23. I am able to discuss at least two theories of racial and/or ethnic identity development.
24. I use racial/ethnic identity development theories to understand my students' problems and concerns.
25. I have assessed my own racial/ethnic development in order to enhance my counseling.

V. Multicultural Assessment
26. I can discuss the potential bias of two assessment instruments frequently used in the schools.
27. I can evaluate instruments that may be biased against certain groups of students.
28. I am able to use test information appropriately with culturally diverse parents.
29. I view myself as an advocate for fair testing and the appropriate use of testing of children from diverse backgrounds.
30. I can identify whether or not the assessment process is culturally sensitive.
31. I can discuss how the identification of the assessment process might be biased against minority populations.

VI. Multicultural Family Counseling
32. I can discuss family counseling from a cultural/ethnic perspective.
33. I can discuss at least two ethnic groups' traditional gender role expectations and rituals.
34. I anticipate when my helping style is inappropriate for an ethnically different parent or guardian.
35. I can discuss culturally diverse methods of parenting and discipline.

VII. Social Advocacy
36. I am knowledgeable about the psychological and societal issues that affect the development of ethnic minority students.
37. When counseling, I consider the psychological and societal issues that affect the development of ethnic minority students.
38. I work with families and community members in order to reintegrate them with the school.
39. I can define "social change agent."
40. I perceive myself as being a "social change agent."
41. I can discuss what it means to take an "activist counseling" approach.
42. I intervene with students at the individual and systemic levels.
43. I can discuss how factors such as poverty and powerlessness have influenced the current conditions of at least two ethnic groups.

VIII. Developing School-Family-Community Partnerships
44. I have developed a school-family-community partnership team or some similar type of group that consists of community members, parents, and school personnel.

(continued)

45. I am aware of community resources that are available for students and their families.
46. I work with community leaders and other resources in the community to assist with student (and family) concerns.
    IX. Understanding Cross-Cultural Interpersonal Interactions
47. I am able to discuss interaction patterns that might influence ethnic minority students' perceptions of inclusion in the school community.
48. I solicit feedback from students regarding my interactions with them.
49. I verbally communicate my acceptance of culturally different students.
50. I nonverbally communicate my acceptance of culturally different students.
51. I am mindful of the manner in which I speak and the emotional tone of my interactions with culturally diverse students.

Supplement 10.2   Additional multicultural resources are provided here for further study and reflection:

Howard, G. R. (1999). *We can't teach what we don't know: White teachers, multiracial schools.* New York: Teachers College.

Obiakor, F. E. (2007). *Multicultural special education.* Upper Saddle River, NJ: Pearson.

Pedersen, P. B. (2004). *110 Experiences for multicultural learning.* Washington, DC: American Psychological Association.

Ridley, C. R. (1995). *Overcoming unintentional racism in counseling and therapy: A practitioner's guide to intentional intervention.* Thousand Oaks, CA: Sage.

Salazar, C. F. (Ed.). (2009). *Group work experts share their favorite multicultural activities: A guide to diversity, competent choosing, planning, conducting, and processing.* Alexandria, VA: American Counseling Association.

Tatum, B. D. (2003). *"Why are all the black kids sitting together in the cafeteria?": A psychologist explains the development of racial identity.* Jackson, TN: Basic Books.

Wardle, F., & Cruz-Janzen, M. I. (2004). *Meeting the needs of multiethnic and multiracial children in schools.* Boston: Pearson.

References

Acosta, F. A., & Cristo, M. H. (1981). Development of a bilingual interpreter program: An alternative model for Spanish-speaking services. *Professional Psychology, 12,* 474–482.

Adams, C. (2008). The scary world of middle school. *Instructor, 117*(6), 44–48.

Adler, A. (1927/2008). *The science of living.* New York, NY: Meredith Press.

Adler, A. (1929/2004). The individual criminal and his cure. In H. T. Stein (Ed.), *The collected clinical works of Alfred Adler: Journal articles 1927–1931* (pp. 111–123). Bellingham, WA: Classical Adlerian Translation Project.

Adler, A. (1929/2006). Education for prevention: Individual psychology in the schools. In H. T. Stein (Ed.), *The collected clinical works of Alfred Adler* (Vol. 11). Bellingham, WA: Classical Adlerian Translation Project.

Akos, P. (2000). Building empathic skills in elementary school children through group work. *Journal for Specialists in Group Work, 25,* 214–223.

Akos, P. (2003). Resiliency in school counseling. *Prevention Researcher, 10*(1), 8–10.

Akos, P., & Galassi, J. P. (2008). Strength-based school counseling: Introduction to the special issue. *Professional School Counseling, 12,* 66–67.

Akos, P., Hamm, J. V., Mack, S. G., & Dunaway, M. (2007). Utilizing the developmental influence of peers in middle school groups. *Journal for Specialists in Group Work, 32,* 51–60.

Akos, P., & Martin, M. (2003). Transition groups for preparing students for middle school. *Journal for Specialists in Group Work, 28,* 139–154. doi:10.1177/0193392203028002005

Akos, P., & Milsom, A. (2007). Introduction to special issue: Group work in K–12 schools. *Journal for Specialists in Group Work, 32,* 5–7.

Aldarondo, F. (2001). Racial and ethnic identity models and their application: Counseling biracial individuals. *Journal of Mental Health Counseling, 23,* 238–255.

Alexander, J. A., & Harman, R. L. (1988). One counselor's intervention in the aftermath of a middle school student's suicide: A case study. *Journal of Counseling & Development, 66,* 283–285.

Allen, K. (2010). A bullying intervention system: Reducing risk and creating support for aggressive students. *Preventing School Failure, 54,* 199–209.

Alvord, M., & Grados, J. (2005). Enhancing resilience in children: A proactive approach. *Professional Psychology: Research and Practice, 36,* 238–245. doi:10.1037/0735-7028.36.3.238.

American Academy of Pediatrics. (n.d.). *Children's health topics: Developmental stages.* Retrieved from http://aap.org/healthtopics/stages.cfm

American Counseling Association. (2005). *ACA code of ethics.* Alexandria, VA: Author.

American Recovery and Reinvestment Act of 2009. Section 14005-6, Title XIV (Public Law 111-5). Retrieved from http://www2.ed.gov/programs/racetothetop/legislation.html

American School Counselor Association. (n.d.). *The ASCA national model: A framework for school counseling programs: Executive summary.* Retrieved from http://www.ascanationalmodel.org/

American School Counselor Association. (2002). *The school counselor and student rights* (Position statement). Alexandria, VA: Author.

American School Counselor Association. (2004a). *ASCA national standards for students*. Alexandria, VA: Author.

American School Counselor Association. (2004b). *Ethical standards for school counselors* (Revised 2010). Retrieved from http://asca2.timberlakepublishing.com//files/EthicalStandards2010.pdf

American School Counselor Association. (2004c). *The professional school counselor and the prevention and intervention of behaviors that place students at risk*. Retrieved from http://asca2.timberlakepublishing.com//files/PS_Prevention%20of%20At-Risk%20Behaviors.pdf

American School Counselor Association. (2005a). *The ASCA national model: A framework for school counseling programs* (2nd ed.). Alexandria, VA: Author.

American School Counselor Association. (2005b). *The professional school counselor and comprehensive school counseling*. Retrieved from http://asca2.timberlakepublishing.com//files/PS_Comprehensive.pdf

American School Counselor Association. (2008a). *The professional school counselor and group counseling* (Position statement). Retrieved from http://asca2.timberlakepublishing.com//files/PS_Group%20Counseling.pdf

American School Counselor Association. (2008b). *The professional school counselor and response to intervention* (Position statement). Retrieved from http://asca2.timberlakepublishing.com//files/PS_Intervention.pdf

American School Counselor Association. (2010). *The professional school counselor and students with special needs* (Position statement). Alexandria, VA.: Author.

Anderson, A. (2009). Connecting families at the middle school level: A single case study (Doctoral dissertation). *Dissertation Abstracts International, 69*. Retrieved from http://gradworks.umi.com/33/15/3315979.html

Arman, J. (2002). A brief group counseling model to increase resiliency of students with mild disabilities. *Journal of Humanistic Counseling, Education & Development, 41*, 120–128.

Aronson, S. M. (2004). Where the wild things are: The power and challenge of adolescent group work. *The Mount Sinai Journal of Medicine, 71*, 174–180.

Arrendondo, P. (1991). Counseling Latinas. In C. C. Lee & B. L. Richardson (Eds.), *Multicultural issues in counseling: New approaches to diversity* (pp. 143–156). Alexandria, VA: American Counseling Association.

Arrendondo, P., Toporek, R., Brown, S., Jones, J. Locke, D. Sanchez, J., & Stadler, H. (1996). *Operationalization of the multicultural counseling competencies*. Alexandria, VA: Association of Multicultural Counseling and Development.

Association of Specialists in Group Work. (1998). (ASGW). *Best practice guidelines*. Retrieved from http://asgw.org/ Association for Specialists in Group Work. (ASGW). (2000). *Professional standards for the training of group workers*. Retrieved from http://www.asgw.org/training_standards.htm

Association for Specialists in Group Work. (ASGW). (2007). *Association of Specialists in Group Work best practice guidelines*. Alexandria, VA: Author.

Astramovich, R. L., & Coker, J. K. (2007). Program evaluation: The Accountability Bridge Model for counselors. *Journal of Counseling & Development, 85*, 162–172.

Astramovich, R. L., Forkner, C. W., & Bodenhorn, N. (2004). In L. E. Tyson, R. Pérusse, & J. Whitledge (Eds.), *Critical incidents in group counseling* (pp. 229–240). Alexandra, VA: American Counseling Association.

Atkinson, D. R., Morten, G., & Sue, D. W. (1998). A minority identity development model. In D. R. Atkinson, G. Morten, & D. W. Sue (Eds.), *Counseling American minorities* (pp. 35–52). Dubuque, IA: W. C. Brown.

Aurelius, M. (c. 150 C.E./2006). *Meditations* (M. Hamond, Trans.). London, UK: Penguin.

Aydlett, A. E. (2008). *Dealing with deployment: A small-group curriculum for elementary and middle school students.* Alexandria, VA: American School Counselor Association.

Baggerly, J., & Parker, M. (2005). Child-centered group play therapy with African American boys at the elementary school level. *Journal of Counseling & Development, 83,* 387–396.

Bandura, A. (1986). *Social foundations of thought and action.* Englewood Cliffs, NJ: Prentice-Hall.

Bandura, A. (1997). *Self-efficacy: The exercise of control.* New York, NY: Freeman.

Bandura, A. (2001). Social cognitive theory: An agentic perspective. *Annual Review of Psychology, 52,* 1–26.

Barlow, A. R. (1981). Gestalt therapy and Gestalt psychology: Gestalt-antecedent influence or historical accident. *The Gestalt Journal, IV*(2). Retrieved from http://www.gestalt.org/barlow.htm

Barlow, S. H., Fuhriman, A. J., & Burlingame, G. M. (2004). The history of group counseling and psychotherapy. In J. L. DeLucia-Waack, D. A. Gerrity, C. R., Kalodner, & M. T. Riva (Eds.), *Handbook of group counseling and psychotherapy* (pp. 3–22). Thousand Oaks, CA: Sage.

Baruth, L. G., & Manning, M. L. (2006). *Multicultural counseling and psychotherapy: A lifespan perspective* (4th ed.). New York, NY: Merrill Macmillan.

Bauer, S. R., Sapp, M., & Johnson, D. (2000). Group counseling strategies for rural at-risk high school students. *High School Journal, 83*(2), 41–50.

Baumberger, J. P., & Harper, R. E. (2007). *Assisting students with disabilities: A handbook for school counselors* (2nd ed.) Thousand Oaks, CA: Corwin Press and American School Counselor Association.

Beck, A. T., Freeman, A., et al. (1990). *Cognitive therapy of personality disorders.* New York, NY: Guilford Press.

Beck, J. S., Liese, B. S., & Najavits, L. M. (2005). Cognitive therapy. In R. J. Frances, S. I. Miller, & A. Mack (Eds.), *Clinical textbook of addictive disorders* (3rd ed.; pp. 474–501). New York: Guilford Press.

Beesley, D. (2004). Teachers' perceptions of school counselor effectiveness: Collaborating for student success. *Education, 125,* 259.

Bemak, F., & Chung, R. C. (2004). Teaching multicultural group counseling: Perspectives for a new era. *Journal for Specialists in Group Work, 29,* 31–41.

Bemak, F., Chung, R. C-Y., & Siroskey-Sabdo, L. A. (2005). Empowerment groups for academic success: An innovative approach to prevent high school failure for at-risk, urban African. *Professional School Counseling, 8,* 377–389.

Benson, P. L. (2003). Developmental assets and asset-building community: Conceptual and empirical foundations. In R. M. Lerner & P. L. Benson (Eds.), *Developmental assets and asset-building communities: Implications for research, policy, and practice* (pp. 19–43). Norwell, MA: Kluwer.

Bent, D. (1996). Rogerian rhetoric: An alternative to traditional rhetoric. In B. Emmel, P. Resch, & B. Tenny (Eds.), *Argument revisited, argument redefined: Negotiating meaning in the composition classroom* (pp. 73–96). Thousand Oaks, CA: Sage. Retrieved from http://people.ucalgary.ca/~dabrent/art/rogchaJap.html

Berg, R. C., Landreth, G. L, & Fall, K. A. (2006). *Group counseling: Concepts and procedures.* New York, NY: Routledge.

Bernes, J., Bernes, K., & Bardick, A. (2011). Externalizing behavior disorders: Supporting students with aggression and violent tendencies. In C. A. Sink (Ed.), *Mental health interventions for school counselors* (pp. 16–34). Belmont, CA: Wadsworth Brooks/Cole.

Betz, N. E. (2004). Contributions of self-efficacy theory to career counseling: A personal perspective. *Career Development Quarterly, 52,* 340–354.

Bierma, J. (2005). *Classroom lesson /units and counseling articles.* Retrieved from http://mis.spps.org/counselors/articles Home.html

Billingsley, A. (1992). *Climbing Jacob's ladder: The enduring legacy of African-American families.* New York, NY: Simon & Schuster.

Bistaman, M. N., & Nasir, R. (2009). An application of Rational Emotive Behavior Therapy in group counseling: A case study on adolescents whose parents were divorced. *European Journal of Social Sciences, 10,* 334–342.

Bitter, J. (2009). The mistaken notions of adults with children. *The Journal of Individual Psychology, 65,* 135–155.

Blakemore, S.-J. (2010). The developing social brain: Implications for education. *Neuron, 65,* 744–747.

Blocher, W.-m. G., & Wade, N. G. (2010). Sustained effectiveness of two brief group interventions: Comparing an explicit forgiveness-promoting treatment with a process-oriented treatment. *Journal of Mental Health Counseling, 32,* 58–74.

Blum, D. J., & Davis, T. E. (2010). *The school counselor's book of lists* (2nd ed.). New York, NY: John Wiley.

Borders, L., & Drury, S. (1992). Comprehensive school counseling programs: A review for policymakers and practitioners. *Journal of Counseling & Development, 70,* 487–498.

Bostick, D., & Anderson, R. (2009). Evaluating a small-group counseling program—A model for program planning and improvement in the elementary setting. *Professional School Counseling, 12,* 428–433.

Bosworth, K., & Walz, G. (2005). *Promoting student resiliency.* Alexandria, VA: American Counseling Association.

Bowen, M. (1998). Counseling interventions for students who have mild disabilities. *Professional School Counseling, 2,* 16–24.

Bradley, C. (2001). A counseling group for African-American adolescent males. *Professional School Counseling, 4,* 370–374.

Bradley, L. J. & Hendricks, C. B. (2008). Ethical decision making: Basic issues. *Family Journal: Counseling and Therapy for Couples and Families, 16,* 261–263.

Brake, K. J., & Gerler, E. R. (1994). Discovery: A program for fourth and fifth graders identified as discipline problems. *Elementary School Guidance and Counseling, 28,* 170–181.

Brasher, K. (2009). Solution-focused brief therapy: Overview and implications for school counselors. *Alabama Counseling Association Journal, 34*(2), 20–30.

Brennan, J., & Brennan, K. (1999). How the M.A.P. club changed perceptions of students with special needs. *Rural Special Education Quarterly, 18*(2), 5–9.

Brigman, G. A., & Campbell, C. (2003). Helping students improve academic achievement and school success behavior. *Professional School Counseling, 7,* 91–98.

Brigman, G., & Early, B. (2001). *Group counseling for school counselors: A practical guide.* Portland, ME: Weston Walch.

Brigman, G. A., & Early Goodman, B. E. (2008). *Group counseling for school counselors: A practical guide* (3rd ed.). Portland, ME: J. Weston Walch.

Brigman, G. A., & Molina, B. (1999). Developing social interest and enhancing school success skills: A service learning approach. *The Journal of Individual Psychology, 55,* 342–354.

Brigman, G. A., Webb, L. D., & Campbell, C. (2007). Building skills for school success: Improving the academic and social competence of students. *Professional School Counseling, 10,* 279–288.

Brinson J. A. (1995). Group work for Black adolescent substance users: Some issues and recommendations. *Journal of Child & Adolescent Substance Abuse, 4*(2), 49–59. doi: 10.1300/J029v04n02_04

Bronfenbrenner, U. (1977). Toward an experimental ecology of human development. *American Psychologist, 32,* 513–531.

Brown, D., & Brooks, L. (Eds.). (2002). *Career choice and development: Applying contemporary theories to practice.* San Francisco: Jossey-Bass.

Brown, N. W. (2004). *Psychoeducational groups: Process and practice* (2nd ed.). New York, NY: Brunner-Routledge.

Brown-Chidsey, R., & Steege, M. W. (2005). *Response to intervention: Principles and strategies for effective practice.* New York, NY: Guildford Press.

Bruce, A. M., Getch, Y. Q., & Ziomek-Daigle, J. (2009). Closing the gap: A group counseling approach to improve test performance of African-American students. *Professional School Counseling, 12,* 450–457.

Burnard, P., Naiyapatana, W., & Lloyd, G. (2006). Views of mental illness and mental health care in Thailand: a report of an ethnographic study. *Journal of Psychiatric & Mental Health Nursing, 13,* 742–749.

Burrow-Sanchez, J., & Lopez, A. (2009). Identifying substance abuse issues in high schools: A national survey of high school counselors. *Journal of Counseling & Development, 87,* 72–79.

Butler, R., & Marinov-Glassman, D. (1994). The effects of educational placement and grade level on the self-perceptions of low achievers and Students with learning disabilities. *Journal of Learning Disabilities, 27,* 325–334.

Callahan, C. M., Cunningham, C. M., & Plucker, J. A. (1994). Foundations for the future: The socio-emotional development of gifted, adolescent women. *Roeper Review, 17,* 99–105.

Campbell, C. A. (2003). Student Success Skills Training: An Adlerian approach to peer counseling. *The Journal of Individual Psychology, 59,* 327–333.

Campbell, C. A., & Brigman, G. (2005). Closing the achievement gap: A structured approach to group counseling. *Journal for Specialists in Group Work, 30,* 1–16.

Capuzzi, D. (Ed.). (2003). *Approaches to group work: A handbook for practitioners.* Upper Saddle River, NJ: Merrill Prentice Hall.

Carey, J. C., & Dimmett, C. (2005, Oct.). The lessons of meta-analysis: Does group counseling with children and adolescents make a difference? Review of Hoag & Burlingame (1997). *School Counseling Research Brief 3.3.* Retrieved from http://www.umass.edu/schoolcounseling/PDFs/Research_Brief_3-3.pdf

Carey, J. C., Dimmitt, C., Hatch, T. A., Lapan, R. T., & Whiston, S. C. (2008). Report of the National Panel for Evidence-Based School Counseling: Outcome Research Coding Protocol and evaluation of Student Success Skills and Second Step. *Professional School Counseling, 11,* 197–206.

Carrell, S. (2000). *Group exercises for adolescents: A manual for therapists* (2nd ed.). Thousand Oaks, CA: Sage.

Carrier, L. A. (1992). *Assisting high school seniors who have not made post graduation plans through the use of individual and group guidance exercises.* Practicum report (ERIC document ED348616). Nova University. Retrieved from http://www.eric.ed.gov/ERICDocs/data/ericdocs2sql/content_storage_01/0000019b/80/12/b5/9a.pdf

Carter, R. T. (1995). *The influence of race and racial identity in psychotherapy: Toward a racially inclusive model.* New York, NY: Wiley.

Cates, J. T., Schaefle, S. E., Smaby, M. H., Maddux, C. D., & LeBeauf, I. (2007). Comparing multicultural with general counseling knowledge and skill competency for students who completed counselor training. *Journal of Multicultural Counseling & Development, 35,* 26–39.

Centers for Disease Control and Prevention. (2005). *Child development.* Retrieved from http://www.cdc.gov/ncbddd/child/default.htm

Chaplin, T. M., Gillham, J. E., Reivich, K., Elkon, A. G. L., Samuels, B., Freres, D. R., Winder, B., & Seligman, M. E. P. (2006). Depression prevention for early adolescent girls: A pilot study of all girls versus co-ed groups. *Journal of Early Adolescence, 26*(1), 110–126.

Chen, M., & Han, Y. (2001). Cross-cultural group counseling with Asians: A stage-specific interactive approach. *Journal for Specialists in Group Work, 26,* 111–128. doi:10.1080/01933920108415732

Cheng, W. D., Chae, M., & Gunn, R. W. (1998). Splitting and projective identification in multicultural group counseling. *Journal for Specialists in Group Work, 23,* 372–387.

Chung, R. C.-Y., & Bemak, F. (2002). The relationship of culture and empathy in counseling. *Journal of Counseling & Development, 80,* 157–158.

Ciborowski, P. (1994). Choosing the military as a career: A group counseling program that addresses issues not presented by recruiters. *School Counselor, 41,* 305–309.

Clark, M., Flower, K., Walton, J., & Oakley, E. (2008). Tackling male underachievement: Enhancing a strengths-based learning environment for middle school boys. *Professional School Counseling, 12,* 127–132.

Coleman, H. L. K. (1998). General and multicultural counseling competency: Apples and oranges? *Journal of Multicultural Counseling and Development, 26,* 147–156.

Collins, S., & Arthur, N. (2010). Culture-infused counselling: A model for developing multicultural competence. *Counselling Psychology Quarterly, 23,* 217–233. doi:10.1080/09515071003798212

Comiskey, P. E. (1993). Using Reality Therapy group training with at-risk high school freshmen. *Journal of Reality Therapy, 12,* 59–64.

Constantine, M. G. (2002). Predictors of satisfaction with counseling: Racial and ethnic minority clients' attitudes toward *counseling* and ratings of their counselors' general and multicultural counseling competence. *Journal of Counseling Psychology, 49,* 255–263.

Constantine, M. G., Miville, M. L., Warren, A. K., Gainor, K. A., & Lewis-Coles, M. E. L. (2006). Religion, spirituality, and career development in African American college students: A qualitative inquiry. *Career Development Quarterly, 54,* 227–241.

Conyne, R. K., Crowell, J. L., & Newmeyer, M. D. (2008). *Group techniques: How to use them more purposefully.* New York, NY: Pearson Merrill/Prentice Hall.

Cook, J. B., & Kaffenberger, C. J. (2003). Solution shop: A solution-focused counseling and study skills program for middle school. *Professional School Counseling, 7,* 116–123.

Cooley, L. (2009). *The power of groups: Solution-focused group counseling in schools.* Thousand Oaks, CA: Corwin Press.

Corey, G. (2008). *Theory and practice of group counseling* (7th ed.). Belmont, CA: Thompson Brooks/Cole.

Corey, J. (2009). *Theory and practice of counseling and psychotherapy* (8th ed.). Belmont, CA: Thompson Brooks/Cole.

Corey, M. S., Corey, G., & Corey, C. (2010). *Groups: Process and practice* (8th ed.). Belmont, CA: Brooks/Cole.

Coy, D. R., & Kovacs-Long, J. (2005). Maslow and Miller: An exploration of gender and affiliation in the journey to competence. *Journal of Counseling & Development, 83*, 138–148.

Crain, W. (2005). *Theories of development: Concepts and applications* (5th ed.). Englewood Cliffs, NJ: Prentice-Hall.

Crespi, T. (2009). Group counseling in the schools: Legal, ethical, and treatment issues in school practice. *Psychology in the Schools, 46*, 273–280.

Crosnoe, R., & Cavanagh, S. (2010). Families with children and adolescents: A review, critique, and future agenda. *Journal of Marriage and Family, 72*, 594–611.

Cummings, C., Gordon, J., & Marlatt, G. A. (1980). Relapse: Strategies of prevention and prediction. In W. R. Miller (Ed.), *The addictive behaviors: Treatment of alcoholism, drug abuse, smoking, and obesity* (pp. 302–337). Oxford, UK: Pergamon Press.

Currie, P. S., & Wadlington, E. M. (2000). *The source for learning disabilities.* East Moline, IL: LinguiSystems.

Curtis, R., Van Horne, J. W., Robertson, P., & Karvonen, M. (2010). Outcomes of a school-wide positive behavioral support program. *Professional School Counseling, 13*, 159–164.

Dalbech, R. (1981). Reality Therapy in school groups. *Journal of Reality Therapy, 1*(1), 14–15.

Davies, D. (2006). Think pink! *Healthcare Counselling & Psychotherapy Journal, 6*, 14–16.

Davis, T., & Osborn, C. (2000). *The solution-focused school counselor: Shaping professional practice.* Philadelphia, PA: Taylor & Francis.

Day, S. X. (2007). *Groups in practice* (2nd ed.). Boston, MA: Houghton Mifflin.

Deck, M., Scarborough, J. L., Sferrazza, M. S., & Estill, D. M. (1999). Serving students with disabilities: Perspectives of three school counselors. *Intervention in School and Clinic, 34*, 150–153.

Delgado, M. (1983). Hispanics and psychotherapeutic groups. *International Journal of Group Psychotherapy, 33*, 507–520.

Delgado, S. (2008). Psychodynamic psychotherapy for children and adolescents: An old friend revisited. *Psychiatry, 5*(5), 67–72.

Delgado-Romero, E. A., Barfield, J., Fairley, B. & Martinez, R. (2005). Using the multicultural guidelines in individual and group counseling situations. In M. G. Constantine & D.W. Sue (Eds.), *Strategies for building multicultural competence in mental health and educational settings* (pp. 29–55). Hoboken, NJ: John Wiley.

DeLucia-Waack, J. (2006). *Leading psychoeducational groups: For children and adolescents.* Thousand Oaks, CA: Sage.

DeLucia-Waack, J., & Donigian, J. (2006). *The practice of multicultural group work.* Belmont, CA: Thompson Brooks/Cole.

del Valle, P., Meachern, A., & Garcia, S. (1999). Using drawings and writings in a group counseling experience with Cuban rafter children, "los balseritos." *Guidance & Counseling, 14*(4), 20–29.

DeRosier, M. E. (2002). *Group interventions and exercise for enhancing children's communication, cooperation, and confidence.* Sarasota, FL: Professional Resource Press.

DeRosier, M. (2004). Building relationships and combating bullying: Effectiveness of a school-based social skills group intervention. *Journal of Clinical Child and Adolescent Psychology, 33*(1), 196–201. doi:10.1207/S15374424JCCP3301_18

de Shazer, S. (1988). Utilization: The foundation of solutions. In J. K. Zieg & S. R. Lankton (Eds.), *Developing Ericksonian therapy: State of the art* (pp. 112–126). Bristol, PA: Milton H. Erickson Foundation, Brunner/Mazel.

de Shazer, S., & Dolan, Y. (2007). *More than miracles: The state of the art of solution-focused brief therapy*. New York, NY: Haworth Press.

Devencenzi, J., & Pendergast, S. (1999). *Belonging: Self and social discovery for children and* Dinkmeyer *adolescents: A guide for group facilitators*. San Luis Obispo, CA: Jalmar Press.

DeVoss, J. A., & Andrews, M. F. (2006). *School counselors as educational leaders*. Boston, MA: Houghton Mifflin.

DeVries, R., & Kohlberg, L. (1987). *Child psychology and childhood education: A cognitive-developmental view*. New York, NY: Longman.

Dimmitt, C., Carey, J. C., & Hatch, T. (2007). *Evidence-based school counseling: Making a difference with data-driven practices*. Thousand Oaks, CA: Sage.

Dinkmeyer, D., & Dreikurs, R. (1963/2001). *Encouraging children to learn* (reprint). New York, NY: Brunner-Routledge Taylor & Francis.

Dinkmeyer, D., & Sperry, J. (1999). *Counseling and psychotherapy: An integrated, individual psychology approach* (3rd ed.). New York, NY: Prentice-Hall.

Dobson, K. S. (2010). *Handbook of cognitive behavioral therapies* (2nd ed.). New York, NY: Guilford Press.

Doremus-Fitzwater, T. L., Varlinskaya, E., & Spear, L. P. (2010). Motivational systems in adolescence: Possible implications for age differences in substance abuse and other risk-taking behaviors. *Brain and Cognition, 72*, 114–123.

Drapela, V. C. (1990). The value of theories for counseling practitioners. *International Journal for the Advancement of Counselling, 13*(1), 19–26.

Dreikurs, R. (1953/1989). *The fundamentals of Adlerian psychology*. (1989). Chicago, IL: Adler School of Professional Psychology.

Drews, A. A., Carey, L. J., & Schaefer, C. E. (2001). *School-based play therapy*. New York, NY: John Wiley.

Drews, A. A., & Schaefer, C. E. (2010). *School-based play therapy* (2nd ed.). New York, NY: John Wiley.

Drucker, C. (2003). Group counseling in the middle and junior high school. In K. R. Greenberg (Ed.), *Group counseling in K–12 Schools: A handbook for school counselors* (pp. 81–96). Boston, MA: Allyn & Bacon.

Dryden, W., Digiuseppe, R., & Neenan, M. (2010). *A primer on rational emotive behavior therapy* (3rd ed.). New York, NY: Research Press.

Duba, C. P., & Mason, J. D. (2009) Using reality therapy in schools: Its potential impact on the effectiveness of the ASCA National Model. *International Journal of Reality Therapy. XXIX*(1), 5–12.

Dykeman, C., & Appleton, V. E. (2002). Group counseling: The efficacy of group work. In D. Capuzzi & D. R. Gross (Eds.), *Introduction to group counseling* (3rd ed., pp. 119–153). Denver, CO: Love.

Echemendía, R. J., & Nuñez, J. (2004). Brief psychotherapy in a multicultural context. In M. J. Dewan, B. N. Steenbarger, & R. P. Greenberg (Eds.), *The art and science of brief psychotherapies: A practitioners guide* (pp. 243–255). Washington, DC: American Psychiatric Publishing.

Ediger, M. (1991). *Excellence in the counseling curriculum*. Retrieved from http://www.eric.ed.gov/PDFS/ED341910.pdf

Edmondson, J. H., & White, J. (1998). A tutorial and counseling program: Helping students at risk of dropping out of school. *Professional School Counseling, 1*, 43–47.

Egan, G. (2007). *Exercises in helping skills* (7th ed.). Belmont, CA: Thomson Higher Education.

Egan, G. (2009). *The skilled helper* (9th ed.). Pacific Grove, CA: Brooks/Cole.

Ehrlich, E., & DeBruhl, M. (1996). *International thesaurus of quotations*. New York,, NY: Harper Perennial.

Elliot, S. (1994). *Group activities for counselors*. Torrance, CA: Innerchoice Publishing.

Ellis, P. H. (2004). White identity development at a two-year institution. *Community College Journal of Research & Practice, 28*, 745–761.

Ellis, A., & Wilde, J. (2001). *Case studies in rational emotive behavior therapy with children and adolescents*. Englewood Cliffs, NJ: Prentice Hall.

Enea, V., & Dafinoiu, I. (2009). Motivational/solution-focused intervention for reducing school truancy among adolescents. *Journal of Cognitive and Behavioral Psychotherapies, 9*, 185–198.

Enfield, G., & Grosser, M. (2008). Picking up coins: The use of video games in the treatment of adolescent social problems. *Popular culture in counseling, psychotherapy, and play-basedinterventions* (pp. 181–195). New York, NY: Springer.

Engberg, J., & Morral, A. R. (2006). Reducing substance use improves adolescents' school attendance. *Addiction, 101*, 1741–1751.

Eppler, C. (2008). Exploring resiliency of parentally bereaved children aged 9–12. *Professional School Counseling, 11*, 189–196.

Eppler, C., Olsen, J., & Hidano, L. (2009). Using stories in school counseling: Brief, narrative techniques. *Professional School Counseling, 12*, 387–391.

Eppler, C., & Weir, S. (2009). Family assessment in K-12 settings: Understanding family systems to provide effective, collaborative services. *Psychology in the Schools, 46*, 501–514.

Erford, B. T. (2010). *Group work in the schools*. Boston, MA: Pearson Education.

Erikson, E. H. (1963). *Childhood and society* (2nd ed.). New York, NY: W. W. Norton.

Erikson, E. H. (1968). *Identity youth and crisis*. New York, NY: W. W. Norton.

Erickson, S., & Feldstein, S. (2007). Adolescent humor and its relationship to coping, defense strategies, psychological distress, and well-being. *Child Psychiatry & Human Development, 37*, 255–271.

Eron, J. B., & Lund, T. W. (1996). *Narrative solutions in brief therapy*. New York, NY: Guildford Press.

Esquivel, G. B. (1998). Group interventions with culturally and linguistically diverse students. In K. C Stoiber & T. R. Kratochwill (Eds.), *Handbook of group intervention for children and families* (pp. 252–267). Needham Heights, MA: Allyn & Bacon.

Esquivel, G. B., & Keitel, M. A. (1990). Counseling immigrant children in the schools. *Elementary School Guidance and Counseling, 24*, 213–221.

Fabian, E., & MacDonald-Wilson, K. (2005). Professional practice in rehabilitation service delivery systems and related system resources. In R. Parker, E. Szymanski, & J. Patterson (Eds.), *Rehabilitation counseling: Basics and beyond* (pp. 55–87). Austin, TX: Pro-Ed.

Farough, S. D. (2006). Believing is seeing. *Journal of Contemporary Ethnography, 35*(1), 51–83.

Fehr, S. S. (2010). *101 interventions in group therapy* (Rev. ed.). New York, NY: Routledge.

Finamore, D. (2008). Little Miss Sunshine and positive psychology as a vehicle for change in adolescent depression. *Popular culture in counseling, psychotherapy, and play-based interventions* (pp. 123–139). New York, NY: Springer.

Fischetti, B. (2010). Play therapy for anger management in the schools. *School-based play therapy* (2nd ed., pp. 283–305). Hoboken, NJ: John Wiley.

Fisher, G. L., & Harrison, T. C. (1993). The school counselor's role in relapse prevention. *School Counselor, 42*, 120–126.

Ford-Harris, D. Y., Schuerger, J. M., & Harris, J. J. (1991). Meeting the psychological needs of gifted Black students: A cultural perspective. *Journal of Counseling & Development, 69*, 577–580.

Forehand, R., Middlebrook, J., Steffe, M., & Rogers, T. (1984). An examination of some trends in child behavior therapy. *Behavioural Psychotherapy, 12*, 203–211. doi: 10.1017/S0141347300010776

Foster, D., & Black, T.G. (2007). An integral approach to counseling ethics. *Counseling and Values, 51*, 221–234.

Freeman, J., & Combs, G. (1996). *Narrative therapy: The social construction of preferred realities*. New York, NY: W. W. Norton.

Freeman, J. C., Epston, D., & Lobovits, D. (1997). *Playful approaches to serious problems: Narrative therapy with children and their families*. New York, NY: W. W. Norton.

Friedman, M., Rholes, W., Simpson, J., Bond, M., Diaz-Loving, R., & Chan, C. (2010). Attachment avoidance and the cultural fit hypothesis: A cross-cultural investigation. *Personal Relationships, 17*(1), 107–126. doi:10.1111/j.1475-6811.2010.01256.x

Froeschle, J., Smith, R., & Ricard, R. (2007). The efficacy of a Systematic Substance Abuse Program for adolescent females. *Professional School Counseling, 10*, 498–505.

Frye, H. N. (2005). How elementary school counselors can meet the needs of students with disabilities. *Professional School Counseling, 8*, 442–450.

Fu Keung Wong, D. (2007). Uncovering sociocultural factors influencing the pathway to care of Chinese caregivers with relatives suffering from early psychosis in Hong Kong. *Culture, Medicine & Psychiatry, 31*(1), 51–71.

Fuertes, J. N., Stracuzzi, T. I., Bennett, J., Scheinholtz, J., Mislowack, A., Hersh, M., & Cheng, D., (2006). Therapist multicultural competency: A study of therapy dyads. *Psychotherapy: Theory, Research, Practice, Training, 43*, 480–490.

Fulton, P. R. (2005). Mindfulness as clinical training. In C. K. Germer, Siegel, R. D., Fulton, P. R. (Eds.), *Mindfulness and psychotherapy* (pp. 55–72). New York, NY: Guilford.

Galassi, J., & Akos, P. (2007). *Strengths-based school counseling*. Mahweh, NJ: Lawrence Erlbaum.

Garrett, M., Garrett, J. T., & Brotherton, D. (2001). Inner circle/outer circle: A group technique based on Native American healing circles. *Journal for Specialists in Group Work, 26*, 17–30.

Gay, G. (1999). Ethnic identity development and multicultural education. *Racial and ethnic identity in school practices: Aspects of human development* (pp. 195–211). Mahwah, NJ: Lawrence Erlbaum.

Geroski, A. M., & Kraus, K. L. (2010). *Groups in schools: Preparing, leading, and responding*. Upper Saddle River, NJ: Pearson.

Gerrity, D., & DeLucia, J. (2007). Effectiveness of groups in the schools. *Journal for Specialist in Group Work, 32*(1), 97–102.

Gibbons, M. M., Borders, L. D., Stephen, J. B., & Davis, P. E. (2006). Career and college planning needs of ninth graders–as reported by ninth graders. *Professional School Counseling, 10*, 168–178.

Gibbs, J. T., & Huang, L. N. (1989). A conceptual framework for assessing and treating minority youth. In J. T. Gibbs & L. Huang (Eds.), *Children of color: Psychological interventions with minority youth* (pp. 1–29). San Francisco, CA: Jossey-Bass.

Gil, E. (1994). *Play in family therapy*. New York, NY: Guilford Press.

Gilbert, A. (2003). Group counseling in an elementary school. In K. R. Greenberg (Ed.),

Group counseling in K–12 schools: A handbook for school counselors (pp. 56–80). Boston, MA: Pearson Education

Gladding, S. T. (1994). *Effective group counseling. ERIC/CASS Digest.* Retrieved from http://www.ericdigests.org/1994/group.htm

Gladding, S. T. (2008). *Groups: A counseling specialty* (5th ed.). Upper Saddle River, NJ. Pearson Prentice Hall.

Glass, S. D. (2010). *The practical handbook of group counseling: Group work with children, adolescents, and parents* (2nd ed.). Victoria, BC: Trafford Publishing.

Glasser, W. (1965). *Reality therapy.* New York, NY: Harper Collins.

Glasser, W. (1990). *The quality school.* New York, NY: Harper Collins.

Glasser, W. (1998). *Choice theory: A new psychology of personal freedom.* New York, NY: Harper Collins.

Glasser, W. (2001). *Counseling with choice theory.* New York, NY: Harper Collins.

Glenn, E. E. (1998). Counseling children and adolescents with disabilities. *Professional School Counseling, 2,* 39–46.

Glosoff, H., & Pate, R. (2002). Privacy and confidentiality in school counseling. *Professional School Counseling, 6,* 20–27.

Goodenow, C., Szalacha, L., & Westheimer, M. (2006). School support groups, other school factors, and the safety of sexual minority adolescents. *Psychology in the Schools, 43,* 573–589.

Grana, R., Black, D., Sun, P., Rohrbach, L., Gunning, M., & Sussman, S. (2010). School disrepair and substance use among regular and alternative high school students. *Journal of School Health, 80,* 387–393. doi:10.1111/j.1746-1561.2010.00518.x

Green, M., & Piel, J. (2010). *Theories of human development: A comparative approach* (2nd ed.). New York, NY: Pearson Education.

Greenberg, K. R. (2003). *Group counseling in K–12 schools.* Boston, MA: Allyn and Bacon.

Greene, R., & Ollendick, T. (1993). Evaluation of a multidimensional program for sixth-graders in transition from elementary to middle school. *Journal of Community Psychology, 21,* 162–176. doi:10.1002/1520-6629(199304)21:2<162:AID-JCOP2290210208>3.0.CO;2-D

Griffin, C. (2010). Transition planning for students with special needs. *District Administration, 46*(2), 52.

Griffin, P., Lee, C., Waugh, J., & Beyer, C. (2004). Describing roles that gay-straight alliances play in schools: From individual support to school change. *Journal of Gay & Lesbian Issues in Education, 1*(3), 7–22.

Guindon, M. (Ed.). (2010). *Self-esteem across the lifespan: Issues and interventions.* New York, NY: Taylor and Francis.

Halperin, D. (2001). The play's the thing: How social group work and theatre transformed a group into a community. *Social Work with Groups, 24*(2), 27–46.

Halverson, S. (2002). Group counseling: Children and adolescents. In D. Capuzzi and D. R. Gross (Eds.), *Introduction to group counseling* (3rd ed., pp. 377–405). Denver, CO: Love Publishing.

Hargrow, A. (2001). Racial identity development: The case of Mr. X, an African American. *Journal of Mental Health Counseling, 23,* 222–237.

Harpine, E. C. (2008). *Group interventions in schools: Promoting mental health for at-risk children and youth.* New York, NY: Springer.

Havighurst, R. J. (1952). *Developmental tasks and education.* New York, NY: David McKay.

Havinghurst, R. J. (1972). *Human development and education.* London: Longmans, Greene.

Heitzman-Powell, L. S., White, R., & Perrin, N. L. (2007). Behavior analysts and counseling: Why Are we not there and how can we get there? *International Journal of Behavioral Consultation and Therapy, 3,* 571–587.

Helms, J. E. (1995). An update of Helms's White and people of color racial identity models. In J. G. Ponterotto, J. M. Casas, L. A. Suzuki, & C. M. Alexander (Eds.), *Handbook of multicultural counseling* (pp. 181–191). Thousand Oaks, CA: Sage.

Henderson, D. A., & Thompson, T. L. (2010). *Counseling children* (8th ed.). New York, NY: Brooks/Cole.

Heppner, P., Heppner, M., Lee, D., Wang, Y., Park, H., & Wang, L. (2006). Development and validation of a Collectivist Coping Styles Inventory. *Journal of Counseling Psychology, 53,* 107–125.

Hernandez, M. (Ed.). (2010). Self-esteem across the lifespan: Issues and interventions. New York, NY: Taylor and Francis.

Hines, P., & Fields, T. (2002). Pregroup screening issues for school counselors. *Journal for Specialists in Group Work, 27,* 358–376.

Hirschfeld, L. A. (1995). *How young children perceive race.* Thousand Oaks, CA: Sage.

Hitchcox, T. (2005). *The body outline: Learning about anger and stress.* Unpublished notes.

Hoag, M. J., & Burlingame, G. M. (1997). Evaluating the effectiveness of child and adolescent group treatment: A meta-analytic review. *Journal of Clinical Child Psychology, 26,* 234–246.

Hoffmann, F. (1975). Use of the Adlerian model in secondary school counseling and consulting. *Individual Psychologist, 12,* 27–32.

Holcomb-McCoy, C. (2004). Assessing the multicultural competence of school counselors: A checklist. *Professional School Counseling, 7,* 178–183.

Huggins, P., Manion, D. W., & Moen, L. (1994). *Building self-esteem in the classroom: Intermediate version.* Longmont, CO: Sopris West.

Hughes, F. P. (2009). *Children, play, and development* (4th ed.). Thousand Oaks, CA: Sage.

Humes, C., & Clark, J. (1989). Group counseling and consultation with gifted high school students. *Journal for Specialists in Group Work, 14,* 219–225. doi:10.1080/01933928908412053.

Hunter, D., & Sawyer, C. (2006). Blending Native American spirituality with individual psychology in work with children. *Journal of Individual Psychology, 62,* 234–250.

Ingram, R. E., & Siegle, G. J. (2010). Cognitive science and the conceptual foundations of cognitive-behavioral therapy: Viva la evolution! In K. S. Dobson (Ed.), *Handbook of cognitive behavioral therapies* (3rd ed., pp. 74–93). New York, NY: Guilford Press.

Iwamoto, D., Creswell, J., & Caldwell, L. (2007). Feeling the beat: The meaning of rap music for ethnically diverse Midwestern college students—A phenomenological study. *Adolescence, 42,* 337–352.

Jackson, K. (2009). Beyond race: Examining the facets of multiracial identity through a life-span developmental lens. *Journal of Ethnic & Cultural Diversity in Social Work, 18,* 309–326. doi:10.1080/15313200903310759.

Jacobs, E., Masson, R., & Harvill, R. (2009). *Group counseling: Strategies and skills* (6th ed.). Pacific Grove, CA: Brooks/Cole.

Jacobs, E., & Schimmel, C. (2005). Small group counseling. In C. Sink (Ed.), *Contemporary school counseling* (pp. 82–115). Boston, MA: Houghton Mifflin.

Jefferson, S. (2002, June). The role of shame in African American racial identity: A bridge to negative affect. *Dissertation Abstracts International, 62.* Retrieved from PsycINFO database.

Johnson, S. K., & Johnson, C. D. (2005). Group counseling: Beyond the traditional. *Professional School Counseling, 8,* 300–400.

Johnson, S. K., Johnson, C. D., & Downs, L. (2006). *Building a results-based student support program.* Belmont, CA: Wadsworth Publishing.

Jong-Un, K. (2006). The effect of a bullying prevention program on responsibility and victimization of bullied children in Korea. *International Journal of Reality Therapy, 26*(1), 4–8.

Kaduson, H. G., & Schaefer, C. E. (2001). *One hundred and one more favorite play therapy techniques.* Lanhan, MD: Rowman & Littlefield.

Karcher, M. J., & Nakkula, M. J. (1997). Multicultural pair counseling and the development of expanded worldviews. In R. L. Selman, C. L. Watts, & L. Hicky Schultz (Eds.), *Fostering Friendship: Pair Therapy for Treatment and Prevention* (pp. 207–227). Hawthorne, NY: Aldine de Gruyter.

Kastner, M., & Neumann, M. (1986). A model combining two psychotherapeutic approaches in group psychotherapy. *Psychotherapy: Theory, Research, Practice, Training, 23,* 593–597. doi: 10.1037/h0085662

Kaufman, R., Herman, J., & Watters, K. (2002). *Educational planning: Strategic, tactical, operational.* Lanham, MD: Scarecrow Press/Rowman & Littlefield.

Kayler, H., & Sherman, J. (2009). At-risk ninth-grade students: A psychoeducational group approach to increase study skills and grade point averages. *Professional School Counseling, 12,* 434–439.

Kelly, V. A., & Juhnke, G. A. (2005). Addictions prevention and interventions within schools. In V. A. Kelly & G. A. Juhnke (Eds.), *Critical incidents in addictions counseling* (pp. 41–46). Alexandria, VA: American Counseling Association.

Kenny, M.C., & McEachern, A. (2009). Children's self-concept: A multicultural comparison. *Professional School Counseling, 12,* 207–212.

Kern, R., & Hankins, G. (1977). Adlerian group counseling with contracted homework. *Elementary School Guidance & Counseling, 11,* 284–290.

Khalsa, S. S. (1996). *Group exercises for enhancing social skills & self-esteem.* Sarasota, FL: Professional Resource Press.

Khantzian, E. (1986). A contemporary psychodynamic approach to drug abuse treatment. *American Journal of Drug and Alcohol Abuse, 12,* 213–222.

Khattab, N., & Jones, C. P. (2007). Growing up girl: Preparing for change through group work. *The Journal for Specialists in Group Work, 32,* 41–50.

Klimstra, T. A., Hale, W. W. III, Raaijmakers, Q. A. W., Branje, S. J. T., & Meeus, W. H. J. (2010). Identity formation in adolescence: Change or stability? *Journal of Youth and Adolescence, 39,* 150–162.

Knesting, K. (2008). Students at risk for school dropout: Supporting their persistence. *Preventing School Failure, 52*(4), 3–10. doi: 10.3200/PSFL.52.4.3-10

Kostelnik, M. J. (1999). Everyone has a culture. In R. E. Lee & S. Emerson (Eds.), *The eclectic trainer* (pp. 147–163). Iowa City, IA: Geist and Russell.

Kress, V., & Hoffman, R. (2008). Empowering adolescent survivors of sexual abuse: Application of a solution-focused Ericksonian counseling group. *Journal of Humanistic Counseling, Education & Development, 47,* 172–186.

Kwan, K. K. (2001). Models of racial and ethnic identity development: Delineation of practice implications. *Journal of Mental Health Counseling, 23,* 269–278.

Kwon, T. (2001). An integrative model for spirituality development in three domains of learning theory. *Dissertation Abstracts International, 61.*

LaFountain, R. M. (1996). Social interest: A key to solutions. *Individual Psychology: Journal of Adlerian Theory, Research & Practice, 52,* 150–157.

LaFountain, R. M., Garner, N. E., &. Eliason, G. T. (1996). Solution-focused counseling groups: A key for school counselors. *School Counselor, 43,* 256–267.

Lam, S. (2005). An interdisciplinary course to prepare school professionals to collaborate with families of exceptional children. *Multicultural Education, 13*(2), 38–42.

Lambert, M. (1992). Psychotherapy outcome research: Implications for integrative and eclectical therapists. *Handbook of psychotherapy integration* (pp. 94–129). New York, NY: Basic Books.

Landreth, G. (2002). *Play therapy: The art of the relationship* (2nd ed.). New York, NY: Brunner-Routledge.

Lansdown, G. (2001). *Promoting children's participation in democratic decisionmaking.* Florence, Italy: UNICEF United Nations Children's Fund Innocenti Research Centre.

Lee, I., & Kelly Jr., E. W. (1996). Individualistic and collective group counseling: Effects with Korean clients. *Journal of Multicultural Counseling & Development, 24*(4), 254–266.

Lee, R., Tiley, C., & White, J. (2009). The Place2Be: Measuring the effectiveness of a primary school-based therapeutic intervention in England and Scotland. *Counselling & Psychotherapy Research, 9,* 151–159. doi:10.1080/14733140903031432

Lee, R., Tiley, C., & White, J. (2009). The Place2Be: Measuring the effectiveness of a primary school-based therapeutic intervention in England and Scotland. *Counselling & Psychotherapy Research, 9,* 151–159. doi:10.1080/14733140903031432

Lee, W. M. L., Blando, J. A., Mizelle, N. D., & Orozco, G. L. (2007). *An introduction to multicultural counseling for helping professionals* (2nd ed.). New York, NY: Routledge.

Leichtentritt, J., & Shechtman, Z. (2010). Children with and without learning disabilities: A comparison of processes and outcomes following group counseling. *Journal of Learning Disabilities, 43,* 169–179.

Lerner, R. M., Lerner, J. V., Almerigi, J. B., & Theokas, C. (2005). Positive youth development: A view of the issues. *Journal of Early Adolescence, 25*(1), 10–16.

Lerner, R. M., von Eye, A., Lerner, J. V., & Lewin-Bizan, S. (2009). Exploring the foundations and functions of adolescent thriving within the 4-H study of positive youth development: A view of the issues. *Journal of Applied Developmental Psychology, 30,* 567–570.

Lewis, J., Arnold, M., House, R., & Toporek, R. (2005). *ACA advocacy competencies.* Retrieved from http://www.counseling.org/Publications/

Liebmann, M. (2004). *Art therapy for groups: A handbook of themes and exercises.* New York, NY: Routledge.

Linden, G. W. (2001). Forward to the reprint. In D. Dinkmeyer & R. Dreikurs, *Encouraging children to learn* (Reprint; pp. x–xii). New York, NY: Brunner-Routledge Taylor & Francis.

Little, S., Akin-Little, A., & Gutierrez, G. (2009). Children and traumatic events: Therapeutic techniques for psychologists working in the schools. *Psychology in the Schools, 46,* 199–205. doi: 10.1002/pits.20364

Lopez, C., & Bhat, C. S. (2007). Supporting students with incarcerated parents in schools: A group intervention. *Journal for Specialist in Group Work, 32,* 139–153.

Lowe, S. (2005). Integrating collectivist values into career counseling with Asian Americans: A test of cultural responsiveness. *Journal of Multicultural Counseling & Development, 33*(3), 134–145. Retrieved from Professional Development Collection database.

Lowenstein, L. (2006). *Creative interventions for children of divorce*. Toronto, Canada: Champion Press.

Mackinlay, E., & Barney, K. (2008). "Move over and make room for Meeka": the representation of race, otherness and indigeneity on the Australian children's television programme Play school. *Discourse: Studies in the Cultural Politics of Education*, 29(2), 273–288. doi:10.1080/01596300801967011.

Malott, K. M., Paone, T. R., Humphreys, K., & Martinez, T. (2010). Use of group counseling to address ethnic identity development: Application with adolescents of Mexican descent. *Professional School Counseling*, 13, 251–266.

Manning, M. L. & Baruth, L. G. (2009). *Multicultural education of children and adolescents* (5th ed.). Boston, MA: Allyn and Bacon.

Mannix, T. (1993). *Social skills activities for special children*. San Francisco, CA: Jossey-Bass.

Mannix, T. (1998). *Social skills activities for secondary students with special needs*. San Francisco, CA: Jossey-Bass.

Marlow, L., Bloss, K., & Bloss, D. (2000). Promoting social and emotional competency through teacher/counselor collaboration. *Education*, 120, 668–674.

Marshak, L. E., Dandeneau, C. J., Prezant, F. P., & L'Amoreaux, N. A. (2009). The school counselor's guide to helping students with disabilities. New York, NY: John Wiley.

Marshall, P. L. (2002). *Cultural diversity in our schools*. Belmont, CA: Wadsworth/Thompson Learning.

Maslow, A. (1965, May). *Self-actualization and beyond*. Proceedings of the Conference on the Training of Counselors of Adults (pp. 107–138). Chatham, MA.

Maslow, A. (1968). *Toward a psychology of being* (2nd ed.). New York, NY: Van Nostrand Reinhold.

Mason, C., & Duba, J. (2009). Using Reality Therapy in schools: Its Potential impact on the effectiveness of the ASCA National Model. *International Journal of Reality Therapy*, 29(1), 5–12.

Mayberry, M. (2006). School reform efforts for lesbian, gay, bisexual, and transgendered students. *Clearing House*, 79, 262–264.

McCabe, P., & Shaw, S. (2010). *Pediatric disorders*. Thousand Oaks, CA: Corwin Press.

McCall-Perez, Z. (2000). The counselor as advocate for English language learners: An action research approach. *Professional School Counseling*, 4, 13–23.

McCarthy, C., Kerne, V., Calfa, N. A., Lambert, R. G., & Guzman, M. (2010). An exploration of school counselors' demands and resources: relationship to stress, biographic, and caseload characteristics. *Professional School Counseling*, 13, 146–158.

McEachern, A., & Kenny, M. (2007). Transition groups for high school students with disabilities. *Journal for Specialists in Group Work*, 32, 165–177.

McGannon, W., Carey, J., & Dimmit, C. (2005, May). The current status of school counseling outcome research. *Monographs of the Center for School Counseling Outcome Research, 2*.

McGuire, J. (2009). A strengths-based approach to building social competence in adolescents with Asperger's syndrome. *Dissertation Abstracts International, 70*. Retrieved from http://gradworks.umi.com/33/56/3356849.html

McIntosh, P. (1989, July/August). White privilege: Unpacking the invisible knapsack. *Peace and Freedom*, 10–12.

McKelvie, W. (1974). An evaluation of a model to train high school students as leaders of Adlerian guidance groups. *Individual Psychologist*, 11(1), 7–14.

McNulty, W. (2008). Harry Potter and the prisoner within: Helping children with traumatic loss. In L.C. Rubin (Ed.),

Popular culture in counseling, psychotherapy, and play-based interventions (pp. 25–42). New York, NY: Springer.

McWhirter, J. J., McWhirter, B. T., McWhirter, E. H., & McWhirter, R. J. (2007). *At-risk youth: A comprehensive response for counselors, teachers, psychologists, and human services professionals* (4th ed.). Belmont, CA: Thompson Higher Education.

Meyer, K. A. (1999). Functional analysis and treatment of problem behavior exhibited by elementary school children. *Journal of Applied Behavior Analysis, 33,* 229–232.

Meyer, R. H. (2006). *When kids grieve: Forever changed.* Presentation at the annual Pennsylvania School Counselor Association Conference. Retrieved from http://www.schoolcounselor.org/files/When%20Kids%20Grieve.pdf

Meichenbaum, D. H. (2007). Stress inoculation training: A preventative and treatment approach. In P. M. Lehrer, R. I. Woolfolk, & W. E. Sime (Eds.), *Principles and practice of stress management* (3rd ed., pp. 497–516). New York, NY: Guilford.

Midgett, T. E., & Meggert, S. S. (1991). A multicultural approach to counselor education. *Journal for Counseling & Development, 70,* 136–141.

Miller, E., & Reid, C. (2009). Counseling older adults: Practical implications. *The professional counselor's desk reference* (pp. 777–787). New York, NY: Springer.

Miller, J., & Garran, A. M. (2008). *Racism in the United States.* Belmont, CA: Thomson Higher Education.

Miller, J. W., Naimi, T. S., Brewer, R. D., & Jones, S. E. (2007). Binge drinking and associated health risk behaviors among high school students. *Pediatrics, 119,* 76–85.

Milsom, A. S. (2002). Students with disabilities: School counselor involvement and preparation. *Professional School Counseling, 5,* 331–338.

Milsom, A. S., & Hartley, M. T. (2005). Assisting students with learning disabilities transitioning to college: What school counselors should know. *Professional School Counseling, 8,* 436–441.

Miranda, A., Webb, L., Brigman, G., & Peluso, P. (2007). Student success skills: A promising program to close the academic achievement gap for African American and Latino students. *Professional School Counseling, 10,* 490–497.

Mistry, J., & Saraswathi, T. (2003). The cultural context of child development. *Handbook of psychology: Developmental psychology* (Vol. 6, pp. 267–291). Hoboken, NJ: John Wiley.

Miville, M. L., Constantine, M. G., Baysden, M. F., & So-Lloyd, G. (2005). Chameleon changes: An exploration of racial identity themes of multiracial people. *Journal of Counseling Psychology, 52,* 507–516.

Mobley, J. A., & Gazda, G. M. (2006). Creating a personal counseling theory. In G. R. Walz, J. Bleuer, & R .K. Yep (Eds.), *VISTAS: Compelling perspectives on counseling* (pp.143–147). Alexandria, VA: American Counseling Association. Retrieved from http://counselingoutfitters.com/vistas/vistas06/vistas06.31.pdf

Molina, B., Brigman, G., & Rhone, A. (2003). Fostering success through group work with children who celebrate diversity. *Journal for Specialists in Group Work, 28,* 166–184. doi:10.1177/0193392203028002007

Molina, B., Monteiro-Leitner, J., Garrett, M., & Gladding, S. (2005). Making the connection: Interweaving multicultural creative arts through the power of group counseling interventions. *Journal of Creativity in Mental Health, 1*(2), 5–15.

Monteiro-Leitner, J., Asner-Self, K. K., Milde, C., Leitner, D. W., & Skelton, D. (2006). The role of the rural school counselor: Counselor, counselor-in-training, and principal perceptions. *Professional School Counseling, 9,* 248–251.

Montgomery, C. (2002). Role of dynamic group therapy in psychiatry. *Advances in Psychiatric Treatment, 8*(1), 34–41.

Moreno, R. (2010). *Educational psychology.* Hoboken, NJ: John Wiley.

Mortola, P. (2001). Sharing disequilibrium: A link between Gestalt Therapy theory and child development theory. *Gestalt Review, 5*(1), 45–56.

Mostert, D., Johnson, E., & Mostert, M. (1997). The utility of solution-focused, brief counseling in schools: Potential from an initial study. *Professional School Counseling, 1*(1), 21–24.

Muller, L. E., & Hartman, J. (1998). Group counseling for sexual minority youth. *Professional School Counseling, 1,* 38–41.

Murphy, J., DeEsch, J., & Strein, W. (1998). School counselors and school psychologists: partners in student services. *Professional School Counseling, 2,* 85–87.

Muth, J. (2005). *Zen shorts.* New York, NY: Scholastic.

Myrick, R. D. (2002). *Developmental guidance and counseling: A practical approach* (4th ed.). Minneapolis, MN: Educational Media.

Myrick, R., & Dixon, R. (1985). Changing student attitudes and behavior through group counseling. *School Counselor, 32,* 325–330.

National Association of Cognitive-Behavioral Therapists. (2009). *Cognitive-behavioral therapy.* Retrieved from http://www.nacbt.org/whatiscbt.htm

National Education Association. (2010). *IDEA/special education.* Retrieved from http://www.nea.org/specialed

Nelson, T. S. (2010). *Doing something different: Solution-focused brief therapy practices.* New York, NY: Routledge.

Nelson-Jones, R. (2000). *Six key approaches to counselling and therapy.* New York, NY: Continuum.

Newsome, D. W., & Gladding, S. T. (2007). Counseling individuals and groups in school. In B.T. Erford (Ed.), *Transforming the school counseling profession* (pp. 168–194). Upper Saddle River, NJ: Pearson Education.

Newsome, W. (2005). The impact of solution-focused brief therapy with at-risk junior high school students. *Children & Schools, 27,* 83–90.

Nicholson, H., Foote, C., & Grigerick, S. (2009). Deleterious effects of psychotherapy and counseling in the schools. *Psychology in the Schools, 46,* 232–237.

No Child Left Behind Act of 2001. *Legislation, regulations, and guidance.* Retrieved from http://www2.ed.gov/about/offices/list/oese/legislation.html#leg

Ochs, N. G. (1994). The incidence of racial issues in white counseling dyads: An exploratory survey. *Counselor Education & Supervision, 33,* 170–177.

O'Hara, M. (2003). Cultivating consciousness: Carl R. Rogers's Person-centered group process as transformative androgogy. *Journal of Transformative Education, 1*(1), 64–79. doi: 10.1177/0095399703251646

Okada, S., Ohtake, Y., & Yanagihara, M. (2010). Improving the manners of a student with autism: The effects of manipulating perspective holders in Social Stories™ - A pilot study. *International Journal of Disability, Development & Education, 57,* 207–219. doi:10.1080/10349121003750927

Oliver, M. (2007). Review of "Breaking through to teens. A new psychotherapy for the new Adolescent." *Journal of Child Psychotherapy, 33,* 122–124.

Page, B. J., & Jencius, M. J. (2009). *Groups: Planning and leadership skills.* Boston, MA: Houghton Mifflin.

Paisley, P. O., & Milsom, A. (2007). Group work as an essential contribution to transforming school counseling, *The Journal for Specialists in Group Work*, 32, 9–17.

Paniagua, F. A. (2005). *Assessing and treating culturally diverse clients: A practical Guide* (3rd ed.). Thousand Oaks, CA: Sage.

Paone, T., Malott, K., & Maddux, C. (2010). School Counselor Collaboration with Language Interpreters: Results of a National Survey. *Journal of School Counseling*, 8(13), 1–30. Retrieved from http://www.jsc.montana.edu/articles/v8n13.pdf

Parette Jr., H., & Hourcade, J. (1995). Disability etiquette and school counselors: A common sense approach toward compliance with the Americans with Disabilities Act. *School Counselor*, 42, 224–232.

Parry, A., & Doan, R. E. (1994). *Story re-visions: Narrative therapy in the postmodern world*. New York, NY: Guilford Press.

Pavlicevic, M. (2003). *Groups in music: Strategies from music therapy*. New York, NY: Jessica Kingsley Publisher.

Pedersen, P. B. (1991). Multiculturalism as a generic approach to counseling, *Journal of Counseling & Development*, 70, 6–12.

Pederson, P. B. (1995). *The five stages of culture shock*. Westport, CT: Greenwood Press.

Pederson, P. B. (2003). Increasing the cultural awareness, knowledge, and skills of culture-centered counselors. In F. D. Harper & J. McFadden (Eds.), *Culture and Counseling* (pp. 31–46). Needham Heights, MA: Allyn & Bacon.

Pedersen, P. B., & Carey, J. C. (2003). *Multicultural counseling in schools: A practical handbook* (2nd ed.). New York, NY: Allyn and Bacon.

Perls, F. S. (1947/1969). *Ego, hunger and aggression*. New York, NY: Vintage Books.

Perls, F. S. (1976). *The Gestalt approach and eye witness to therapy*. New York, NY: Bantam Books.

Perls, F. S., Hefferline, R., & Goodman, P. (1951/1994). *Gestalt therapy: Excitement and growth in the human personality*. Highland, NY: Gestalt Journal Press.

Pérusse, R., Goodnough, G., & Lee, V. (2009). Group counseling in the schools. *Psychology in the Schools*, 46, 225–231.

Peterson, J. S. (1993). *Talk with teens about self and stress: 50 guided discussions for school and counseling groups*. Minneapolis, MN: Free Spirit Publishing.

Piaget, J., & Inhelder, B. (1966/2000). *The psychology of the child*. New York, NY: Basic Books.

Picklesimer, B. K., Hooper, D. R., & Gineter, E. J. (1998). Life skills, adolescents, and career choices. *Journal of Mental Health Counseling*, 20, 272–282.

Pijl, S., Skaalvik, E., & Skaalvik, S. (2010). Students with special needs and the composition of their peer group. *Irish Educational Studies*, 29(1), 57–70.

Polster, E., & Polster, M. (1973). *Gestalt therapy integrated: Contours of theory and practice*. New York, NY: Random House.

Pope, M. (1999). Applications of group career counseling techniques in Asian cultures. *Journal of Multicultural Counseling & Development*, 27, 18–30.

Portman, G. L., & Portman, T. A. A. (2002). Empowering Students for Social Justice (ES²J): A Structured Group Approach. *Journal for Specialists in Group Work*, 27, 16–31.

Portman, T. A. (2003). Multicultural competencies and group work: A collectivist view. In G. Roysircar, D. Singh Sandhu, & V. E. Bibbins, Sr. (Eds.), *Multicultural competencies: A guidebook of practices* (pp. 141–147). Alexandria, VA: Association for Multicultural Counseling and Development.

Poulin, F., & Chan, A. (2010). Friendship stability and change in childhood and adolescence. *Developmental Review, 30,* 257–272.

Pound, P. (2009). Choice Theory and psychoeducation for parents of out-of-competition adolescent athletes. *International Journal of Reality Therapy, 29*(1), 34–37.

Power, F. C., Higgins, A., & Kohlberg, L. (1989). *Lawrence Kohlberg's approach to moral education.* New York, NY: Columbia University Press.

Pyle, K. R. (2007). *Group career counseling: Practices and principles.* Broken Arrow, OK: National Career Development Association.

Quintana, S. M. (1998). Children's developmental understanding of ethnicity and race. *Applied and Preventive Psychology, 7,* 27–45.

Randall, V. (1997). Gifted girls: What challenges do they face? *Gifted Child Today, 20,* 42–49.

Reeves, D. (2008). *What is a psychotherapy process oriented group?* Retrieved from http://www.goodtherapy.org/blog/therapy-group/

Remley, T. P. Jr., & Herlihy, B. (2009). *Ethical, legal, and professional issues in counseling* (3rd ed.). Upper Saddle River, NJ: Pearson Education.

Ripley, V. V., & Goodnough, G. E. (2001). Planning and implementing group counseling in a high school. *Professional School Counseling, 5,* 62–65.

Ritter, K. Y. (1978). The use of growth-groups as a critical ingredient in counselor training. *International Journal for the Advancement of Counselling, 1,* 295–302. doi: 10.1007/BF00120551

Roaten, G. K., & Schmidt, E. A. (2009). Using experiential activities with adolescents to promote respect for diversity. *Professional School Counseling, 12,* 309–314.

Robbins, R., Tonemah, S., & Robbins, S. (2002). Project Eagle: Techniques for multi-family psycho-educational group therapy with gifted American Indian adolescents and their parents. *American Indian and Alaska Native Mental Health Research, 10*(3), 56–74.

Rogers, C. R. (1951/2007). *Counseling and psychotherapy.* Cambridge, MA: Riverside Press.

Rogers, C. R. (1958). The characteristics of a helping relationship. *Personnel and Guidance Journal, 37,* 6–16.

Rogers, C. R. (1961/1989). *On becoming a person: A therapist's view of psychotherapy.* New York, NY: Houghton-Mifflin.

Rogers, C. R. (1965). *Client-centered therapy.* Boston, MA: Houghton Mifflin.

Rollnick, S., & Miller, W. R. (1995). What is motivational interviewing? *Behavioural and Cognitive Psychotherapy, 23,* 325–334.

Rose, S. D. (1998). *Group work with children and adolescents: Prevention and intervention in school and community systems.* Thousand Oaks, CA: Sage.

Rowe, W., & Atkinson, D. (1995). Misrepresentation and interpretation: Critical evaluation of White racial identity development models. *The Counseling Psychologist, 23,* 364–367. doi:10.1177/0011000095232011

Rowell, L. (2006). Action research and school counseling: Closing the gap between research and practice. *Professional School Counseling, 9,* 376–384.

Rowley, W. (2000). Expanding Collaborative Partnerships Among School Counselors and School Psychologists. *Professional School Counseling, 3,* 224–228.

Rutter, P. A., & Leech, N. A. (2006). Sexual minority youth perspectives on the school environment and suicide risk interventions: A qualitative study. *Journal of Gay & Lesbian Issues in Education, 4,* 77–91.

Ryba, K., & And, O. (1995). Computers empower students with special needs. *Educational Leadership, 53,* 82–84.

Salazar, C., & Abrams, L. (2005). Conceptualizing identity development in members of marginalized groups. *Journal of Professional Counseling: Practice, Theory, & Research, 33*(1), 47–59. Retrieved from PsycINFO database.

Saldaña, L. (2008). Metaphors, analogies, and myths, oh my! Therapeutic journeys along the Yellow Brick Road. In L.C. Rubin (Ed.), *Popular culture in counseling, psychotherapy, and play-based interventions* (pp. 3–23). New York, NY: Springer.

Sanders, J. R., & Sullens, C. D. (2005). *Evaluating school programs* (3rd ed.). Thousand Oaks, CA: Corwin Press.

Sapp, M. (2009). *Psychodynamic, affective, and behavioral theories to psychotherapy.* Springfield, IL: Charles Thompson Publisher.

Satterly, B. A., & Dyson, D. A. (2005). Educating all children equitably: A strengths-based approach to advocacy for sexual minority youth in schools. *Contemporary Sexuality, 39,* i–viii.

Scarborough, J. L., & Gilbride, D. D. (2006). Developing relationships with rehabilitation counselors to meet the transition needs of students with disabilities. *Professional School Counseling, 10,* 25–33.

Schlozman, S. (2000). Vampires and those who slay them: Using the television program *Buffy the Vampire Slayer* in adolescent therapy and psychodynamic education. *Academic Psychiatry, 24,* 49–54.

Schmidt, J. (2009). Review of "Using superheroes in counseling and play therapy." *Smith College Studies in Social Work, 79,* 87–92. doi:10.1080/00377310802634905

Seligman, M. E., Reivich, K., Jaycox, L., & Gillham, J. (1995). *The optimistic child.* Boston, MA: Houghton Mifflin.

Sendak, M. (1963). *Where the wild things are.* New York, NY: Harper Collins.

Senn, D. S. (2004). *Small group counseling for small children.* Chapin, SC: Youthlight.

Shechtman, Z. (2007). *Group counseling and psychotherapy with children and adolescents: Theory, research, and practice.* Mahwah, NJ: Lawrence Erlbaum.

Shechtman, Z., & Gluk, O. (2005). An investigation of therapeutic factors in children's groups. *Group Dynamics: Theory, Research, and Practice, 9,* 127–134. doi:10.1037/1089-2699.9.2.127

Shechtman, Z., & Pastor, R. (2005). Cognitive-behavioral and humanistic group treatment for children with learning disabilities: A comparison of outcomes and process. *Journal of Counseling Psychology, 52,* 322–336. doi:10.1037/0022-0167.52.3.322

Shen, Y. (2007). Developmental model using Gestalt-play versus cognitive-verbal group with Chinese adolescents: Effects on strengths and adjustment enhancement. *Journal for Specialists in Group Work, 32,* 285–305. doi:10.1080/01933920701431784

Sherrod, M. D., Getch, Y. Q., & Ziomek-Daigle, J. (2009). The impact of positive behavior support to decrease discipline referrals with elementary students. *Professional School Counseling, 12,* 421–427.

Shoffer, M., & Briggs, M. (2001). An interactive approach for developing interprofessional collaboration: Preparing school counselors. *Counselor Education and Supervision, 40,* 193–202.

Silver, S. & Green, R. (2001). *A guide to New York's child protective services system.* Retrieved from http://assembly.state.ny.us/comm/Children/20011016/htmldoc.html

Simcox, A., Nuijens, K., & Lee, C. (2006). School counselors and school psychologists: Collaborative partners in promoting culturally competent schools. *Professional School Counseling, 9,* 272–277.

Sink, C. A. (2009). School counselors as accountability leaders: Another call for action. *Professional School Counseling, 13,* 68–74.

Sink, C. A. (Ed.). (2011). *Mental health interventions for school counselors.* Belmont, CA: Brooks/Cole Wadsworth Publishing.

Sink, C. A., & Devlin, J. R. (2011). Student spirituality and professional school counseling: Definitional Issues, opportunities, and challenges. *Counseling and Values, 85,* 130–148.

Sink, C. A., & Mvududu, N. (2010). Statistical power, sampling, and effect sizes: Three keys to research relevancy. *Counseling Outcome Research and Evaluation, 1,* 1–18.

Sink, C. A., & Stroh, H. R. (2006). Practical significance: Use of effect sizes in school counseling research. *Professional School Counseling, 9,* 401–411.

Sink, C. A., Thompson, C., & Risdal, J. (2007, November). *Evaluation of year three (2006–2007) of Highline School District's Elementary School Counseling Grant* (Tech. Rep.). Burien, WA: Highline School District, Research Department.

Sink, C. A., & Zuber, A. (2005). *Hang time evaluation survey.* Unpublished test. Seattle Pacific University, WA.

Skinner, B. F. (1984). The operational analysis of psychological terms. *The Behavioral and Brain Sciences, 7,* 547–581.

Sklare, G. B. (2005). *Brief counseling that works: A solution-focused approach for school counselors and administrators* (2nd ed.). Thousand Oaks, CA: Corwin and American School Counselor Association.

Smead, R. (1990). *Skills for living: Group counseling activities for young adolescents* (Vol. 1). Champaign, IL: Research Press.

Smead, R. (1995). *Skills and techniques for group work with children and adolescents.* Champaign, IL: Research Press.

Smead, R. (2000). *Skills for living: Group counseling activities for young adolescents* (Vol. 2). Champaign, IL: Research Press.

Smith, E. J. (1991). Ethnic identity development: Toward the development of a theory within the context of majority/minority status. *Journal of Counseling & Development, 70,* 181–188.

Smith, T. B., Chin, L., Inman, A. G., & Findling, J. H. (1999). An outreach support group for International students. *Journal of College Counseling, 2,* 188–190.

Sommers-Flanagan, R., Barrett-Hakanson, T., Clarke, C., & Sommers-Flanagan, J. (2000). A psychoeducational school-based coping and social skills group for depressed students. *Journal for Specialists in Group Work, 25,* 170–190.

Sonstegard, M. A., Bitter, R. B., & Pelonis, P. (2004). *Adlerian group counseling and therapy: Step-by-step.* New York, NY: Brunner-Routledge.

Springer, D., Lynch, C., & Rubin, A. (2000). Effects of a solution-focused mutual aid group for Hispanic children of incarcerated parents. *Child & Adolescent Social Work Journal, 17,* 431–442. doi: 10.1023/A:1026479727159

Staton, A., & Gilligan, T. (2003). Teaching school counselors and school psychologists to work collaboratively. *Counselor Education and Supervision, 42,* 162–176.

Steen, S., & Kaffenberger, C. (2007). Integrating academic interventions into small group counseling in elementary school. *Professional School Counseling, 10,* 516–519.

Stein, H. T. (2006). Basic principles of classic Adlerian psychology. In H. T. Stein (Ed.), *The collected clinical works of Alfred Adler* (Vol. 11, Appendix A). Bellingham, WA: Classical Adlerian Translation Project.

Stephens, D., Jain, S., & Kim, K. (2010). Group counseling: Techniques for teaching social skills to students with special needs. *Education, 130*, 509–512.

Stone, C. B. (2005). *Ethics and law: School counseling principles.* Alexandria, VA: American School Counselor Association.

Stone, C. B., & Dahir, C. (2005). *The transformed school counselor.* Belmont, CA: Wadsworth.

Stone, C., & Dahir, C. (2011). *The transformed school counselor* (2nd ed.). Belmont, CA: Wadsworth.

Stormer, G., & Kirby, J. (1969). Adlerian group counseling in the elementary school: Report of a program. *Journal of Individual Psychology, 25*, 155–163.

Stroh, H. R., & Sink, C. A. (2002). Applying APA's learner-centered principles to school-based group counseling. *Professional School Counseling, 6*, 71–78.

Studer, J., & Quigney, T. (2003). An analysis of the time spent with students with special needs by professional school counselors. *American Secondary Education, 31*, 71–83.

Sue, D., & Sue, D. W. (1991). Counseling strategies for Chinese Americans. In C. C. Lee & B. L. Richardson (Eds.), *Multicultural issues in counseling* (pp. 19–90). Alexandria, VA: American Counseling Association.

Sue, D. W., Arrendondo, P., & McDavis, R .J. (1992). Multicultural counseling competencies and standards: A call to the profession. *Journal of Counseling & Development, 70*, 477–486.

Sue, D. W., & Sue, D. (1999). *Counseling the culturally different: Theory and practice* (3rd ed.). New York, NY: John Wiley.

Sue, D. W., & Sue, D. (2007). *Counseling the culturally diverse* (5th ed.). New York, NY: John Wiley.

Sugai, G. (n.d.). *School-wide positive behavior support and response to intervention.* Retrieved from http://www.rtinetwork.org/Learn/Behavior/ar/SchoolwideBehavior

Sun, C. (2007). The impact of inclusion-based education on the likelihood of independence for today's students with special needs. *Journal of Special Education Leadership, 20*, 84–92.

Sunde Peterson, J., & Ray, K. E. (2006). Bullying and the gifted: Victims, perpetrators, prevalence, and effects. *The Gifted Child Quarterly, 50*, 148–170.

Super, D. E. (1990). A life-span, life-space approach to career development. In D. Brown, L. Brooks, & Associates (Eds.), *Career choice and development: Applying contemporary theories to practice* (2nd ed., pp. 197–261). San Francisco, CA: Jossey-Bass.

Sweeney, D. S., & Homeyer, L. E. (Eds.). (1999). *The handbook of group play therapy.* San Francisco: Jossey-Bass.

Sweeney, T. J. (2009). *Adlerian counseling and psychotherapy: A practitioner's approach* (5th ed.). New York, NY: Routledge.

Sweeney, T. J., & Witmer, J. (1991). Beyond social interest: Striving toward optimum health and wellness. *Individual Psychology: Journal of Adlerian Theory, Research & Practice, 47*, 527–540.

Tarver-Behring, S., & Spagna, M. (2004). Counseling with exceptional children. *Focus on Exceptional Children, 36*(8), 1–12.

Taylor, J. V. (2005). *Salvaging sisterhood.* Chapin, SC: Youthlight.

Taylor, J. V., & Trice-Black, S. (2010). *Girls in real life situations, grades 6-12: Group counseling activities for enhancing social and emotional development.* Champaign, IL: Research Press.

Taylor, R. (1995). *African American youth: Their social and economic status in the United States.* Westport, CT: Praeger.

Terrell, F., & Terrell, S. (1984). Race of counselor, client sex, cultural mistrust level, and premature termination from counseling among Black clients. *Journal of Counseling Psychology*, 31, 371–375.

Tessier, D. M. (1982). A group counseling program for gifted and talented students. *Pointer*, 26, 43–46.

Thompson, C. L., & Henderson, D. A. (2007). *Counseling children* (7th ed.). Belmont, CA: Brooks/Cole.

Tice, D. M., Bratslavaky, R. F., & Baumeister, R. F. (2001). Emotional distress regulation takes precedence over impulse control: If you feel bad, do it! *Journal of Personality and social psychology*, 80, 53–67.

Tomlinson-Clarke, S., & Clarke, D. (2010). Culturally focused community-centered service learning: An international cultural immersion experience. *Journal of Multicultural Counseling & Development*, 38, 166–175.

Trolley, B., Haas, H., & Patti, D. (2009). *The school counselor's guide to special education*. Thousand Oaks, CA: Corwin Press.

Trumbull, E., & Rothstein-Fisch, C. (2008). Cultures in Harmony. *Educational Leadership*, 66(1), 63–66. Retrieved from Professional Development Collection database.

Tuckman, B., & Jensen, T. (1977). Stages of small group development. *Group and Organizational Studies*, 2, 19–27.

Turner, S. L. (2007). Introduction to special issues: Transition issues for K–16 students. *Professional School Counseling*, 10, 224–227.

U.S. Department of Education. (2001). *Public law print of PL 107-110, the No Child Left Behind Act of 2001*. Retrieved from http://www2.ed.gov/policy/elsec/leg/esea02/index.html

U.S. Department of Education. (2004). *Building the legacy: IDEA 2004*. Retrieved from http://idea.ed.gov/explore/home

U.S. Department of Education. (2010a). *Characteristics of the largest 100 public elementary and secondary school districts in the United States: 2007–2008 statistical analysis report*. Washington, DC: National Center for Educational Statistics.

U.S. Department of Education (2010b). *Essential components of RTI: A closer look at response to intervention*. Washington, DC: Author.

Van Ausdale, D., & Feagin, J. R. (2000). *The first r: How children learn race and racism*. New York, NY: Rowman & Littlefield.

Venkatesh, S. (2006). *Group counseling*. Retrieved from http://changingminds.org/articles/articles/group_counseling.htm

Vernon, A. (1998). *The passport program: A journey through emotional, social, cognitive, and self-development*. Champaign, IL: Research Press.

Vernon, A., & Davis-Gage, D. (2010). Theoretically based group counseling models used in counseling and psychotherapy groups. In B. T. Erford (Ed.), *Group work in the schools* (pp. 224–235). New York, NY: Pearson.

Villalba, J. A. (2007). Incorporating wellness into group work in elementary schools. *Journal for Specialist in Group Work*, 32, 31–40.

Walker, B. A., Reis, S. M., & Leonard, J. S. (1992). A developmental investigation of the lives of gifted women. *Gifted Child Quarterly*, 36, 201–206.

Walsh-Bowers, R. (1992). A creative drama prevention program for easing early adolescents' adjustment to school transitions. *The Journal of Primary Prevention*, 13(2), 131–147. doi:10.1007/BF01325071

Walter, S., Lambie, G., & Ngazimbi, E. (2008). A Choice Theory counseling group succeeds with middle school students who displayed disciplinary problems. *Middle School Journal*, 40(2), 4–12.

Watson, S., & Gresham, F. (Eds.). (1998). *Handbook of child behavior therapy*. New York, NY: Plenum Press.

Watts-Jones, D. (2002). Healing internalized racism: The role of a within-group sanctuary among people of African descent. *Family Process, 41,* 591–602.

Webb, L. D., & Brigman, G. (2006). Student Success Skills: Tools and strategies for improved academic and social outcomes. *Professional School Counseling, 7,* 112–120.

Webb, L. D., Brigman, G., & Campbell, C. (2005). Linking school counselors and student success: A replication of the student success skills approach targeting the academic social competence of students. *Professional School Counseling, 8,* 407–413.

Webb, L. D., & Myrick, R. D. (2003). A group counseling intervention for children with attention deficit hyperactivity disorder. *Professional School Counseling, 7,* 108–115.

Wells, G. (2006). Language experience of children at home and at school. In J. Cook-Gumperz (Ed.), *The social construction of literacy* (pp. 76–109). New York, NY: Cambridge University Press.

Whiston, S. C., & Aricak, O. T. (2008). Development and initial investigation of the School Counseling Program Evaluation Scale. *Professional School Counseling, 11,* 253–261.

Whiston, S. C., Tai, W. L., Rahardja, D., & Eder, K. (2011). School counseling outcome: A meta-analytic examination of interventions. *Journal of Counseling & Development, 89,* 37–55.

Whiston, S. C., & Quinby, R. F. (2009). Review of school counseling outcome research. *Psychology in the Schools, 46,* 267–272.

Whiston, S. C., & Sexton, T. L. (1998). A review of school counseling outcome research: Implications for practice. *Journal of Counseling & Development, 76,* 412–426.

White, M., & Epston, D. (1990). *Narrative means to therapeutic ends.* New York, NY: W. W. Norton.

White, J. L., & Parham, T. A. (1990). *The psychology of Blacks: An African-American perspective.* Englewood Cliffs, NJ: Prentice-Hall.

White, S. W., & Kelly, F. D. (2010). The school counselor's role in school dropout prevention. *Journal of Counseling & Development, 88,* 227–235.

Wilkerson, K. (2009). An examination of burnout among school counselors guided by stress-strain-coping theory. *Journal of Counseling & Development, 87,* 428–437.

Wilson, S. J. (2003, November). *Family programs to prevent antisocial behavior: Results from* meta-analysis. Paper presented at the annual conference of the American Evaluation Association, Reno, NV.

Winslade, J. M., & Monk, G. (2007). *Narrative counseling in schools: Powerful & brief* (2nd ed.). Thousand Oaks, CA: Sage.

Winters, K. C., Leitten, W., Wagner, E., & Tevyah, T. O. (2007). Use of brief interventions for drug abusing teenagers within a middle and high school setting. *Journal of School Health, 77,* 196–206.

Woldt, A. L., & Toman S. M. (2005). *Gestalt therapy: History, theory, and practice.* Thousand Oaks, CA: Sage.

Wong, C., & Cho, G. E. (2005). Two-headed coins or Kandinskys: White racial identification. *Political Psychology, 25,* 699–720.

Woodard, S. (1995). Counseling disruptive black elementary school boys. *Journal of Multicultural Counseling & Development, 23,* 21–28.

Wubbolding, R. (2000). *Reality therapy for the 21st century.* Philadelphia, PA: Brunner-Routledge.

Wubbolding, R. (2007). Glasser quality school. *Group Dynamics: Theory, Research, and Practice, 11,* 253–261. doi:10.1037/1089-2699.11.4.253.

Yalom, I. (1995). *Theory and practice of group psychotherapy* (4th ed.). New York, NY: Basic Books.

Young, S., & Holdorf, G. (2003). Using solution focused brief therapy in individual referrals for bullying. *Educational Psychology in Practice, 19,* 271–282. doi: 10.1080/0266736032000138526.

Yu, A., & Gregg, C. H. (1993). Asians in groups: More than a matter of cultural awareness. *Journal for Specialists in Group Work, 18,* 86–93.

Zhou, Z., Siu, C., & Xin, T. (2009). Promoting cultural competence in counseling Asian American children and adolescents. *Psychology in the Schools, 46,* 290–298. doi:10.1002/pits.20375.

Zimmerman, J. L., & Dickerson, V. C. (1996). *If problems talked: Narrative therapy in action.* New York, NY: Guilford Press.

Zinck, K., & Littrell, J. M. (2000). Action research shows group counseling effective with at-risk adolescent girls. *Professional School Counseling, 4,* 50–59.

Ziomek-Daigle, J., & Manalo, M. (2010). Understanding differences in the schools. J. R. Studer & J. F. Diambra (Eds.), *A guide to practicum and internship for school counselors-in-training* (pp. 161–177). New York, NY: Routledge/Taylor & Francis Group.

Subject Index

A

ABCD worksheet, 50

ACA Advocacy Competencies, 123–124

Academic and social skills small group
  activities useful for later sessions, 223
  assertiveness training, 221–222
  basic format and procedures, 219
  confidentiality guideline, 220
  content of group meetings, 220–221
  "delaying" strategy, 221
  early stages, 221–222
  go-around technique, 222
  initial session, 220–221
  intergroup communication and personal
    sharing, 221
  leadership effect, 222
  math skill learning, 223
  middle stages, 222
  objectives, 219
  "one-down" position in group, 221
  "pretest" evaluation questionnaire, 221
  productivity development activities,
    221–222
  reading strategies, 222
  relaxation and visualization exercise, 221
  sample evaluation form, 224
  social strength developing activity, 222
  student pregroup self-evaluation, 219

Academic/educational development groups,
  19–20
  academic success, empowerment for, 26
  group objectives, 24
  school success skills, 26
  study skills and tutoring combo, 25

ADHD students, group counseling
  intervention for, 22

Adlerian theory/individual psychology, 36–39

Adolescent groups, facilitation. *See* High
  school groups, efficacy and
  practice at

Alateen (Alanon for teenage populations), 239

Alcoholics Anonymous (AA), 233, 239

American Recovery and Reinvestment Act of
  2009, 11

American School Counselor Association
  (ASCA) Position statement, 108–109

Anger management, 177

Anger Survey (Bierma, 2005), 181–182

ASCA National Model, 43, 101, 189
  accountability, 7
  broader perspective, 6
  delivery system, 7
  management system, 7
  primary objectives, 6
  supporting pillars, 7

ASCA's National Standards for School
  Counseling Programs, 7

ASGW group model, 13

ASGW Professional Standards, 12

ASGW's *Professional Standards for the
  Training of Group Workers*, 12

Asperger's syndrome, 233

ASSIST curriculum, 201

B

Behavioral theory, 53–55

Behaviorism, 53–54

Behavior problems reduction, suggestions,
  154–155

Bullying, 235–236

C

Career development groups, 20
  military as a career, 28
  postsecondary planning, 27
  school-to-work (or postsecondary
    education/training)
    transition groups for high school students
    with disabilities, 29

Choice theory (CT), 45, 48–49

Clinic-based psychotherapy groups, 14

Cognitive-based theories and related
  counseling methods, 47–53

Cognitive-behavioral therapy (CBT), 19,
  33, 47
  related groups with K–12 students, 52–53

Comprehensive school counseling programs
  (CSCP), 6–7, 31, 101